Y0-DEZ-406

Blood Technologies, Services, and Issues

Blood Technologies, Services, and Issues

**OFFICE OF TECHNOLOGY
ASSESSMENT TASK FORCE**

Lawrence H. Miike, Project Director
Denise M. Dougherty, Analyst
Jeffrey Stryker, Analyst
Anne M. Guthrie, Analyst

American Red Cross Blood Services,
 Missouri-Illinois Region
New York Blood Center
Emily B. Rossiter, Regulatory Resources, Inc.
Elaine Power, University of California, Berkeley
Jerrold B. Grossman, New York Blood Center
Victor Schmitt, American Red Cross Blood
 Services
James L. Tullis, M.D., New England Deaconess
 Hospital
Peter Tomasulo, South Florida Blood Services

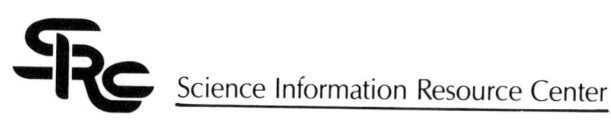

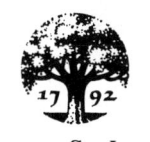

Science Information Resource Center

**J.B. LIPPINCOTT COMPANY
PHILADELPHIA**

London   Mexico City   New York   St. Louis   São Paulo   Sydney

Authorized Hardbound Edition, 1988

Science Information Resource Center
East Washington Square
Philadelphia, Pennsylvania 19105

Publisher's Note:

This permanent edition includes the complete text of the Office of Technology Assessment Special Report entitled *Blood Policy and Technology*. Under the direction of the OTA Project Staff, and with the help of a distinguished Advisory Panel and reviewers from industry and academia and experts in blood banking and transfusion technology, nineteen Author/Contractors conducted new research and reviewed and distilled much valuable existing material.

Science Information Resource Center is a cooperative venture of J.B. Lippincott Company and Hemisphere Publishing Corporation, subsidiaries of Harper & Row, Publishers, Inc., New York.

Library of Congress Cataloging-in-Publication Data
   Blood technologies, services, and issues.
   Originally published: Blood policy & technology. Washington, D.C.: Congress of the U.S., Office of Technology Assessment: For sale by the Supt. of Docs., U.S. G.P.O., [1985].
   Includes bibliographies and index.
   1. Blood—Transfusion—Government policy—United States. 2. Blood banks—Government policy—United States. I. Miike, Lawrence H. II. United States. Congress. Office of Technology Assessment. III. Title.
[DNLM: 1. Blood Banks. 2. Blood Preservation. 3. Blood Transfusion. 4. Health Policy. WH 460 B6355 1985a]
RM171.B 1988 362.1'784'0973 87-26401
ISBN 0-397-53001-3

Foreword

Posttransfusion hepatitis, inefficiencies in blood collection and distribution, payment for blood donations, and the cost of blood products are subjects that, from time to time, have focused attention on the Nation's blood services system. In response, tests have been developed for detecting carriers of transfusion-related hepatitis. Transfusions with the individual components of blood instead of whole blood have become accepted therapy and also resulted in more efficient use of blood donations. Improved technologies have extended the storage life of blood, and improved methods of collection have enabled large-scale processing of plasma so that its component proteins could be extracted. One result of this progress was increased availability of Factor VIII, the antihemophilic factor, which has allowed hemophiliacs to lead nearly normal lives.

In sum, improvements in blood banking and transfusion medicine in the late 1970s and early 1980s have resulted in a stable and safer blood supply. Recent developments, however, create uncertainties. Transfusion-related cases of acquired immunodeficiency syndrome (AIDS) have threatened the safety of the blood supply and the equanimity that has been the foundation of the voluntary blood donor system. Recombinant DNA technologies are being applied to the production of plasma proteins, and other technologies are under development for the production of the cellular components of blood. Legislation of prospective payment by diagnosis-related groupings for Medicare patients' hospital care has begun to exert pressure on blood center revenues as hospitals seek ways to pare costs. Organ and tissue transplants have been increasing, raising questions in the blood banking community about its role in these new types of tissue banks. These developments led the House Committee on Energy and Commerce to request that the Office of Technology Assessment (OTA) conduct an assessment of blood policy and technologies.

In preparing this report, OTA staff drew upon the expertise of members of the study advisory panel, chaired by Louanne Kennedy; members of the OTA Health Program Advisory Committee, chaired by Sidney S. Lee; representatives from industry, academia and the public; and experts in blood banking and transfusion medicine, blood research and development, and health policy. Key OTA staff involved in the preparation of the report were Lawrence Miike, Denise Dougherty, Jeffrey Stryker, and Anne Guthrie.

JOHN H. GIBBONS
Director

Blood Policy and Technology Advisory Panel

Louanne Kennedy, *Chair*
Baruch College/Mt. Sinai School of Medicine
New York, NY

Alvin W. Drake
- Professor of Systems Science and Electrical Engineering
- Massachusetts Institute of Technology
- Cambridge, MA

Thomas C. Drees
- Los Angeles, CA

Tibor J. Greenwalt
- Director
- Paul I. Hoxworth Blood Center
- University of Cincinnati Medical Center
- Cincinnati, OH

Sylvia Drew Ivie
- Director
- National Health Law Program
- Los Angeles, CA

Aaron Kellner
- President
- New York Blood Center
- New York, NY

Sidney S. Lee
- President
- Milbank Memorial Fund
- New York, NY

James W. Mosley
- Los Angeles County Department of Health Services
- Los Angeles, CA

Sharon Perkins
- Coordinator, Donor Program
- Fairfax Hospital
- Falls Church, VA

Michael B. Rodell
- Vice-President
- Regulatory and Technical Affairs
- Ethical Products Division
- Revlon Health Care Group
- Tarrytown, NY

Rosemary Stevens
- Professor of History and Sociology of Science
- University of Pennsylvania
- Philadelphia, PA

Scott N. Swisher
- President's Council
- American Red Cross
- Washington, DC

Martin J. Valaske
- Medical Director
- Medical Faculty Associates
- George Washington University Medical Center
- Washington, DC

William D. White
- Associate Professor
- Department of Economics
- University of Illinois at Chicago
- Chicago, IL

Theodore Zimmerman
- Professor
- Departments of Immunology and Basic and Clinical Research
- Scripps Clinic and Research Foundation
- La Jolla, CA

Wolf Zuelzer
- Silver Spring, MD

OTA Project Staff—Blood Policy and Technology

Roger Herdman, *Assistant Director, OTA*
Health and Life Sciences Division

Clyde J. Behney, *Health Program Manager*

Lawrence H. Miike, *Project Director*

Denise M. Dougherty, *Analyst*
Jeffrey Stryker, *Research Analyst*
Anne M. Guthrie, *Research Assistant*

Virginia Cwalina, *Administrative Assistant*
Beckie Erickson, *Secretary/Word Processor Specialist*
Brenda L. Miller, *Word Processor/P.C. Specialist*

Contractors

Richard Kahn, Ph.D., Robert Allen, Ph.D., Joseph Baldassare, Ph.D., Pamela Cheetham, M.P.H., American Red Cross Blood Services, Missouri-Illinois Region

Johanna Pindyck, M.D., Suzanne Gaynor, R.N., Robert Hirsch, M.D., Mercy Kuriyan, M.D., Robert Reiss, M.D., Theodore Robertson, M.D., Martin Stryker, Ph.D., Alan Waldman, Ph.D., Kenneth Woods, Ph.D., New York Blood Center

Emily B. Rossiter, Regulatory Resources, Inc.

Elaine Power, University of California, Berkeley

Jerrold B. Grossman, New York Blood Center; Victor Schmitt, American Red Cross Blood Services

James L. Tullis, M.D., New England Deaconess Hospital

Peter Tomasulo, South Florida Blood Services

Contents

Chapter — *Page*

1. Introduction and Summary ... 3
2. Overview ... 33
3. The Blood Services Complex ... 51
4. Blood Technologies ... 79
5. Current Issues ... 99
6. Alternative Technologies ... 133
7. Future Directions ... 175

Appendixes — *Page*

A. The Blood Resources Program, Division of Blood Diseases and Resources, National Heart, Lung, and Blood Institute ... 191
B. Glossary of Acronyms and Terms ... 203
C. Acknowledgments and Health Program Advisory Committee ... 208
References ... 213
Index ... 239

1. Introduction and Summary

Contents

	Page
Introduction	3
Summary	4
The Blood Services Complex	4
Cost of Blood Products	7
Availability	8
Safety	10
Issues and Points to Consider	12
AIDS	13
Cost of Blood Products	17
Containment of Health Care Costs	18
Alternatives and Substitutes for Blood Products	20
Appropriate Use	22
Coordination of Blood Resources	23
Voluntary v. Commercial	25
Conclusion	26

TABLE

Table No.	Page
1. Worldwide Demand for Plasma Fractions, by Product, 1978	10

LIST OF FIGURES

Figure No.	Page
1. Collection of Whole Blood in 1971, 1979, and 1980	5
2. U.S. Transfusions of Blood and Components, 1971-80	6
3. Disposition of Domestically Collected Plasma, 1983	7

1. Introduction and Summary

INTRODUCTION

A decade ago, national interest in assuring an adequate and safe blood supply resulted in a pronouncement by the Federal Government of a National Blood Policy (NBP), with the four general goals of improving supply, quality, accessibility, and efficiency. Among the policies that were to be implemented were the adoption of an all-voluntary blood collection system, resource sharing and regionalization of blood collection and distribution, and programs to assure appropriate use.

In addition, information systems were to be developed on a continuing basis to monitor: 1) the whole blood collection system for transmissible diseases and transfusion mishaps to aid in improving the effectiveness of the blood banking system; and 2) the source plasma and plasma fractionation sector to determine the sufficiency of domestic sources of plasma fractions, develop future positions on the relationships between plasmapheresis and plasma fractionation and whole blood banking, and determine the degree of interdependence between the United States and other countries with respect to plasma and plasma products. Adherence to the highest attainable standards for blood products were to be achieved through Federal regulatory authority, and research on all aspects of blood products was to be supported.

Despite a flurry of legislative activity preceding the announcement of the National Blood Policy, no legislation was actually enacted. The announcement of the NBP by the Secretary of the Department of Health, Education, and Welfare (DHEW, the precursor to the present Department of Health and Human Services, DHHS) became the focal point around which blood banking policy has evolved over the past decade.

Following announcement of the National Blood Policy, the Federal Government accepted, and partially funded, a private sector plan to establish an American Blood Commission (ABC) to implement "the lion's share" of the NBP. A number of factors have inhibited the ABC's effectiveness in implementing the NBP: the Commission had no enforcement power; its long-range financial support was dependent on the blood resource organizations which were already involved in the functions that ABC was expected to influence; and many of the factors that contribute to improvements in blood resources (e.g., development of new technologies) were outside ABC's reach. However, ABC succeeded in providing a forum in which blood banking issues could be openly discussed, and much of the conflict among blood bankers of a decade ago is gone today.

ABC, because it was initiated in response to the call for a National Blood Policy, has been the NBP's most visible activity. Because the National Blood Policy represented a pluralistic, private sector approach instead of a central, Government-directed approach, its primary contribution over the past decade has been its acceptance as a general guiding principle by both the private and public sectors, infusing a sense of common purpose into all contributors to our blood resources. The Policy may have been sufficiently general in purpose so that few interest groups felt seriously threatened by it. Whatever its real or imagined impact, however, many of the problems areas identified over a decade ago have shown substantial improvement.

Of course, other problems remain or have arisen since the NBP was announced, and, for the first time, technologies are being developed that could replace many, if not eventually all, of the products currently obtainable only from human blood. Some of these new products, especially the major derivatives (albumin and antihemophilic factor) currently extracted from plasma, may be commercially available before the end of the 1980s.

This study was conducted at the request of the House Committee on Energy and Commerce. The committee pointed out that questions remain concerning donor screening and selection, the appropriate Federal reaction to the changing pattern of blood-related transmissible diseases, the efficiency and coordination of blood banking systems, emerging and future technologies for blood-function substitution, and whether there is a constructive role for a National Blood Policy.

Progress in blood resources over the past decade, and current and future technologies, are the subjects of this report. The rest of this chapter summarizes the major issues in blood banking policy and focuses on specific points within each issue area that deserve continuing attention.

Chapter 2 presents a brief overview of Federal interest in maintaining and improving the Nation's blood resources, the blood products used in therapeutic applications, the donors who provide blood, and Federal activities in blood resources.

Chapter 3 describes the blood services complex; the voluntary, whole blood and blood components sector; and the commercial plasma and plasma derivatives sector.

Chapter 4 describes the blood technologies: technologies for blood collection and processing; and plasma fractionation technologies.

Chapter 5 discusses current issues: the impact of AIDS on blood collection and use; coordination of blood resources; the impact of health care cost containment efforts on blood resources; and issues of appropriate use of blood products.

Chapter 6 provides a look at alternative technologies: alternative sources and substitutes for blood products.

Chapter 7 considers future directions for blood banking: voluntary v. commercial approaches; and tissue and organ banking and blood centers' interests in these activities.

SUMMARY

The Blood Services Complex

The structure of the blood resources system remains nearly the same as it was 10 years ago, but it is very different in terms of the products, services, and technologies offered. The system continues to consist of two essentially different sectors: 1) a largely voluntary whole blood and components sector, and 2) a largely commercial source plasma and plasma derivatives sector. (Products separated from whole blood [red cells, platelets, cryoprecipitate, and fresh-frozen, single-donor plasma] are usually referred to as "components," while products derived from plasma [albumin, Factors VIII and IX, the immune globulins] are called "derivatives.")

Three types of facilities are involved in the voluntary sector: 1) community and regional blood centers which collect and distribute blood to hospitals in circumscribed geographic areas, 2) hospital blood banks which both collect and transfuse whole blood and components, and 3) hospitals which primarily store and transfuse blood but do not collect it. These facilities are represented by several organizations with overlapping memberships.

The American Red Cross (ARC) has 57 regional centers operating under a single Federal license. These Red Cross regional centers cover about half the geographic area of the United States and collect about half of the Nation's whole blood. The institutional members of the American Association of Blood Banks (AABB), including members who belong to the Council of Community Blood Centers (CCBC), collect another 45 percent of the Nation's blood. In 1980, seven ARC regional centers and all but two CCBC centers also belonged to the AABB, as did 1,977 blood collecting hospitals. One hundred and one community blood centers were members only of AABB and did not belong to CCBC. Approximately 2 percent of blood was collected through 16 unaffiliated blood centers.

The trend has been for hospital blood banks to play less of a role in blood collections. In 1971, 69 percent of the blood collected came from regional and community blood centers (555). By 1980 these centers collected 88 percent of the total, increasing to 91 percent in 1981 (29). The increasing predominance of regional and community centers has been attributed to their ability to collect blood through constant mobile collections. In 1980, nearly 70 percent of whole blood collections was through mobile units.

Whole blood collections have been able to keep up with increasing demand while paid whole blood donations have decreased significantly (fig. 1). The ability to meet increased demand has occurred through increased recruitment, improved inventory management, technologies that have increased the storage life of blood and its components, and a large increase in the use of blood components instead of whole blood. Between 1971 and 1980, whole blood collections increased from 8.8 million to 11.15 million units per year, while whole blood and red cell losses decreased from 2.44 million to 1.15 million units, an improvement in losses from 28 to 10 percent of blood collected. Out of the 11.15 million units collected in 1980 (fig. 1), 14.8 million units of blood components were transfused, exclusive of blood that was outdated or lost (fig. 2).

The source plasma sector, on the other hand, is largely commercial and has two main components: 1) collectors, or plasmapheresis centers; and 2) fractionators. Not-for-profit blood banks and blood centers also play a part in the commercial plasma industry when they sell recovered or salvaged plasma (plasma recovered after components have been removed from whole blood, or salvaged after whole blood has outdated) to fractionators; when they contract with commercial firms to fractionate their plasma into derivatives which they then market themselves; or, in one case, when they fractionate and market their own products. Approximately 45 percent of the Red Cross' recovered plasma is fractionated by commercial fractionation companies, and 17 to 20 percent of the plasma derivatives sold in the United States is sold by the voluntary sector (primarily the Red Cross and the New York Blood Center).

Figure 1.—Collection of Whole Blood in 1971, 1979, and 1980

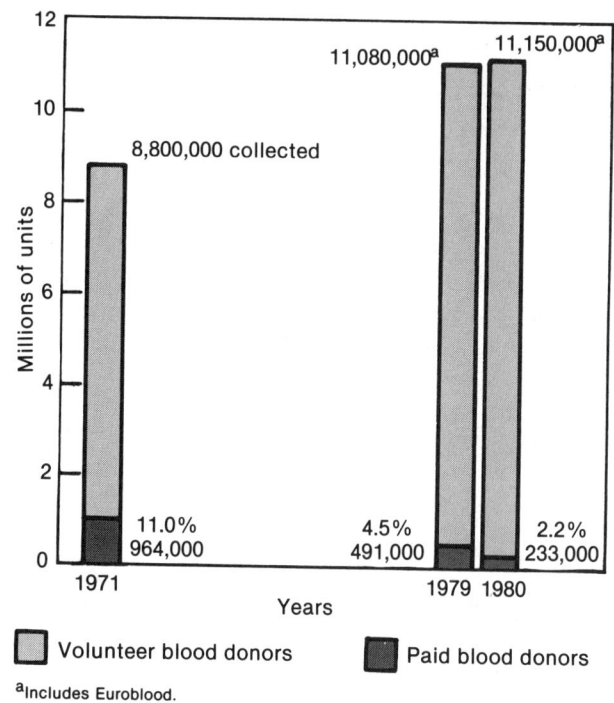

1971: 8,800,000 collected; 11.0% 964,000 paid
1979: 11,080,000[a]; 4.5% 491,000 paid
1980: 11,150,000[a]; 2.2% 233,000 paid

Volunteer blood donors | Paid blood donors

[a]Includes Euroblood.

SOURCE: Surgenor and Schnitzer/ABC, 1983.

There are 336 source plasma centers licensed by the Food and Drug Administration (FDA), 317 of which are commercially operated, and 19 of which are operated by community or Red Cross blood centers. More than 90 percent of the source plasma centers are owned by 30 companies which market biological products. Some of these biological companies are in turn subsidiaries of larger corporations (e.g., Sera-Tec Biologicals, owned by the Rite-Aid Corp., operates nine centers in the East and Midwest, most of which are located near college campuses).

Plasma collected by commercial plasmapheresis centers is either sold to U.S. fractionators who separate it into a number of products (primarily albumin, Factor VIII [antihemophilic factor] and immune globulins), or exported to fractionators in Europe, Japan, or South America. The way plasma is provided from plasmapheresis centers to fractionators varies. Four fractionation com-

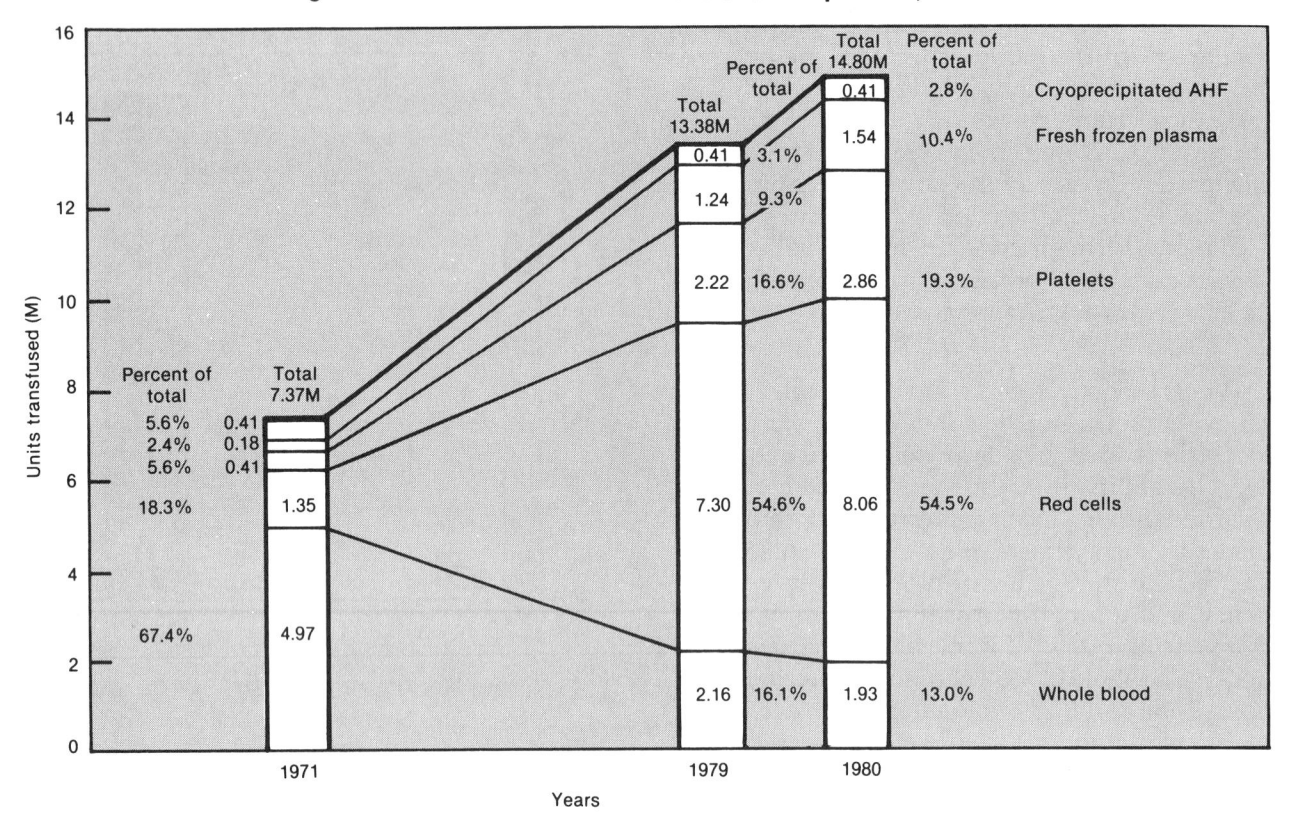

Figure 2.—U.S. Transfusions of Blood and Components, 1971-80

SOURCE: Surgenor and Schnitzer/ABC, 1983.

panies "self-source"; i.e., they run their own source plasma centers. Ninety-eight U.S. source plasma centers (30 percent) are owned by fractionation companies. In addition, most of the other centers contract annually with fractionators to provide a certain amount of plasma, although there is some "spot buying." Recovered plasma (from whole blood) is either contracted for, or marketed through the efforts of nine major brokers. Both the brokers and the for-profit source plasma centers are members of the American Blood Resources Association (ABRA), a nonprofit trade association organized in 1972 to represent the interests of businesses engaged in the collection, manufacturing, or distribution of certain biological products—in particular, plasma for further manufacturing.

The market for source plasma is largely controlled by four pharmaceutical companies (Hyland Therapeutics, Cutter Laboratories, Alpha Therapeutics, and Armour), which are in turn subsidiaries of major corporations (Travenol, Bayer, Green Cross of Japan, and Revlon, respectively). Each commercial fractionator accounts for about 1 million of the 4 million liters fractionated commercially in the United States annually (459). In addition, the nonprofit New York Blood Center operates its own plant, with a capacity to fractionate 300,000 liters per year from plasma recovered from its own donors and from a portion of Red Cross donors.

The U.S. source plasma collection industry is the most important contributor to worldwide plasma fractionation. The approximate disposition of both source and recovered plasma collected in the United States at the present time is shown in figure 3. About 1.3 million of the 6 million liters of source plasma produced is exported, in addition to the export of plasma derivatives manufactured in the United States. Some 5.5 million of the 12.5-million-liter worldwide manufacturing capacity in 1978 was in the United States.

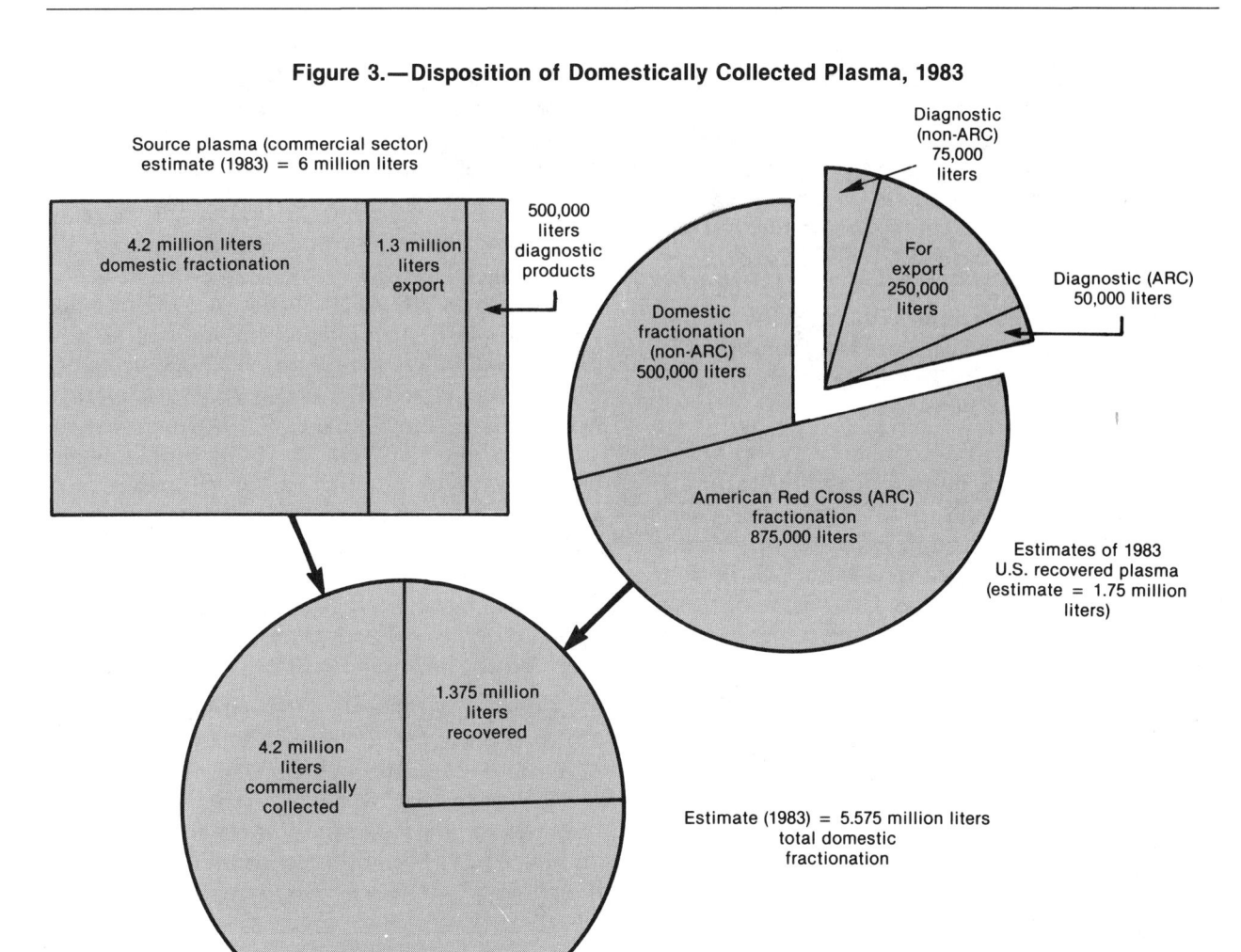

Figure 3.—Disposition of Domestically Collected Plasma, 1983

Source plasma (commercial sector) estimate (1983) = 6 million liters
- 4.2 million liters domestic fractionation
- 1.3 million liters export
- 500,000 liters diagnostic products

Domestic fractionation (non-ARC) 500,000 liters
American Red Cross (ARC) fractionation 875,000 liters
Diagnostic (non-ARC) 75,000 liters
For export 250,000 liters
Diagnostic (ARC) 50,000 liters

Estimates of 1983 U.S. recovered plasma (estimate = 1.75 million liters)

4.2 million liters commercially collected
1.375 million liters recovered

Estimate (1983) = 5.575 million liters total domestic fractionation

SOURCE: Understanding Plasma, *Plasma Quarterly*, 1984.

Of the 7.0-million-liter capacity outside the United States, about 5 million liters were in the commercial sector, and about 2.0 million liters in the voluntary sector. But there were only about 77 plasma fractionation firms worldwide outside the United States (439) and commercial plants outside the United States operate at about 60 percent capacity, compared to about 85 to 90 percent in the United States (459). Increasing amounts of the albumin and antihemophilic factor (Factor VIII) produced in the United States are used abroad. In 1984, it is estimated that approximately one-third of the albumin and one-half of the Factor VIII produced in the United States will be consumed in foreign countries (see table 19). The U.S. fractionation industry currently supplies about 70 percent of Factor VIII, 70 percent of albumin, and lesser amounts of the gamma globulin used in the world. Thus, much of the plasma and plasma derivatives used worldwide comes from U.S. sources.

Costs of Blood Products

Blood collection and transfusion facilities have not developed an industrywide uniform method of allocating costs to each step in the collection and transfusion process. Further, most of the available data are on charges or prices, not on costs.

In 1980, the average cost to a community blood center for the collection of one unit of whole blood was nearly $46, but costs varied widely, with a standard deviation of over $15. Most of these costs are allocated to red cells (see, e.g., 142). In 1980, the average community blood center red cell processing fee was about $32, while the average total hospital charge for a unit of red cells was about $89. Processing fees charged for whole blood and packed red cells are less than the cost per unit of blood collected because costs are also allocated to other components.

There are wide variations in the fees charged to hospitals by blood collectors and by hospitals to patients. For example, in 1983, processing fees for whole blood charged to hospitals by American Red Cross regions ranged from $28 (in San Juan, PR) to $59 (in San Jose, CA). Some of these differences can be explained by differences in costs between geographic areas, but blood centers can allocate more costs to one component than to others (as in the case of red cells), and also factor into their charges such program expenses as personnel training, research support, and capital costs for new buildings and equipment. There are also substantial variations in hospital charges for red cells (the only component for which hospital data are available), with standard deviations from a quarter to a third of the mean (576).

In addition to the processing fee charged by the blood center, hospital charges might include an additional processing fee, a nonreplacement charge if a replacement policy is still in effect, a laboratory charge, an infusion charge, and other charges. Total charges are usually higher at collecting than at noncollecting hospitals, with higher processing fees and nonreplacement fees accounting for the higher total charges (576). (Latest available data on hospital charges are for 1980, and such charges have undoubtedly risen since then.)

Increases in blood costs have generally not exceeded increases in total health care costs. From 1980 to 1982, national health expenditures increased an average of 15 percent per year, while blood center processing fees increased 7 percent (for CCBC members) and 12 percent (for Red Cross regions). Increases in hospital charges for blood, on the other hand, appear closer to increases in hospital charges in general, although it is difficult to draw conclusions with information from only 2 years.

As for costs of plasma derivatives, 1984 retail prices for Factor VIII (including heat-treated products) ranged from $0.09 to $0.26 per unit in the United States (99,464). Needs vary for mild, moderate, and severe hemophiliacs, but assuming an average consumption of 50,000 units per year (293), Factor VIII could cost the average hemophiliac from $4,500 to $13,000 per year. In addition, from 10 (99) to 15 (76) percent of hemophiliacs have inhibitors to Factor VIII and require a special form of coagulation product, anti-inhibitor coagulant complex, which can cost from $0.70 to $1.00 per unit (99). Factor IX Complex, used for hemophilia B patients, costs from $0.05 to $0.10 per unit. Products for hemophiliacs are more costly in foreign countries.

In the United States, a 250-milliliter bottle of albumin costs approximately $32. The price of albumin has not been challenged per se, but its use instead of less expensive crystalloid alternatives for volume restoration has been questioned, and there have been other longstanding questions over the proper use of albumin.

Availability

The trend in collection and distribution of blood components has been toward centralization; i.e., toward the establishment of community and regional blood centers and away from hospital blood banks individually providing for their own needs. Blood components, especially the cellular ones, still have relatively short storage lives; whole blood and red cells have 35 days (with preservative solutions recently approved for 49 days), and platelets up to 5 days (5-day storage bags have recently been approved, increased from 3-day bags). Thus, the regionalization of blood resources has been primarily oriented toward maximum use of a perishable product, and purchasers (predominantly hospitals) have been less concerned over the price they paid than the assurance that they could obtain blood components as needed. That is, the cost to hospitals could be passed on to patients and their insurors; so availability, and not price, was the primary factor in purchasing blood components. (The implications of present health care cost containment measures and their effect on price-consciousness are discussed below.) Regionalization of blood resources has proceeded on this basis, including the American Blood Commission's regionalization recognition program.

Blood banks, whether as regional centers or as part of a hospital, have also kept their stocks in approximate balance with demand by sharing between banks with surpluses and those with shortages. There is apparently much undocumented ad hoc sharing by blood banks both within regions and between regions, and there are also two national sharing programs, one run by the American Association of Blood Banks, and another by the American Red Cross.

Periodic attempts to combine these two systems into a single system, with the American Blood Commission as the mediator, have been unsuccessful. One reason is that, despite a Department of Justice opinion that a resource sharing agreement would not violate Federal anti-trust legislation, the American Red Cross has expressed fear that it would be liable to a civil suit if it were to sign a formal nationwide resource sharing agreement. For example, representatives of the plasma derivatives industry have objected to limiting a resource sharing agreement to voluntarily collected blood. On the other hand, there are no systematic deficiencies which can be clearly identified which would be resolved by a single sharing system. Blood banks have their own informal networks and use both of the national systems on an as-needed basis. In addition, sharing can and does take place on a regular, planned basis between blood banks with chronic shortages and those which have a consistent surplus.

It is not possible to estimate what the minimal amount of sharing should be between blood service regions to determine whether regions are collecting their "fair share" of the blood components they need and use; i.e., whether they are adequately self-sufficient. Blood collection regions have been established reflecting past blood collection organization efforts, the distribution of hospitals in the region, as a compromise between competing local collectors, etc. They have not been established on the basis of assuring that the population base from which blood is collected is the same population as the users of those blood products. Nor would that be possible, given the widespread population that modern medical centers draw from. Similarly the majority of donors are under 40, while the majority of users are older people, and blood collected from small cities and towns is used in large cities.

In conclusion, there do not seem to be systematic problems with availability in the voluntary whole blood sector. Imbalances between supply and demand have been met both within and between regions by a combination of ad hoc and organized methods of sharing. Price has not played much of a role, but indications are that it is becoming increasingly important as purchasers come under prospective payment systems and can no longer pass on all the costs of their purchases.

Because the plasma derivatives sector is part of the pharmaceutical industry its distribution networks are similar to those for the marketing of prescription drugs. Thus, the commercial sector presents a different picture from that of blood components, although, as in the voluntary sector, availability of products does not seem to be a problem. The national plasma derivatives market is intertwined with the international market, and both profit and nonprofit companies and organizations are involved. Because of the increased use of red cell concentrates instead of whole blood, the voluntary sector has become a significant supplier of plasma and plasma derivatives, accounting for about 20 percent of the plasma derivatives sold in the United States. The American Red Cross (which contracts with commercial fractionators to produce derivatives from Red Cross plasma) markets its own products, as do the New York Blood Center, and laboratories run by the States of Michigan and Massachusetts. In addition, both the Swiss and Dutch Red Cross sell some albumin in the U.S. market. The New York Blood Center and the American Red Cross also sell Factor VIII, and the Massachusetts Biologics Laboratory is the sole producer in the United States of herpes zoster immune globulin.

Following the establishment of the plasma fractionation industry in World War II to produce albumin in mass volume, albumin for civilian use became the principal product of the industry. This "driving force" role was briefly taken over by the immune globulins in the 1950s, then by the coagulation proteins (principally Factor VIII) toward the end of the 1960s as techniques to extract coagulation proteins in mass volumes were perfected. At the present time, coagulation proteins, being the most profitable, are the principal desired product of the fractionation industry, and albumin is a "byproduct" although still the largest in terms of volume and total sales (see table 1). Hyperimmune globulins against specific diseases have been developed in addition to general immune serum globulins that contain a mixture of antibody types.

Albumin marketing is much like that for basic commodities or generic drugs. The market is sensitive to price changes, a high level of competition exists, and product choice is related more to the price, source of service, packaging, and other inducements than to the quality of a particular manufacturer's product. All manufacturers' products must meet FDA standards.

Distribution outlets for the coagulation proteins vary from region to region, but most large urban areas have at least one major hemophilia treatment center that routinely stocks them. As home care of hemophiliacs increases, patients are beginning to be able to have these products supplied directly to them on prescription. Packaging, auxiliary supplies (e.g., infusion sets), availability, as well as price and brand name loyalty have begun to determine which manufacturer's products are purchased. In addition, some manufacturers provide financial assistance in the form of reduced prices for insured hemophiliacs. Product availability may be an issue, however, for those who are uninsured or live in remote areas.

Sellers of both albumin and the coagulation proteins have central distribution or supply networks, and volume purchasing, often by organized groups of purchasers, on an annual bidding basis, is fairly prevalent. Immune globulins are routinely distributed by pharmaceutical distributors, hospital supply companies and blood centers, as well as directly by manufacturers to the numerous hospitals, nursing homes, physicians, and clinics that prescribe these preparations. Annual bidding is not as common as for albumin and the coagulation proteins, but is increasing.

In sum, regional shortages and surpluses in the voluntary sector have been handled through sharing programs between regions, but there is much ad hoc sharing between blood banks outside the organized intra- and interregional programs. Technological improvements in storage methods have also enhanced availability. Price and other competitive aspects of supplying a product have not been important factors but may become so with the implementation of programs to contain health care costs through prospective payment systems.

In contrast, the major plasma derivatives are marketed nationally and internationally, with no apparent advantages in price and quality of the nonprofit products over the commercial ones. Excess plasma from greater use of red cell concentrates instead of whole blood has led to nonprofits becoming increasingly involved in the plasma derivatives industry. Product availability seems to be an issue only for hemophiliacs, as a consequence of inadequate resources or geographic inaccessibility to treatment.

Safety

Although recent attention on the safety hazards of blood transfusions has focused on acquired immunodeficiency syndrome (AIDS), individuals have a much greater chance of contracting some form of hepatitis from transfusions of blood components and some plasma derivatives than they do of contracting AIDS, despite a number of med-

Table 1.—Worldwide Demand for Plasma Fractions, by Product, 1978 (in monetary value)

Albumin/PPF	41%
Intravenous gamma globulin	23
Hyperimmune globulins	14
Factor VIII concentrate	13
Immune serum globulin	8
All others	1
Total	100%

SOURCE: International Federation of Pharmaceutical Manufacturers, 1980.

ical advances and the decrease in paid whole blood donors. Laboratory tests for hepatitis B have greatly increased in sensitivity over the past decade; as a consequence, there has been a dramatic reduction in posttransfusion hepatitis B cases. (Hepatitis A is rarely transmitted by blood because the individual's blood usually contains the virus only during the clinical stage, during which the individual is unlikely to donate blood and which is easily detected during routine donor screening procedures.) However, by the late 1970s, a new type of transfusion-associated hepatitis was found.

This form of hepatitis has been named non-A, non-B hepatitis, because it is distinctly different from both hepatitis A and B. Five to eighteen percent of Americans who receive five or more units of transfused blood develop non-A, non-B hepatitis (271a). Currently, approximately 90 percent of all posttransfusion cases of hepatitis is due to non-A, non-B hepatitis, and 10 percent due to hepatitis B (558). No etiologic agent(s) has so far been identified, although a retrovirus has recently been implicated as the cause of non-A, non-B hepatitis. Therefore, there are no specific tests for non-A, non-B hepatitis at present.

Efforts to prevent infection can occur at the following stages of blood processing: 1) donor screening, to prevent collection of potentially contaminated units; 2) laboratory testing of collected units, to detect contaminated units; and 3) inactivation or removal of micro-organisms, to destroy infectious agents prior to use.

Screening of donors may begin by selection of populations with a low prevalence of transmissible diseases. Preference for voluntary over paid donors was based, in addition to ethical considerations, on the lower prevalence of hepatitis and other transmissible diseases in voluntary donors. The exclusion of intravenous drug abusers is based on the same considerations, and recent decisions to ask homosexual and bisexual men with multiple partners to refrain from donating, due to the high incidence of AIDS in this group, were similarly motivated.

Individual donor screening is also carried out. Each prospective blood or plasma donor, whether voluntary or paid, is subjected to screening by medical history and selected physical and laboratory examinations. Prospective donors are questioned for signs and symptoms of disease and a history of exposure to disease. Laboratory tests to determine whether or not the collected unit may transmit infection may be specific or nonspecific. Specific tests, such as the test for hepatitis B surface antigen, which is required of all blood and plasma donors, detect the infectious agent itself or some element of it. Nonspecific tests, such as the screening for syphilis that is also required of all blood and plasma collections, usually measure a response of the body which may occur in several disease states, one of which includes the disease in question. They have obvious limitations but may be useful until specific tests can be developed. Other examples of nonspecific tests are measurement of the liver enzyme, alanine aminotransferase (ALT), used by a few blood centers to screen for carriers of non-A, non-B hepatitis, and the T-lymphocyte helper:suppressor ratio, which was initiated at the Stanford Medical Center to screen for AIDS. The presence of antibodies to hepatitis B **core** antigen (as contrasted to the presence of hepatitis B **surface** antigen, which is indicative of the presence of the **active** virus) has been used by some blood centers to screen donors for AIDS, because it is believed that those individuals who have been exposed to hepatitis B may also have a higher risk for exposure to AIDS.

To be useful, laboratory tests should be: 1) able to be performed easily, rapidly, and on a large scale to permit testing of the large number of units collected to prepare perishable blood products; 2) sensitive enough to detect a large proportion of contaminated units; 3) specific enough not to have incorrectly positive reactions in most noninfected units; 4) able to detect a disease of health importance to the recipient population; and 5) targeted at a disease which occurs frequently enough to warrant screening of all donated units (434). Of the tests mentioned above, the specific test for hepatitis B surface antigen is the only test that satisfies all these criteria.

Early attempts to prevent AIDS from entering the blood supply were reminiscent of early methods oriented toward hepatitis B and current attempts to screen out hepatitis non-A, non-B carriers. One of the principal stimuli for a National Blood Policy was the risk of hepatitis B. Donor screening methods, directed both at groups with high incidences of hepatitis and at individuals, plus the labeling of blood as being derived from "paid" or "voluntary" donors, were the principal methods of screening for hepatitis B until very sensitive laboratory tests to detect the presence of the hepatitis B surface antigen were developed and applied to every unit of blood and plasma collected. In the case of non-A, non-B hepatitis, donor screening remains the primary line of defense, with a few blood centers using the nonspecific ALT test in addition. This is similar to strategies to screen for AIDS; specific classes of donors have been excluded, physical examinations in high risk areas look for some of the preclinical signs of AIDS such as general enlargement of the lymph nodes, and a few blood centers have used surrogate tests for AIDS. (A specific blood test for the presumed AIDS agent, human T-cell lymphotropic virus, type III (HTLV-III), will be available in early 1985.)

In addition to screening through donor exclusion and laboratory testing, some transmissible infections can be prevented by treatment of the blood product to remove or inactivate infectious agents. Currently, the most important of these methods is pasteurization. (The cellular elements of blood cannot withstand this treatment, which is applicable only to some of the plasma derivatives.) Albumin, which is widely used for blood volume expansion and other medical purposes, can be heated to 60° C for 10 hours, which inactivates hepatitis viruses and appears to inactivate other viruses as well. Thus, FDA requires that all albumin preparations be pasteurized in this manner.

Prior to the AIDS problem, concentrates of the clotting factors (e.g., Factor VIII) had not been subject to pasteurization because of inactivation of the clotting factors. However, recent advances in heat processing of Factor VIII in the presence of stabilizers have been accomplished, with evidence of inactivation of some type of viruses but with some loss in potency of the preparations (162). All four commercial manufacturers of Factor VIII have recently received FDA approval to market these products. Claims of reduced hepatitis transmission from heat-treated products, based on chimpanzee studies, are currently under study, with the hope that pasteurization will also inactivate other viral agents, such as the presumed virus(es) for AIDS. (Current research suggests that the presumed AIDS agent, HTLV-III, is inactivated by this process.)

ISSUES AND POINTS TO CONSIDER

Currently, three areas of primary concern in blood resources development and maintenance are at issue, none of which were major issues a decade ago when a National Blood Policy was enunciated. These issues are: 1) the impact of AIDS on blood collection and use, 2) the impact of efforts to contain health care costs and the related issue of the costs of blood products, and 3) alternative sources and substitutes for blood products. AIDS is having an immediate impact, health care cost containment portends possible fundamental changes in the near future, and new and emerging technologies have the potential in the not too distant future to profoundly affect the present source plasma and plasma fractionation and voluntary whole blood industries.

In contrast, the primary issues a decade ago, in addition to that of safety, were: 1) coordination of blood resources (including disagreement over community v. individual responsibility for blood donations, and the desirability of Federal intervention in the blood supply); 2) appropriate use; 3) voluntary v. commercial approaches; and 4) information systems to monitor blood resources. These are still issues today, although they been pushed into the background by AIDS, cost containment, and alternative sources. Furthermore, continuing activities in these areas are likely to be influenced by what happens in the three current primary issue areas.

AIDS

In some sense, the safety issues associated with AIDS and blood products are but an extension of the safety issues of a decade ago, when hepatitis B was the primary disease that was transmitted through blood. Hepatitis continues to be the primary blood-transmitted disease, with non-A, non-B hepatitis replacing hepatitis B as the primary transmitted disease. The experience with non-A, non-B hepatitis is very similar to that with AIDS, with the difference that it has not captured the public's attention as AIDS has. Of the risks associated with blood products, transfusion recipients and users of coagulation proteins are much more likely to contract non-A, non-B hepatitis or hepatitis B than AIDS. Hemophiliacs, however, are a special class even though their rates of hepatitis are higher than their risk of contracting AIDS, because of their great use of coagulation proteins and the high incidence of AIDS among them.

Publication in January 1984 by Centers for Disease Control (CDC) researchers of their conclusion that there were cases of AIDS associated with transfusions (143) caused consternation in blood resources circles. But at a February 1984 meeting, convened by CDC, of representatives of blood banks and other groups interested in transfusion-associated AIDS, there was agreement that the evidence that AIDS could and had been transmitted through blood products was conclusive enough that no further studies need be conducted to prove/disprove the association. Rather, studies to quantify and clarify the risks were needed. Even before this, however, AIDS was already suspected as being due to some type of transmissible agent such as a virus, and procedures had been adopted in an attempt to reduce the risk of blood-related AIDS. Furthermore, it was already known in 1982 that hemophiliacs were among the groups that were at increased risk for AIDS, with their heavy use of clotting factors as the suspected mode of transmission.

In March 1983, the FDA, in consultation with the major blood banking and plasma derivative organizations, the National Hemophilia Foundation, the National Gay Task Force, the Centers for Disease Control, and the National Institutes of Health (NIH), issued recommendations to initiate: 1) educational programs to inform persons at increased risk of AIDS to refrain from blood or plasma donation, 2) expanded medical screening of blood and plasma donors to identify individuals with early signs or symptoms of AIDS, 3) examination of source plasma donors for lymph node enlargement, and 4) measurement of body weight of source plasma donors prior to each donation to detect unexplained weight loss. Some blood banks began to introduce procedures which allow donors to privately indicate whether or not their blood donations should be used for transfusions, because such individuals may be especially reluctant to acknowledge their homosexuality or use of injectable drugs before their peers at school, business or community blood drives.

As part of public information campaigns about the risks of AIDS, the Public Health Service and blood banking organizations included warnings about who should refrain from donating blood and also tried to allay groundless fears that AIDS could be contracted by simply donating blood. For source plasma collectors, FDA made additional recommendations that plasma collected in geographic areas of high risk for AIDS not be used to manufacture coagulation proteins. And the National Hemophilia Foundation issued guidelines for the use of cryoprecipitate, Factor VIII and Factor IX complex, including the preferential use of cryoprecipitate in some circumstances.

As of May 1984, the FDA Blood Products Advisory Committee was also studying the issue of whether specific surrogate tests should be instituted for all whole blood and plasma collections and had also recommended that a pilot study be conducted to measure the effectiveness of procedures by which plasma donors could privately indicate that their plasma should not be used in the manufacture of coagulation products (as had been adopted by a number of blood banks for whole blood donations).

All four commercial manufacturers, the Red Cross, and the New York Blood Center withdrew lots of Factor VIII (and related lots of Factor IX Complex) upon being informed that a donor(s) whose plasma had been used in the preparation of those lots had developed AIDS. (Donor records must be kept for at least 5 years, and matchups of AIDS cases with donor lists had been made.) The largest of these voluntary market withdrawals involved enough Factor VIII to represent 500 patient-years of treatment (434).

As noted, all four commercial manufacturers also subsequently developed heat-treatment (pasteurization) methods with claims of reduced infectivity of hepatitis viruses, the hope being that the process would also affect the presumed AIDS virus. These pasteurization methods have reduced the potency of the clotting factor preparations (the reason why previous preparations could not be pasteurized), but apparently not enough to markedly affect their efficacy.

Surrogate laboratory tests for AIDS have also been extensively discussed, and some blood banks have instituted them. The tests are of two types: 1) detection of abnormalities associated with AIDS or the preclinical stages of the disease, and 2) evidence of past infections with diseases that have a high incidence in the same population groups that are at increased risk for AIDS. However, conditions other than AIDS can lead to abnormal test results in tests of the first type. For example, Stanford University Blood Bank began to test all blood donations for T-lymphocyte helper:suppressor ratios (445). About 1 to 2 percent of collections have been positive, but such individuals are not permanently deferred from donating, since short-term virus infections can also cause an abnormal ratio.

The Irwin Memorial Blood Bank in San Francisco instituted a test for antibodies to hepatitis B core antigen (as did Cutter Laboratories for its source plasma donors) which reveals past infection with hepatitis B and expects that donor deferrals will increase by 5 to 7 percent. (Cutter expected a positive test rate of 15 percent and planned to use this plasma only for production of albumin and immune globulins, which are not implicated with AIDS.)

AIDS also kindled interest among patients and physicians for autologous and directed donations. Autologous donations, where a patient "banks" his/her own blood prior to elective surgery, was always considered the safest of transfusions. However, it could pose problems for the management of blood if it were to be more widely applied. Surgeons often prefer not to use it, medical personnel may be exposed to health risks because the blood is not tested for hepatitis, and autologous blood may outdate if surgery is postponed. Individual blood banks have allowed the use of directed donations either to ease patients' fears or in response to pressures from patients and their physicians. Directed donations, however, have been opposed by most blood bankers because of the potential for disruption of the blood collection and distribution system if widely adopted, and because of a lack of evidence that such donations are indeed safer than anonymous donations.

In April 1984, the Secretary of DHHS announced that researchers had identified the AIDS virus and developed technologies to mass-produce a blood test which would become "widely available within about 6 months," and would "identify AIDS victims with essentially 100 percent certainty" (256). A few days later, DHHS announced a request for applications to produce and distribute such a test, with requests to be submitted within 10 days of the announcement (181). Thus, whether the Secretary's promise to provide a reliable test for AIDS can be kept will be known soon, and if the test is provided it should alleviate much of the pressure to adopt some type of surrogate test—and may again turn directed donations into a nonissue in the blood community.

But questions raised as a result of the donor screening methods developed against AIDS, use of surrogate tests, and interest in directed donation programs will not be completely moot even if a highly specific test for AIDS is available soon.

Points to Consider

Evaluation of Donor Screening Criteria.—*One of the first steps taken by the blood community in attempting to keep AIDS out of the blood* *supply was to exclude classes of people who were deemed at high risk for AIDS.* The impact of this policy has been especially felt by the gay male community. (Young males have always been among the principal, if not the largest, groups of blood donors.) Intravenous drug abusers have always been one of the excluded blood donor groups, and exclusion of recent Haitian immigrants can be likened to policies which exclude donors who have recently arrived from areas with high incidences of infectious diseases which can be transmitted through blood donations.

An evaluation of the exclusion of gay males is needed, not only to confirm whether or not this policy has indeed led to decreased AIDS transmission through blood, but also to confirm whether or not such an exclusionary, stigmatizing policy is justified by the results.

There are two measures of whether or not this policy has worked. First is an assessment of the process; i.e., whether or not the donor population has indeed changed, with fewer young to middle-aged males in the donor base. This would be especially significant in areas of high incidences of AIDS, where the implementation of this policy has been actively pursued. This evaluation would also include the effectiveness of providing avenues of private communications by donors to indicate whether or not their blood should be used for transfusions.

Second would be an evaluation of whether or not exclusion of gay males has in fact resulted in a reduction of blood-transmitted cases of AIDS. The time between transfusion and onset of illness has ranged from 10 to 43 months, with an average of about 24 months (143). Cases of blood-transmitted AIDS that were diagnosed through the end of 1984, would have resulted from transfusions of blood which were donated prior to instituting the donor exclusion policies, which began in early 1983. If donor exclusion policies have made a difference, the effect should not begin to appear until late 1984.

These evaluations could also be tied to the expected development of highly specific laboratory tests for AIDS. As those expected tests are instituted and evaluated, a reassessment of current donor screening policies could help determine whether or not they should continue, be modified, or be eliminated.

These evaluations were discussed at the February 1984 meeting of blood bankers convened by CDC, but no decisions were made. CDC sees its primary role as risk assessment, not risk management. Therefore, thought was given to the role of the blood banking organizations in the evaluation of donor screening.

Individual blood centers have instituted variations on the basic donor screening recommendations, such as different ways to allow donors to withdraw their donations in private. Several of these centers have ongoing evaluations of these efforts, and the blood organizations (AABB, ARC, CCBC) could coordinate these efforts or mount a centralized research effort. Thus, *blood organizations could be encouraged to conduct evaluations of donor screening and its impact on blood-transmitted AIDS.*

The alternative to a blood banking organization-directed evaluation is to direct Federal agencies to evaluate donor screening and its impact on blood-transmitted AIDS. Federal agencies could play the primary role in evaluating donor screening, with cooperation and/or contracting with the voluntary organizations or directly with a consortium of blood centers to perform the actual study. A possible locus for this Federal role could be the National Center for Health Services Research instead of CDC, NIH, or FDA, since the latter agencies are oriented more toward epidemiological field work and basic and applied biomedical research. It is conceivable that FDA could sponsor the evaluation because of its regulatory responsibilities.

Congress could advise the Department of Health and Human Services as to its priorities in this evaluation as against other evaluations of blood-transmitted AIDS, or it could provide separate funds. The evaluation could also be expanded to address the broader question of the continued need for donor screening methods specific to AIDS once a specific laboratory test for AIDS is in place.

Identification of Suspected AIDS-Carrying Donors and Recipients of Their Blood Donations.—*CDC has gathered and continues to accumulate information on AIDS cases in general and on donors who have been implicated with cases suspected to be blood transfusion related, although they are now doing so with a coded system, making donors anonymous even to CDC until tracing is required.* While some health departments have a policy to inform the local blood center as new cases of AIDS are diagnosed in order to match their names with blood donor lists (e.g., the San Francisco health department and Irwin Memorial Blood Bank), blood donations are not necessarily limited to the current city of residence, particularly with the mobility associated with modern life. One issue, then, has been: *should the names of AIDS patients be made available, to what extent, and to whom?* For example, should all State health departments be notified? Should all blood banks be notified, so that they can match the list of names with their donor registries?

Finding donors who actually have had AIDS has been the exception. Most of the "suspected" donors have not been found to actually have AIDS; they either belong to a high-risk group (e.g., are gay males) or have nonspecific laboratory abnormalities (e.g., reversed T-lymphocyte helper:suppressor ratios) or physical signs that could be AIDS related (e.g., enlarged lymph nodes). The use of a test for HTLV-III will also identify persons who have been exposed to the presumed AIDS agent and who may or may not be carriers of the virus. *Should these donors be treated in the same way as confirmed AIDS patients, insofar as releasing their names is concerned?*

An even more vexing problem has been in dealing with patients who received blood components from donors who are suspected in the blood-transfusion AIDS cases. Should they be told, or should that information be passed on only to the blood bank which provided the blood, or to the patient's personal physician, leaving it up to his/her judgment to inform the patient? Since *monitoring of these recipients of suspected AIDS-contaminated blood is important in determining the epidemiological characteristics of the disease*—e.g., its rates of infectivity, morbidity, and mortality—it does not seem practical to design such monitoring activities without informing the patients.

These issues were addressed at the February 1984 CDC meeting, a subsequent March 1984 meeting of the National Heart, Lung, and Blood Institute's AIDS Working Group, and another meeting of the AIDS Working Group in late May 1984. This latter meeting also included medical ethicists to see how such studies could be reconciled with the ethical problems. A previous assessment of "Confidentiality in Research on AIDS" had been completed by The Hastings Center, but the focus of that assessment was on assuring the confidentiality of AIDS victims, and not to the issue above—i.e., how to approach the question of monitoring other recipients of suspected AIDS-contaminated blood, and who should be informed.

Laboratory Tests for AIDS.—*Current surrogate tests lead to exclusion of far more donors than are ever expected to actually have or develop AIDS, and seem to have been instituted more to allay patients' and physicians' fears rather than in hopes of decreasing exposure to AIDS.* Besides increasing costs due to the expense of testing, discarding of blood after collection, lost donors, and the need to recruit additional donors, the psychic costs to donors labeled as suspect have been subordinated in order to reduce the psychic costs of potential and actual recipients and their physicians. Given the public apprehension surrounding AIDS, this situation can be expected to continue. For example, testing for past infections with hepatitis B (anti-HBc) is expected to exclude about 6 percent of current voluntary donors and 15 percent of commercial source plasma donors, and apparently this cost is not viewed as too high for the psychic benefit it is expected to produce.

The criterion used in decisions to institute these programs appears to be whether the added costs can be handled, not whether in fact AIDS will be reduced. *However, these decisions seem entirely compatible with public reaction to the threat of AIDS* in the blood supply. The risk is very small, but the fear is great, *and the perception that something is being done is important to public confidence.*

A highly accurate, AIDS-specific test should decrease the perceived need for adopting any of the surrogate tests that have been proposed, but reassuring the public will probably mean that these tests *can also be expected to be applied far beyond the application that would be scientifically justified.* For example, hepatitis B testing is justified on the basis of its incidence and severity, and the search for a test for non-A, non-B hepatitis is also justified on that basis. On the other hand, the continued requirement for testing for syphilis of all whole blood and plasma collections has been questioned because of its low cost effectiveness. The syphilis testing example, however, points to the fact that safety has been the primary concern, and it can be expected to take priority once an AIDS-specific test is available.

Thus, it can be expected that the test for HTLV-III will be a requirement for all blood and plasma collections, regardless of the relative degree of risk among blood banks and geographic areas. Even if not required for all, blood banks and plasma collectors will feel compelled to perform the test anyway because of the public confidence factor and the threat of lawsuits. It should also be reasonable to expect that plasma fractionators, because of the pooling of plasma from thousands of donors, may be required to test for AIDS a second time when they receive plasma from blood banks and source plasma centers (this is currently being discussed in FDA for the test of active hepatitis B, the HBsAg test, which is currently required only at the time of donation).

Such additional testing will further raise the costs of blood and plasma products, but the advent of cost containment measures will exert pressures in the opposite direction; i.e., it can no longer be assumed that blood testing (and other processing) costs can be passed on to purchasers. The circumstances surrounding AIDS will most likely compel nationwide adoption of tests that are developed, *but the additional costs of such testing should provide incentives to reassess all of the tests that have been adopted over the years to improve safety.* Among these are the requirements for syphilis testing and for blood typing each time a donor gives blood (blood types do not change).

Directed Donations.—Interest in directed donations increased with AIDS and has been implemented in some of the areas with a high incidence of AIDS (e.g., Los Angeles, San Francisco). Such interest may diminish with the availability of an accurate and sensitive test for AIDS, but individual blood centers may maintain directed donations for individual patients indefinitely. A serious problem may arise, however, *if organizations press for directed donations.* In this case, *entire sets of blood might be tied up and have the potential for disrupting the present, well-balanced system of blood supplies. The potential scope is great: a third of those who donate regularly do so to contribute to a company blood drive* (25).

Costs of Blood Products

Charges for blood products vary considerably but are generally not considered to be a national problem because they account for only about 1 percent of total health care costs and because increases in charges do not appear to have exceeded increases in overall health care costs. However, the costs of blood products may cause hardships for two types of consumers: hemophiliacs and public hospitals.

Points to Consider

Coverage for Hemophiliacs' Care.—The situation for hemophiliacs has improved dramatically since passage of Public Law 94-63 in 1975. The law provided funding for the creation of comprehensive hemophilia treatment centers, 23 of which have since been created. A recent survey of about half of those centers found that conditions had markedly improved for the 3,705 patients seen in the fifth year of the program. Compared to the year before the programs had started, the costs of total care, including rates of hospitalization, had been reduced, and unemployment among hemophiliacs was lower. The proportion of patients with third-party coverage had also grown, both because employment of hemophiliacs increased as a result of better treatment, and because health care workers at the centers have helped patients arrange for coverage. However, the survey of treatment centers represented only those hemophiliacs with access to comprehensive treatment centers, probably half of the hemophiliac population. In addition, third-party payments may not cover the plasma derivatives needed for prophylactic treatment, which can cost $13,000 per year for a severe hemophiliac.

Medicare does not, and private insurers often do not, cover the costs of the needed blood products on an outpatient basis, because plasma derivatives are considered to be pharmaceuticals. Distributors of coagulation proteins sometimes disregard copayment requirements for their hemophiliac clients. Coverage is further complicated by the fact that unlike the End-Stage Renal Disease Program under Medicare, which recognizes patients with end-stage renal disease as being totally disabled and thus eligible for Medicare coverage for dialysis and transplants, hemophiliacs can receive Medicare coverage only through a case-by-case determination. State plans to cover hemophiliacs exist but vary widely in comprehensiveness, and hemophiliacs have been known to relocate in search of better benefits, disassociating themselves from important family and community ties. *Thus, opportunities exist for improving health care provisions for hemophiliacs, if not by creating a special program for them, then by providing coverage for blood products on an outpatient basis.*

Costs of Blood for Public Hospitals.—As for many other products and services the purchase of blood is a problem for public hospitals. Blood centers feel obliged to deliver needed blood products to public hospitals regardless of the fact that they may not be paid, and public hospital bills are often written off as uncollectible (420). Thus, the costs of blood for public hospitals are partially underwritten by hospitals which can pay the prices that blood centers charge. This situation is somewhat analogous to the sources and users of blood itself—suburban, rural, and middle-class urban residents already support inner cities by providing much of the needed blood. *As cost containment measures pressure hospitals to reduce overall per patient costs, pressure on blood centers to lower or not increase their charges may make it difficult for them to continue absorbing losses from their public hospital clients.*

Containment of Health Care Costs

The diagnosis-related grouping (DRG) method of payment for Medicare is now in the process of implementation. Under previous cost reimbursement, there were few incentives for hospitals to be price-conscious in purchasing blood products, reliability of sources being their primary criterion.

Higher charges for whole blood and red cells were associated with hospitals that collect part of their blood requirements v. those hospitals that did not (576). While no comparable hospital blood bank cost data were available, it seems reasonable to assume that at least part of the higher charges was due to higher costs. For example, regional blood centers have been found to have economies of scale for total costs. Under cost reimbursement, there was no incentive for hospitals to rely more on regional blood centers, but under fixed reimbursement rates management will have to reassess its arrangements for blood supplies. Even for hospital blood banks with costs lower than those of regional blood centers, other factors may lead to greater dependence on the regional center. These include the possibility of duplication of services, competition for blood donors, inventory control and outdating, and greater need for blood because of expanded and new services (189).

Another factor is the trend in ownership in both for-profit and nonprofit hospitals toward multihospital chains, which are introducing corporate management practices and volume purchases, thereby inserting hospital management more into the traditional relationships between hospital blood banks/transfusion services and regional blood centers. These developments mean that hospital management will be taking a close look at the cost effectiveness of purchasing blood from regional centers versus maintaining complete blood banking operations, although it has been argued that because blood is such a small portion of a patient's bill, such reviews may not occur for some time (534).

However, a move toward greater dependence on regional centers may be tempered by the need to generate income to support remaining blood banking activities. For example, with a fixed overhead in running hospital blood banks, hospitals may look toward additional services to generate income, such as platelet collections and therapeutic apheresis. Another opinion is that it is more cost effective for hospitals to collect their own blood, but that it has been more convenient to purchase it from a blood center (140).

Finally, one blood banker predicted that blood centers would expand even more and hospital blood banks would eventually close. The blood center has freedom from hospital cost control, and has a distinct advantage when it comes to research opportunities, since the blood center does not have the external controls that are found in hospitals (90).

Clearly, what will actually happen is still quite speculative, but some indications of the influence of cost containment measures are beginning to emerge. Limits were placed on hospital payment rates to provide them with incentives to be cost-conscious, including not only the services they performed, but also the purchases they made. While capital costs have been excluded from the DRG payment system by the current legislation, purchases of supplies have not. One blood center has been told by one of its hospitals that it would not accept any price increases in 1984 (196). In addition, the president of the ABC has expressed concern that hospitals are now shopping around for blood supplies on the basis of price, even using the AABB Clearinghouse at times in preference to their usual regional blood center sources (383).

Points to Consider

Financing of Blood Center Operations.—Blood centers use their revenues for their operating, research, and capital costs. Predictability of demand (and related revenues) for their products has been made easier by the regional systems that have developed over the past decade. Ad hoc and formal sharing of blood between blood centers with shortages and surpluses have also contributed to a fairly predictable stream of revenue. Furthermore, as availability/convenience has been the controlling factor instead of price under previous cost reimbursement for hospital services, the prices that blood centers have quoted have generally been what they received.

Some price competition is now appearing for blood products, either through requests to hold prices level or through purchases from less expensive sources. *Some blood bankers have already suggested that the service (processing) fee be treated as a pass-through, leaving under DRGs those costs of typing patients, cross-matching and all of the other services provided by the hospital for the patient* (120). Whatever the merits of such a proposal, it is premature at this point. Very good reasons would have to be provided without opening the door for other health care sectors to clamor for such an exclusion. This does not mean, however, that these concerns should be dismissed. *One area of concern is the research and training programs conducted by blood centers, and capital costs for new or improved facilities.* The Red Cross, because of the large reserves it has accumulated from blood revenues, could help some of its centers to maintain their research and training programs, but independent blood centers do not have this cushion to fall back on.

One reason for proceeding with caution before reaching the conclusion that cost restraints will significantly affect the present supply system *is the underlying assumption that price competition will (or could) develop into a significant purchasing factor.* The system is, after all, based on a system of voluntary donations. While regions with surpluses and those with shortages are part of the system, and spot purchases at better prices than available at the regional blood center may occur, *competitive purchases in the kinds of volumes that would endanger a region's blood center are not highly probable.* In order to do so, competing blood centers and blood banks may have to collect blood far beyond their needs and would have to justify to their donors why they are doing so. Increased revenues would hardly be accepted as a valid reason. Thus, hospitals may augment their major purchases by "spot buying" on the basis of price, and the real impact on blood centers may be to make them more cost conscious in their operations.

Current Supply and Distribution Systems.—The same considerations apply to the effect of cost containment measures on the collection and distribution systems that have been nurtured over the past decade, with the blood center at the hub (regionalization). *If publicized, overcollection of blood for the purpose of increasing revenues would threaten the blood center/donor relationship. As long as voluntary donors are the basic source of blood components, collection centers should not be able to increase their supplies for the purpose of competing for sales outside their existing distribution channels without threatening the relationship that has been so carefully nurtured over the years.* Thus, current indications of price shopping may be a temporary phenomenon, or an activity that will continue only at the margin.

Alternatives and Substitutes for Blood Products

Recent advances in biotechnology, particularly in the field of recombinant DNA technology, have suddenly raised the prospect that alternative sources for some blood products can be available by the end of the 1980s. The gene for albumin was cloned a few years ago, and many recombinant DNA companies have publicly claimed to have both recombinant yeast and bacterial strains carrying the human albumin gene. Most companies appear to have this project on hold for the present, due to problems of scaleup to mass production, purification of the resulting product, and questions over whether a recombinant albumin could be priced competitively with albumin from human sources. Many of the technical problems facing commercialization of recombinant albumin are unique. Not until those problems are solved will recombinant albumin be capable of meeting worldwide demand for albumin.

Developing recombinant DNA sources for Factor VIII was initially a much more difficult process, because the protein is much larger than albumin, and bacteria are incapable of producing the entire molecule because of the complexity of the gene. One company (Genetics Institute) announced in December 1983 that it had cloned part of the gene for Factor VIII, and several other companies have given the impression that they were close to testing recombinant Factor VIII in clinical trials.

These claims were met with skepticism, given the complexity of the molecule and its gene, and the instability of the biologically active protein. However, in April 1984, Genentech announced that it had succeeded in cloning the entire Factor VIII gene, and used a mammalian cell to produce the protein, thereby bypassing many of the problems inherent with bacteria or yeast as the cellular host. Genentech also claimed that it had tested the product and found it biologically active. Thus, technologies for producing both albumin and Factor VIII, the foundations of the plasma derivatives industry, are rapidly being developed. There are, however, some hurdles to be overcome before these products will be commercially available. These include development of techniques for production on a commercial scale, completion of tests of safety and efficacy, and approval by FDA for marketing. There is also the danger that litigation to resolve patent disputes may be quite protracted, delaying commercial availability of new products until claims of priority are resolved.

Other potentially useful plasma proteins not presently produced by the plasma derivatives industry or produced only on a small scale are also under exploration or testing by recombinant DNA companies. However, the activities necessary for developing other useful protein products are different from those used to develop Factor VIII and albumin. Small markets, and the unexplored clinical utility of these proteins, may mean that companies will not devote resources to their development.

True cellular substitutes for blood are much further away. Two products, perfluorochemicals and hemoglobin solutions, have been under development for a number of years, but still face safety and efficacy hurdles before they will become available. Even if and when they do become available, however, they will not be true substitutes for red blood cells, but will be only partial substitutes which can be used in place of red cells in special circumstances. Platelet substitutes are much further away, although there is growing interest in this field. White blood cell substitutes do not seem to be needed, given the doubtful need for them now from human blood.

The approach of developing cellular substitutes on a synthetic basis may be ultimately supplanted by cell culture techniques. Both red cells and platelets come from common progenitor "stem" cells found in bone marrow (and a small amount circulating in blood). If cell lines could be developed which both proliferate in massive amounts and can be controlled to differentiate into the desired cell types (red cells and platelets), a true alternative source of blood cells will have been accomplished. Given the rapid advances in cell culture techniques (e.g., hybridoma technology for the production of monoclonal antibodies) and understanding of cellular functions, it is not science fiction to assume that production of red blood cells and platelets from "stem" cells will eventually become a reality.

Nearly all of the work on developing recombinant DNA sources of plasma proteins is being conducted by biotechnology companies, some in conjunction with the parent corporations of the large fractionators of plasma (e.g., Green Cross of Japan, Baxter-Travenol). Most of the work on (partial) red cell substitutes has been performed by academic investigators or at military research institutes, although an array of commercial organizations has also been interested, ranging from plasma fractionation companies and large industrial concerns to small biotechnology firms. Most of the work on hemoglobin solutions has been sponsored by the military in its search for a battlefield resuscitation fluid. The company most closely associated with the other major class of partial red cell substitutes, perfluorochemicals, is Green Cross of Japan and its American subsidiary, Alpha Therapeutics (purchased a few years ago by Green Cross, and one of the four major plasma fractionators in the United States).

Points to Consider

Impact on the Plasma Derivatives Industry.— As an industry whose primary products are Factor VIII and albumin, *the plasma derivatives sector is obviously vulnerable to inroads or eventual takeover of the market by recombinant DNA sources of the two principal plasma proteins that are marketed. Moreover, monoclonal antibodies may also replace the third principal part of the plasma derivatives market, the immune globulins.* In the past few years, the plasma derivatives market has shifted more toward collection of antibodies toward specific diseases, collectively known as the "hyperimmune" globulins. Monoclonal antibodies would be more effective than even these hyperimmune globulins, because they would be composed of single antibodies, not a mixture with a high titer of one antibody as is the case for plasma from sensitized donors.

The large plasma fractionators have been positioning themselves so they will be able to switch to the new sources of plasma proteins, and it is likely that they will continue to be the major producers, or at least continue as the major marketers, of these new sources of plasma proteins. However, *some destabilization of the plasma derivatives industry is inevitable, with possible difficulties in providing other, less profitable, derivatives such as Factor IX Complex.* Source plasma centers are especially vulnerable, since their sole role is in providing the raw material, human plasma, from which current plasma proteins are extracted. While the upshot for albumin may be a desired decline in its use because of questions of its appropriateness, there is some concern about how Factor IX will be provided to the relatively small population that needs it. In addition, the clinical utility of other plasma proteins may be harder to explore. Factor IX, for example, was "discovered" in the process of fractionating plasma for Factor VIII.

When and how this impact on plasma collectors and fractionation products will occur is not predictable at this time, although some impact seems inevitable. Even if recombinant DNA and monoclonal antibody sources of plasma proteins are phased in gradually, there could be large dislocations in the plasma derivatives industry. Many source plasma collection centers and some fractionation plants could close. The price and perhaps even availability of some of the plasma proteins would also be affected, not only because of competition from alternative sources, but also because of the nature of the processes in the plasma derivatives industry where the extraction of marketable proteins from plasma is done in successive steps, linking the costs of each plasma fraction product to the costs of the others.

Impact on the Voluntary Whole Blood Sector.—The voluntary sector could also experience negative consequences as a result of shifting plasma protein production to nonhuman sources. *The whole blood and plasma sectors are now interrelated* to a significant extent because of excess plasma capacity in whole blood collections, which has been sold to plasma fractionators or converted to plasma derivatives independently (New York Blood Center) or by contract (Red Cross). This interrelationship is *a direct consequence of the increased volume of whole blood that has been separated into components over the past decade.* Currently, the voluntary sector accounts for about 20 percent of the plasma derivatives market, and significant revenues would be lost. Possible consequences are increased prices for blood components because of lost income from plasma sales; increased collection of specific components (i.e., red cells, platelets), or at least attempts to make component-specific collections more cost effective; and increased transfusion therapy activities by blood centers to generate other sources of revenues.

Impact on Consumers.—Development of alternatives to human blood products has both positive and negative implications for consumers, particularly hemophiliacs. While recombinant antihemophilic factor (and other nonhuman-derived products) would be free of infectious agents, nonhuman alternatives will be more expensive, at least in the short run. In addition, *less profitable products* such as Factor IX Complex *may not be produced, or may become exorbitantly expensive, and the clinical utility of trace proteins may not be explored by commercial firms.* Thus, additional public support for hemophiliacs and for research on trace proteins in plasma may be necessary.

Appropriate Use

There is wide agreement that blood products are overused, but little data exist by which to evaluate the extent of overuse, in many cases because scientific precision is lacking as to when a component or derivative should be administered. Estimates of the extent of overuse are high: 20 to 25 percent for red blood cells (204), as much as 90 percent for albumin (8), and 95 percent for fresh-frozen plasma (457).

Initially, the focus was on the use of whole blood instead of red cell concentrates. Currently, questions continue on overuse of red cells and have focused especially on albumin, and fresh-frozen, single-donor plasma.

One of the most controversial areas concerning red cells is the matter of the "transfusion trigger," the hemoglobin level which is considered the point at which transfusion is required. For example, women naturally have lower hematocrits than men, but surgeons use the same support and ceiling hematocrit levels to indicate transfusions for both sexes. Iron-deficiency anemia continues to be among the leading reasons for transfusions (202), even though it rarely warrants transfusions.

The dramatic increase in the use of fresh-frozen plasma over the last decade has led to concerns that its uses are often vague and without scientific basis and that other products are available that are as effective and safer (567).

Even the growing use of platelets has been questioned; for example, their prophylactic use in patients with malignancies (see, e.g., 481), the practice of treating the "platelet count" rather than the patient, and the use of pheresis platelets over platelet concentrates.

Despite workshops and the development of guidelines for albumin use in the mid to late 1970s, its use continues and production continues to increase. Per capita use of albumin differs markedly from country to country, even in countries similar in levels of medical sophistication (388).

A key element of inappropriate use is that criteria for clinical use are often unclear. Past attempts to change medical practice in this area have been largely educational, using such methods as seminars, handbooks of suggested practices, and textbooks. These attempts appear to have been largely unsuccessful, although systematic data on specific uses of blood products are lacking.

Points to Consider

Direct Attempts to Improve Use.—The NHLBI's Division of Blood Diseases and Resources has instituted a program of "Transfusion Medicine Academic Awards" through which recipients will work with medical schools to incorporate transfusion medicine into the curriculum. Thus, *one method is to build up a specialty base in transfusion medicine.*

Some blood centers have attempted to modify the practices of physicians directly. For example, at Puget Sound Blood Center in Seattle, requests for more than eight units of a blood component must be cleared through a blood center consultant before the blood is released. This is made possible because Puget Sound maintains a central crossmatching laboratory, and all orders for blood and blood products are received and reviewed in that lab. Most blood centers supply blood in volume to hospitals and are not aware of individual clinical practices. Thus, *another method is for blood centers to have more control over the use of their products.*

A third method is to monitor use through hospital transfusion committees and pharmacy committees (for plasma derivatives), but such committees have been largely regarded as ineffective.

Indirect Effects on Improved Use.—The threat of AIDS has made patients and their physicians more cautious in their use of blood products, and perhaps this effect will outlive the current threat. A more sustained limiting factor, however, is the widely accepted need to curb health care costs and the implementation of the prospective payment diagnosis-related grouping system for Medicare that was recently enacted. *The prospective payment method is likely to have the effect of revitalizing hospital transfusion and pharmacy committees' monitoring* of physicians' use of blood products in attempts to stay within the limits of payments on a DRG basis.

Coordination of Blood Resources

Regionalization is not acknowledged by all to be the best approach to managing blood supplies, and a recurring question is the benefit gained from participation in the American Blood Commission's regionalization recognition program. Another recurring debate centers on the issue of centralized blood services v. hospital-based services, or some combination of the two. On the whole, within any region of the country, a patient who needs blood will receive it, but there still remain the questions of efficiency and cost. There are many groups operating within each region. Should the plurality of the present system be left as is, because it produces acceptable products at a sufficient level, or is there a better organizational framework for provision of blood at lower cost?

The need for resource sharing, on the other hand, is not seriously debated. The need for a *single* resource sharing system has been the issue, given the existence of two parallel, though largely successful systems, run by the American Association of Blood Banks and the American Red Cross. Without a single national sharing system, regions with blood shortages are able to meet their needs. Individual blood centers contract with other blood centers outside of the formal mechanisms of the AABB or ARC, as well as within them. In some regions, there are even local clearinghouses which serve functions similar to the AABB.

Other issues concerning coordination of blood resources revolve around the need for a blood credit system, and the need for the American Blood Commission or some similar organization.

Points to Consider

Regionalization.—As discussed previously under cost containment, there are some indications that hospitals are shopping around for blood products on the basis of price, going outside their usual suppliers and even using the AABB Clearinghouse. Some blood bankers are concerned enough that they have suggested that the service (processing) fee for blood from blood banks be treated as a cost pass-through. However, the observation was made that it is hard to see how blood centers could explain to their donors why they should greatly increase their sales to hospitals outside their normal distribution channels, and why therefore donations should also greatly increase. Thus, sales of excess capacity could be justified, but increasing capacity in the face of existing surpluses would be hard to explain to the blood center's donors, assuming that blood center donors (or community representatives) are kept informed of the disposition of the blood they donate.

Sharing and the Blood Credit System.—*One interesting aspect of AABB's Clearinghouse is that the blood credit/replacement system is alive and well, at least among blood banks, and to a lesser extent, for individuals.* In addition to coordinating the movement of blood and blood components, the Clearinghouse transfers credits between blood banks and between regions where such programs exist. In 1983, 47 percent of the transactions coordinated by the Clearinghouse were for actual shipments of blood, including blood shipped for replacement. The remaining transactions consisted of issuing and/or transferring blood credits (25 percent) and payment of nonreplacement fees (28 percent). Individuals giving blood in one region may receive credit for their donation in another area of the country, thereby canceling nonreplacement fees for themselves or in the name of another patient. *The American Red Cross may not want to be involved in a single resource sharing system because it would mean participating in the AABB's system, which, although only partially, involves a credit system.* The American Red Cross withdrew from the AABB Clearinghouse in 1976 in an attempt to put more fully into practice its philosophy of "community responsibility."

Cost-consciousness on the part of corporations, many of whom are beginning to self-insure for health care because of rising costs over the past decade, and the costs that they incur for company-sponsored blood drives which are usually conducted during business hours, may combine to provide a continued stimulus for these corporations to maintain the blood credit system. Thus, it is not unreasonable to ask whether or not *cost-consciousness may lead to increased demand for a blood credit system or for discounts on blood costs, such as on processing fees.* Over the past 10 years, the use of blood credits has declined, but an increase in their use is obviously not viewed negatively by all. Payment of the nonreplacement fee goes to the blood bank, not to any donor, and would be a welcome source of income. Donors only benefit when they or their immediate families are treated in a hospital which is part of a credit system, usually within a year of the donation.

Discounts on processing fees, instead of maintenance/revival of a nonreplacement fee, would benefit transfusion recipients directly, if only modestly. However, there is a wide array of health insurance plans, and they treat blood costs in a variety of ways. Patients would directly benefit only if such costs were part of their deductible or coinsurance requirements. Moreover, administration of such a discount system could be extremely complex. The blood credit system can result in lack of coordination for individual patients who give blood at a center where no credits are given, yet who receive transfusions at hospitals where replacement fees are charged. *It may be necessary for the blood banking community to take a stand on whether blood credits should increase again, or conflict between the representative organizations may be renewed.*

American Blood Commission.—The impact of the American Blood Commission on coordination of blood resources is difficult to evaluate. ABC was unable, for example, to get the blood collecting organizations to take a unified stand on the blood credit system, or to finalize a single resource sharing agreement. Similarly, its attempt at establishing a National Blood Data Center met with mixed reviews. However, many credit it with reducing the conflict between the AABB and ARC which 10 years ago threatened to lead to Federal takeover of blood collection and distribution. ABC today receives no Federal funds, and is dependent on member fees and private donations. Both membership and private donations have recently declined, leaving ABC facing an annual deficit for the first time since its inception. *It is not clear what could be done to stabilize ABC, but many believe its demise would mean the attenuation of constructive dialog between the blood collecting organizations.*

Voluntary v. Commercial

A continuing issue in the use of blood-derived products is that of voluntary v. commercial sources. This was a critical issue in the whole blood sector a decade ago, with the result that commercial whole blood collections have been effectively eliminated. Currently, the distinction between voluntary and paid whole blood donations has been maintained through the labeling of blood components as being derived from a "paid donor" or "voluntary donor." This labeling is applicable to whole blood, red cells, platelets, single donor plasma, and cryoprecipitate, but does not apply to source plasma or plasma derivatives. Donor and laboratory screening tests have been applied over the last decade, with the result that there are no substantial differences in the safety of plasma derivatives whether they are derived from voluntary or commercial sources. One reason is the necessary pooling of large amounts of plasma from individual donors for the efficient processing of plasma into plasma derivatives.

But the availability of products that are derived from human tissues may also be influenced by criteria other than whether or not the market has resulted in a safe, readily available product. Canada, for example, in 1980, amended its national policy of a voluntary blood supply by extending its nonprofit policy to fractionation products. Currently, the only major import is Factor VIII, at the rate of 20 million to 22 million activity units per year. Other products imported in relatively small amounts are specific immunoglobulins to varicella zoster, hepatitis B, tetanus and rabies, and the activated Factor IX Complex. Canadian Red Cross (CRC) meets all requirements for blood and blood components, and CRC plasma sources supply all albumin, normal Factor IX Complex, pooled immune serum globulins, and about 20 million activity units of Factor VIII. Canada also has developed a collection system oriented toward maximum preservation of plasma coagulation proteins so that 95 percent of its whole blood collections can be processed and the plasma frozen within 12 hours (147).

The Canadian experience shows that a voluntary system can meet nearly all blood needs, but other factors make it unlikely that a policy will be pursued in the United States to make the voluntary sector the exclusive or even dominant collector of plasma as well as whole blood.

Points to Consider

Can the Voluntary Sector Provide All Blood Products?—It has been estimated that voluntary whole blood collections would have to triple to meet U.S. production of plasma derivatives (165). U.S. plasma sources, however, also supply a large part of the world market, and not as much plasma would be needed to supply the U.S. market alone. But sales abroad have been claimed to help to lower prices in the United States, whatever one's position is on the morality of this situation.

Whether the voluntary sector would want the responsibility of serving the United States and part of the world markets then becomes the question. Aside from the problems of establishing and maintaining an adequate donor base, costs for starting up or retooling plasma fractionation plants are substantial.

New technologies make the future prospects of the plasma derivatives industry sufficiently doubtful that no planned movement toward a voluntary system can be expected. *By the end of the century, there is a real chance that plasma as a source of current biological proteins will be replaced by recombinant DNA and monoclonal antibody technologies.* For the first time, there are real prospects that *the longstanding controversy over commercial plasma donors may be solved— not through implementation of a deliberate, contested public policy, but through advances in technology which could make the voluntary v. commercial policy debate moot.*

Blood centers themselves do not see the plasma sector as their future, but are instead looking toward organ and tissue banking and their related technologies, such as tissue typing, as their growth areas.

CONCLUSION

The past decade has been a contentious one for the blood resources community, but the results have been generally gratifying, and the blood community's internal conflicts have generally been out of the public's eye— perhaps indicating public satisfaction with and commitment to the informal system even while internal battles continued.

The "National Blood Policy" which has guided development of our blood services complex over the past decade was not codified in law but was an expression of commitment, backed by specific activities that used the Policy as a general guiding principle. The establishment of a Blood Program in the National Heart, Lung, and Blood Institute, represented by the NHLBI's Division of Blood Diseases and Resources, and the strengthening of safety and efficacy standards through establishment of a blood products division in the Office of Biologics Research and Review (previously the Bureau of Biologics) provided the primary instruments through which Federal policy could be formulated, implemented, and maintained. In the initial years of the NBP, there was a direct fiscal relationship between the Federal and private sectors through major support of the private sector body, the American Blood Commission, which was established in order to provide for continued, decentralized management of blood resources. Federal interest at the central policy level within the Department of Health and Human Services slowly faded away, leaving the Blood Division at NHLBI and the Office of Biologics Research and Review as the primary Federal participants in continuing with the objectives of the National Blood Policy, and improving the biomedical base of blood resources and the safety and effectiveness of blood products.

OTA concludes from this broad review of blood policy and technology that the policies implemented over the past decade have been successful in assuring a safe and available blood supply. This has occurred despite continuing internal conflicts; e.g., whether or not to maintain a credit system, other differences between the major organizations involved in blood collection, and commercial v. nonprofit operations. Conflicts of these types seem inevitable in the pluralistic system which evolved, should not come as a surprise, and should not be the basis for judging whether or not the policies of the past decade have been successful.

The current situation presents new challenges. AIDS has shaken the public's confidence in blood supplies far beyond its actual risk to blood recipients, yet no widespread shortages have resulted, and both donors and blood collection organizations have generally responded to the challenge. It remains to be seen if AIDS will have a long-lasting effect on blood resources. In addition, blood suppliers and users face additional pressures because of continually escalating health care costs and recent economic policies instituted to deal with them. And on top of all of this, truly new technologies have emerged which have a high probability of replacing some blood products by the end of the 1980s, and if not yet making human-derived blood products obsolete, represent the first real steps toward that event.

Given the overall success of the past decade and the transitional nature of present circumstances, the prudent course would be to continue with the cooperative arrangements that have been established over the past years and to monitor key developments to anticipate when particular adjust-

ments need to be made. In the previous section, OTA has identified what it considers as the key issues and enumerated some of the points that need to be considered in determining future actions in these issue areas. The following chapters provide background information and more detailed discussions of these and related issues.

Some of these issues involve actions in which the Federal Government is expected to take the leading role, such as in assurances of safety, although the private sector is also deeply involved and needs and wants to participate in such actions. Other areas, such as use of the blood credit or nonreplacement fee, involve differences in philosophy about how much responsibility individuals should have in providing blood resources and what rewards they should have for doing so. *Thus, Federal participation involves resolving or reconciling these differences among the different collection organizations and their clientele,* should any decision be made to modify the course of developments in the blood field.

Still other areas involve consequences of Federal policies directed at even larger problems— the continually escalating costs of health care and recent legislation to "cap" these costs through prospective payment mechanisms—whose purpose was to impose exactly the kinds of cost-saving behavior which hospitals apparently are beginning to exhibit, and over which the blood community is so concerned. The architects of these broader policy changes in health care financing are aware of the negative consequences in particular circumstances—e.g., their effects on research and training programs and capital acquisitions. Such consequences also need to be explored in the blood resources area, but simply shielding blood products from these cost containment efforts is no answer. *Federal action might also be considered in the areas of support for biomedical research and studies to determine appropriate use of blood products, and improved coverage for hemophiliacs.*

A decade ago, developing a data system for blood resources was a major objective of the National Blood Policy. The efforts subsequently undertaken under the sponsorship of the American Blood Commission and financed primarily by the Blood Resources Program at NHLBI did not meet expectations. In retrospect, one problem was the general nature of the data and the inability to find sponsors to continue the data collection. In other words, the data may have been informative and useful in understanding the general contours of the blood services complex, but they were not useful to organizations interested in information that could help them in their operations. Thus, there is general agreement that future data collections should be much more targeted.

The problem with collecting data which would be useful to the operations of organizations is the issue of who should be responsible for collecting it, and the relevance of those types of data for public policy illumination and formulation. Another problem is that, while specialized data sets are the most useful, they also tend to be fragmented, and some type of coordination needs to be arranged. For example, both the American Red Cross and members of the American Association of Blood Banks are involved in data collection on a daily basis, and much of this data would be useful for public policy purposes. In fact, much of this information is used for determining policy within those organizations, and the organizations are willing to share a large amount of this information, although as health care provision becomes more competitive as a consequence of cost containment efforts, much of this information is coming to be regarded as proprietary. Other information sources can be found in the data systems that are being organized to monitor the effects of the Medicare prospective payment system, which have the potential to provide more specific information on use and costs than have been possible previously.

Monitoring functions which include coordination of data sources require a capacity for sustained activities, and the problem is in identifying who can and should assume this function. The Federal Government's primary data collection organization in the health field, the *National Center for Health Statistics,* can collect comprehensive data on specific issues, but the kinds of data needed to help formulate policy in the issue areas identified above are of a different type. *The National Center for Health Services Research* can also conduct policy-relevant research, but it too, lacks the capacity for sustained and coordinated activities. *The Office of the Assistant Secretary for Health* is the logical choice for such data coordination and policy formulation, but it is preoccupied with immediate issues and functions more as the receiver rather than as the gatherer of information. *FDA and NIH*, which are the primary Federal agencies involved in blood resources on a sustained basis, could be given that responsibility, but their primary responsibilities are in circumscribed areas of the blood services area—assuring safety and efficacy and resource building—and the net effect would be what has happened in the past; i.e., they can be required to fund such activities, but would not be able to assume the primary Federal role in determining overall blood resources policy.

The private sector could conduct these activities, and in fact would argue that they are already doing much of it. Federal funds could again be provided, as it was for the data collection efforts and early general support of the American Blood Commission. Two problems would recur, however. First, is the question of whether any single private sector organization would be recognized by the diverse interests in the blood services complex as a legitimate policymaking body, instead of serving primarily as a policy debating forum. Second is the question of how sustainable Government funding could be.

If there are no obvious answers as to who could assume both a monitoring and policy formulation role, or on the even more limited role of monitoring developments in blood resources, perhaps a different approach should be taken. Just as the emphasis on data needs has shifted from the general to the specific, *a more practical and useful approach might be to have periodic appraisals that monitor specific issues to see: 1) what happens in these issue areas over time, 2) whether the issues identified initially continue as the primary ones, and 3) what new issues arise.* Thus, one approach is to formulate a set of questions and use them as guidelines for narrowing the issues, to see how these questions are resolved, and how public policy can contribute to their resolution. The issues and points to consider that have been enumerated above represent one attempt to delineate those questions, based on the broad overview represented by this report.

Certain policies could be extracted from this approach. For example, *oversight hearings* could be structured around the identified issues, with both private organizations and Federal agencies contributing information to further clarify the issues and to suggest approaches to their resolution. Periodic hearings or other methods of followup could then take place to follow the course of events. For example, *the National Academy of Sciences could be requested to review these issues periodically, or the Federal Department of Health and Human Services could be required to reassess them in reports to Congress as is often required for other policy issues. Specific issues could be examined in detail by any of the congressional support agencies. A restatement of the National Blood Policy could also be constructed to provide general guidance—as its original formulation a decade ago has done. Within any of these approaches, specific actions could be taken as the need arises, either by legislative action, by administrative changes in the operations of Federal agencies, or by voluntary actions by the private sector.*

In conclusion, in the decade since the National Blood Policy was announced, blood resources have become safer and more available, despite continuing differences among participants in the blood services complex. This should not be surprising, given the decentralized, pluralistic approach that was continued under the NBP. Today, AIDS, cost-consciousness, and radically new technologies have significantly affected the blood services complex and portend changes that will most likely be even more significant. These changes are occurring rapidly; over the short time that this report was prepared, the cause of AIDS has been apparently identified and tests for its detection are under development, and the entire gene for Factor VIII has been cloned, adding to the already available gene for albumin.

The transition that the blood services complex is currently undergoing, as represented by these events, calls for a policy of focused monitoring and adjustments to particular circumstances as the need arises. Policy formulation can proceed both with specific actions and general guidelines. General guidelines can be provided either implicitly through oversight hearings and other methods of communicating Congress' priorities to the blood services community, or through a restatement of the National Blood Policy and actions commensurate with that reorientation.

2. Overview

Contents

	Page
Part 1: History of Federal Interest	33
Part 2: Blood and Blood Products	36
Part 3: The Blood Donor	38
Risk for Donors	39
Part 4: Federal Activities	41
Introduction	41
Payment for Blood Products and Services	42
National Institutes of Health	43
Food and Drug Administration	45

LIST OF TABLES

Table No.	Page
2. Ten Policies and Six Critical Issues in Support of National Blood Policy Goals	35
3. Blood Components and Plasma Derivatives in Therapeutic Use	37
4. FDA Statutory Authority to Regulate Blood Products and Blood Banking Technologies	45
5. Blood Products Recalls, June 1975 to November 1983	46
6. Significant Deviations Leading to Plasma Center Suspensions, Oct. 1, 1979 to Aug. 31, 1981	46
7. Types of Numbers of Blood Processing Errors, 1981-82	47
8. New Blood Products and Procedures Approved by FDA in the Past Two Years (approx. 1982-83)	47
9. Blood Products and Related Technologies in the Approval Process as of Early 1984	48

2. Overview

PART 1: HISTORY OF FEDERAL INTEREST

Federal interest in assuring an adequate and safe blood supply has a long history. President Truman called blood a "critical national resource vital to the country's well-being and security." The Federal Government regulates blood banking (as do State governments), monitors the safety and efficacy of blood products, and promotes research on blood diseases and resources.

In the 1960s, scientists recognized the correlation between high rates of posttransfusion hepatitis and blood obtained from paid donors. Cardiac surgery and other advances in medical care increased the use of whole blood for transfusion, and with this increased use came increased concern for the safety of blood transfusions. Separation of whole blood into components and the use of platelets and plasma derivatives became increasingly widespread. One result of this heightened interest in blood was the establishment of a National Blood Resources Program at the National Heart and Lung Institute in 1967. In 1972, the program was reconstituted as the Division of Blood Diseases and Resources in the expanded National Heart, Lung, and Blood Institute (NHLBI), where it still operates.

In the early 1970s, there was a surge of public interest that prompted Federal policymakers in both the executive and legislative branches to review the Nation's blood program. This round of debate was sparked largely by the publication of *The Gift Relationship* by Professor Richard Titmuss, a British scholar and student of social welfare policy. Professor Titmuss excoriated the commercial market for whole blood in the United States on both safety and ethical grounds. His book received much attention in the news media and inspired a television documentary which highlighted the hepatitis problem and featured pint after pint of blood being poured down the drain to dramatize the wastage problem.

During this time period, over 40 bills designed to regulate blood resources were introduced in the 92d Congress, including H.R. 11828, introduced by Representative Victor V. Veysey, which proposed that a National Blood Bank Program be located in the Department of Health, Education, and Welfare (DHEW, the predecessor to the current Department of Health and Human Services, or DHHS) (485). Simultaneously, the increasing input of private sector health organizations prompted the executive branch to take a stand on the blood issue.

President Nixon's annual health message to the Congress in March 1972 described blood as a "unique national resource," and he subsequently charged a DHEW task force with the assignment of developing a safe, fast, and efficient nationwide blood collection and distribution system.

In May 1972, monitoring of blood resources was transferred from the National Institutes of Health (NIH) to the Food and Drug Administration (FDA). Since that time, FDA's Bureau of Biologics (currently renamed the Office of Biologics Research and Review) has been the principal regulator (States also play a regulatory role) of blood collection, processing, testing, and marketing. As a result of this change, all blood banking in the country, not just interstate blood trade, came under direct Federal regulation.

Following extended examination and debate, including the DHEW Task Force Report which found that: 1) the supply of blood was sometimes inadequate, 2) the quality of blood was uneven and reliance on commercial blood was contributing to a high rate of hepatitis, 3) gross inefficiencies existed, and 4) the cost of blood therapy was a burden to many people, a National Blood Policy (NBP) was enunciated by the Federal Government in 1973. There were four goals underlying the National Blood Policy (180):

1. *Supply*. A supply of blood and blood products adequate to meet all of the treatment and diagnostic needs of the population of this country.
2. *Quality*. Attainment of the highest standard of blood transfusion therapy through full application of currently available scientific knowledge, as well as through advancement of the scientific base.
3. *Accessibility*. Access to the national supply of blood and blood products by everyone in need, regardless of economic status.
4. *Efficiency*. Efficient collection, processing, storage, and utilization of the national supply of blood and blood products.

The National Blood Policy was broken down into 10 specific policies, along with six issues which were to be examined critically. Prominent among the policies were adoption of an all-voluntary blood collection system, coordination of charges and costs for blood services, and regionalization of blood collection and distribution. Critical examinations of the nonreplacement fee, the plasmapheresis industry, and standards of care for hemophiliacs and other special groups were also recommended (table 2).

A number of Federal and private sector initiatives were undertaken in order to begin implementing the National Blood Policy. In 1974, DHEW accepted the private sector plan to establish an American Blood Commission (ABC), which was to implement "the lion's share" of the National Blood Policy (180). The National Heart, Lung, and Blood Institute provided partial funding for ABC activities until recently, when the existing contract expired (ABC may still apply to NIH for funding of specific projects, but on a competitive basis). ABC now depends on membership fees and donations, and it has been experiencing difficulty in retaining some of its organizational members.

There were no direct government actions to ban the sale of whole blood and plasma, although steps were taken to regulate the safety of plasma products and discourage the use of commercial whole blood. FDA became increasingly involved in regulating the plasma industry, building on its initial involvement which had begun during the late 1960s (506). In 1973, FDA's Bureau of Biologics published additional standards for source plasma and required all plasmapheresis operating facilities to file an application for licensure of both their establishments and products; a formal compliance program began in mid-1977. FDA oversight over the plasmapheresis industry was relaxed somewhat in 1977, when responsibility for annual inspections was transferred from the Bureau of Biologics to FDA field investigators and supervisors (506).

No Federal efforts were made to ban commercial plasma collections. Regulators realized that the demand for plasma supplies could not be met by the existing voluntary sector. Since the collection of whole blood and preparation of blood components were largely in the province of the voluntary sector, an FDA rule was implemented in 1977 to identify the source of whole blood and its components (red cells, platelets, single-donor plasma, cryoprecipitate). This action was taken on the basis that available data indicated a greater risk of transmission of hepatitis with the use of blood and blood components from paid donors. Under this regulation (21 CFR sec. 606.120(b)(2)), whole blood and its components are labeled as collected from a "paid donor" or "volunteer donor." The regulations state that a paid donor is a person who receives monetary payment for a blood donation, while a volunteer donor is a person who does not receive such payment. Other benefits that are not readily converted to cash, such as time off from work and cancellation of nonreplacement fees, are not considered as monetary payment. These labeling requirements do not apply to source plasma or plasma derivatives, since plasma derivatives produced from plasma obtained from paid or volunteer donors are considered to be equally at risk for transmission of infectious agents.

Steps were also taken to assure that hemophiliacs were afforded access to care. The Public Health Service Act of 1975 (Public Law 94-63): 1) established Federal funding for comprehensive hemophilia diagnostic and treatment centers, and 2) authorized funds for projects to develop and expand blood derivative operations in the event the Secretary of DHEW found that there was an

Table 2.—Ten Policies and Six Critical Issues in Support of National Blood Policy Goals

Ten policies:
1. Efforts toward an all-volunteer system for blood and blood components were encouraged, fostered, and supported.
2. The establishment of a system for the collection and analysis of all relevant information concerning plasmapheresis, plasma fractionation, and the flow of plasma and plasma products within the United States and other countries was to be encouraged, fostered, and supported. This information was believed necessary to determine the sufficiency of domestic sources of plasma fractions; develop future positions on the relationships between plasmapheresis and plasma fractionation and whole blood banking; and develop a degree of interdependence between the United States and other countries with respect to plasma and plasma products.
3. Continuing data and information collection and processing systems to describe all elements and functions in the blood banking sphere on a continuing basis. The purpose of this policy was to acquire fundamental information on the nature and transmission of diseases by blood and blood products and the occurrence of transfusion mishaps, as well as to design and create changes which would enhance the effectiveness of the blood banking system.
4. Resource sharing and areawide cooperation in the collection, processing, distribution, and utilization of blood.
5. Ample donations were to be assured through encouraging: a) improved accounting and reporting systems to identify the relationship between costs and charges; and b) public and health professional education.
6. Educational and other programs to assure appropriate use.
7. Adherence to the highest attainable standards for blood products, including plasma derivatives, through use of or extension of Federal regulatory authorities were to be employed.
8. Research, including systems analysis and other management approaches to extend shelf life, and to identify and control diseases transmittable by blood.
9. Insurance benefits for the service aspects of blood components and both the acquisition and service aspects of plasma derivatives. The acquisition costs of plasma derivatives were to be covered in recognition that commercial acquisition may still be necessary.
10. The Secretary of Health, Education, and Welfare was to be responsible for implementing this policy.

Six[a] critical issues to be examined:
1. The adequacy of any proposed implementation action in meeting the extraordinary demands for blood that may arise in national and regional emergencies.
2. The appropriateness of the replacement fee in an all-voluntary system.
3. Systems approaches to the integration of various functions and segments of the blood banking industry.
4. Regionalization of blood services management.
5. Appropriate inducements and authorities, whether existing or to be sought, necessary to exclude commercial acquisition of whole blood or blood components.
6. Special problems of accessibility for hemophiliacs and others with continuing or extraordinary needs for blood or blood products.

[a]A seventh issue was stated as "other issues relevant to the four principal goals."
SOURCE: *Federal Register*, Mar. 8, 1974.

---

insufficient supply of blood derivatives available to meet the treatment needs of hemophiliacs. A contractor's report to DHEW (554) projected that sources of supplies of antihemophilic factor and prothrombin complex were adequate to meet hemophiliacs' needs through and beyond the authorization period, so the treatment centers were established but projects to develop and expand blood derivative operations were not funded.

The nonreplacement fee became an issue when the American Red Cross, in order to make its practices conform to its philosophy of community responsibility, withdrew from the AABB National Clearinghouse system, which used blood credits and nonreplacement fees. The lack of cooperation between the three major blood supply organizations (American Red Cross, American Association of Blood Banks [AABB], and the Council of Community Blood Centers [CCBC]) led to concerns over the possibility of blood shortages in some regions, and to the introduction of two bills in Congress (S. 1610, introduced by Senator Schweiker in 1979; and S. 140, introduced by Senator Hatch in 1981). The Schweiker and Hatch bills would have eliminated the nonreplacement fee and provided donors with a discount on the charge for blood when they were patients.

The nonreplacement fee was also the focus of concern that Medicare was overpaying for blood (546). Medicare guidelines require that patients pay a three-unit blood deductible by either replacing or paying for the first three units of blood transfused. A General Accounting Office (GAO) investigation found that billing and replacement practices of blood banks and hospitals had caused substantial Medicare overpayments for blood and blood products, that blood banks had prevented the use of blood replacement credits to reduce blood fees whenever Medicare would pay the fees, and that hospitals charged nonreplacement fees to Medicare patients for blood supplied by community blood banks that charged only processing fees.

In addition to improved monitoring practices, one of GAO's recommendations was that the Health Care Financing Administration (HCFA) undertake a study of the relationship between the costs and charges for blood. Such a study has not been conducted by HCFA. (In addition to a blood replacement fee, there are fees for blood processing, typing and crossmatching, and for transfusion services, which are charged whether or not a blood replacement fee is imposed. In 1980, for example, average total charges for transfusing a unit of red cells was $88.17, including an average replacement fee, when charged, of $27.98 (576).)

Other Federal interests in the issues surrounding blood services delivery have come in the form of support for a variety of basic and applied research, principally from the Division of Blood Diseases and Resources of the National Heart, Lung, and Blood Institute (556). Most recently, the same division has begun efforts to improve the appropriate use of blood products (e.g., the "Transfusion Medicine Academic Awards"). Current activities of the Federal Government with respect to blood services, policy and technology are set forth in part 4 of this chapter.

PART 2: BLOOD AND BLOOD PRODUCTS

Blood is a mixture of specialized cells suspended in plasma, which itself is a complex liquid containing proteins, nutrients, salts, and hormones. Blood has many functions, including transport of oxygen and nutrients to body tissues, removal of carbon dioxide and other wastes, and transfer of hormonal messages between organs. It also plays a major role in the body's defenses, inhibiting invasion and spread of organisms by transporting antibodies and infection-fighting cells to the sites of infection. Albumin, the principal protein found in plasma, helps maintain blood volume by maintaining an osmotic gradient (oncotic pressure) between the vascular system and surrounding tissue, and serves as the carrier molecule for fatty acids and other small molecules (467). A complex clotting system to prevent blood loss involves both cellular (i.e., platelets) and protein elements of blood.

In blood banking terminology, "components" refers to products separated from whole blood and consist of the various types of blood cells, plasma, and special preparations of plasma. Components are usually separated from single whole blood donations, using a sterile system of plastic bags attached to the collection bag.

"Derivatives" refers to products derived from the chemical fractionation of plasma to concentrate selected blood proteins. Plasma from many donors is pooled prior to chemical fractionation in order to yield sufficient amounts of the final concentrated material for cost-effective production.

Blood components and plasma derivatives and their general indications for use in medical therapy are listed in table 3.

Hazards associated with therapeutic use derive primarily from immunologic incompatibility between donor and recipient and from transmissible diseases. Incorrectly typed and crossmatched blood or mislabeled blood can lead to reactions ranging from transient fever and chills to death. More subtle incompatibilities that may not be uncovered in routine typing and crossmatching may lead to sensitization of the recipient and hypersensitivity reactions from subsequent transfusions.

Infections of various types can occur through collection of blood from donors whose blood contains the infectious agent or from contaminants introduced in the collection, processing, or transfusing procedures. Syphilis was one of the first bacterial diseases known to be transmitted through

Table 3.—Blood Components and Plasma Derivatives in Therapeutic Use

Components and their therapeutic use:
Whole blood: Replacement of large volume blood loss.
Packed red cells: Anemia; provision of oxygen-carrying capacity.
Leukocyte-poor red cells: As for packed red cells; used in patients with reactions to leukocytes.
Frozen red cells: As for packed red cells; used in patients with more severe reactions to leukocytes; provision of rare red cells.
Platelets: Platelet deficiency; platelet function abnormalities.
Fresh-frozen plasma: Multiple coagulation factor deficiencies (indications under review).
Single-donor plasma: Uncommon use.
Cryoprecipitate: Provision of Factor VIII, von Willebrand's factor, fibronectin, fibrinogen.
Leukocytes: Bacterial infections in immunocompromised patients (rarely used).

Derivative:
Albumin: Plasma volume expansion.
Immune serum globulin: Infection prevention (immunodeficiency states, travelers).
Hyperimmune gamma globulin (e.g., Varicella Zoster immune globulin, Hepatitis B immune globulin): Prevention of specific infections.
Factor VIII (antihemophilic factor): Factor VIII replacement in hemophilia A.
Factor IX Complex: Factor IX replacement in hemophilia B.
Anti-Inhibitor Coagulant Complex: Hemophilia A patients with high levels of Factor VIII inhibitor.

SOURCE: J. Pindyck, S. Gaynor, R. Hirsch, et al., "Prevention of Infection Transmission by Transfusable Blood, Blood Components or Plasma Derivatives," 1984.

blood, but in general, bacterial contamination is not a problem in modern blood banking. Protozoal diseases such as malaria and sleeping sickness can also be transmitted through blood, but most of these diseases are not endemic to the United States, and a history of travel to endemic areas or exposure to the disease that is uncovered during the medical screening of blood donors has effectively kept these diseases out of the blood supply.

Viruses are the major class of infectious agents that are transmitted through blood. Of these, hepatitis B and non-A, non-B hepatitis are the most prevalent. Surveys of blood donors show a frequency of hepatitis B of 5 to 7 percent. In the 1970s, development of increasingly more sensitive laboratory tests for the detection of hepatitis B that are now applied to every blood donation resulted in a dramatic reduction of posttransfusion hepatitis B cases. However, a new form of hepatitis (non-A, non-B) appeared, which, although no agent(s) has been isolated, is presumed to be a virus.* Currently, 5 to 18 percent of Americans who receive five or more units of transfused blood develop non-A, non-B hepatitis (271b). About 90 percent of all post-transfusion cases of hepatitis are non-A, non-B, and about 10 percent are due to hepatitis B (558).

Other viruses are relatively common in the general population and normally are of no consequence in transfusions. One exception is cytomegalovirus, which can cause infections in premature infants and immunosuppressed recipients, such as kidney or bone marrow transplant recipients. Other viruses are fairly common but not known to lead to transfusion-related disease (e.g., Epstein-Barr virus, the agent for infectious mononucleosis), while other, recently discovered rare viruses could be theoretically transmitted through transfusions. AIDS, which is now accepted as being transmittable through blood, is now considered to be of viral etiology (i.e., the retrovirus—HTLV-III) (256).

All blood components and some plasma derivatives are capable of transmitting viral infections. Components are stored either at room temperature (platelets), in cold storage (whole blood, red cells), or frozen (red cells, plasma), and none of these processes inactivate viruses. Of the plasma derivatives, only albumin (and a related product, plasma protein fraction) and immune serum globulin (ISG) appear to be free of active viruses. Albumin is heated for 10 hours at 60° C in the presence of stabilizers to help maintain the structure of albumin, and this pasteurization inactivates viruses. Inactivation of viruses in immune serum globulin appears to be due to two factors: 1) the cold ethanol fractionation method appears to precipitate ISG in a fraction separate from the fraction containing viruses (61); and 2) ISG contains many antibodies against many viruses, which may diminish or destroy their infectivity (217).

Until recently, virus inactivation for the plasma-derived clotting factors had not been available be-

---

*A retrovirus has now been implicated as the cause of non-A, non-B hepatitis (493).

cause heat treatment caused loss of function. Heat-treated clotting Factor VIII, however, has recently been licensed by the FDA. It is not known how much Factor VIII activity is lost in the heat treatment process, and, since a balance has to be maintained between loss of function and inactivating viruses, the conditions under which these products are heated may not inactivate all viruses. (Current research suggests that the presumed AIDS agent, HTLV-III, is inactivated by this process.)

Other methods of inactivating viruses include heating the derivative in the dry state (529), using detergents and organic solvents instead of heat (447), or neutralizing viruses by the addition of antibodies, a method which requires the use of specific antibodies against each type of virus to be inactivated (100). The Netherlands Red Cross is reportedly producing derivatives containing specific antibodies against hepatitis B virus (373).

PART 3: THE BLOOD DONOR

Approximately 8 million people, representing about 3.5 percent of the population or about 10 percent of those eligible to give, donate blood in a year. There are no nationwide sources of data which profile blood donors. Nevertheless, many individual blood banks and donor recruitment centers have conducted studies to find out who constitutes their pool of donors, by characteristics such as age, sex, race, socioeconomic and occupational status, as well as by geographical location (e.g., urban, suburban, and rural). From these studies has emerged a picture of the "typical" blood donor: a white, middle-class male family member who gives at his place of work. The prevalence of male donors is a worldwide phenomenon, and it has been estimated that between 60 and 70 percent of all those donating blood in the United States are male (291).

Mobile blood collections have traditionally taken place in corporate and institutional settings, where relatively well-educated, middle-class white males are most likely to be found. This picture may be changing. Women have entered the work force in increasing numbers and hence are more likely to be subject to recruitment and to have convenient opportunities to donate.

Members of minority groups, and blacks in particular, may be harder to motivate (450), with speculation that it may be due to mistrust of the health care system in general, or existence of a sociocultural gulf between donation officials and potential minority donors. Blood bankers have attempted to overcome some of these hurdles by special recruitment tactics. These efforts include involving leaders and spokespersons for minority groups in recruitment efforts and reaching out to cohesive minority fraternal, social and civic groups. Churches, which have long been a mainstay of recruitment drives, are particularly fertile grounds for such efforts.

Lower socioeconomic status may also compromise the willingness to give, in view of the finding that altruism is almost always at the top of the list of reasons for donating. Donors invoke altruistic reasons even when participating for the purpose of blood credits/replacements or being paid (49,71,409). Even scholars who have questioned the depth and the validity of altruism as a motivating force have concluded that, because it is a socially accepted motivation and one most often verbalized, it should continue to form the basis for appeals for donors (417,433).

There are certain physical limitations that are applied to potential donors. In general, any healthy person who weighs more than 110 pounds and is between the ages of 17 and 66 can be a blood donor. The upper age limits are imposed by blood collection agencies and are subject to some exceptions, while the lower age limits are imposed by State law. Blood donors who weigh less than 110 pounds are rejected because the standard amount of whole blood collected (450 ml) amounts to too great a percentage of their blood volume, a loss which could result in a serious hypotensive episode. Pregnant women are excluded from donating, as is anyone who has undergone major surgery in the preceding 6 months.

Many States have made statutory exceptions to the age of majority (usually 18) by allowing 17 year olds to donate. This allows entry into high school, which is not only a convenient donation site, but also inculcates youngsters with an understanding of the need for blood donors. The cutoff for those aged 66 or older has attracted some criticism. Critics argue that a more rational end point would be based not on age alone, but rather on health status, weight, and donation history. By these measures, many older people can give blood safely into their later 60s and 70s.

Physical limitations aside, most donations appear to be influenced by motivational and situational circumstances. Both donors and nondonors are aware of the need for blood, and personal experiences with the need for blood is distributed widely throughout the population (35). But many who claim they intend to donate do not actually follow through, and the "slippage" between those who say they will donate and those who actually do so may be as high as 60 to 65 percent (192). This general acknowledgment of the need for blood and its contrast with those who actually donate have led to criticisms of generalized appeals through the mass media to donate blood. Much of the efforts of recruitment officials has involved generalized announcements of the continued need for blood donors. These most commonly take the form of television or radio public service announcements, often showing celebrities in the act of giving blood or recipients whose lives have been saved through transfusions. Such advertising campaigns, geared toward raising awareness of the need for blood, are ineffective in helping to overcome fears of donating, and suggestions have been made that advertising dollars may be better spent in allaying such fears.

More frequent and convenient donation opportunities, rather than knowledge of the need for blood, are correlated with increased donation rates (35). Observing others donating increases the chances that a person will also donate. Social and peer pressure can be an important force in donor motivation, especially regarding first-time donors, who often report to the donor site accompanied by friends (132,133). And the existence of an identifiable patient in need heightens awareness and the feeling of an obligation to give, even when the specific patient in need is identified anonymously (e.g., "a young mother with children") (489).

Most of the research on blood donors has focused on the motivations and characteristics of donors, not on factors involving the donation setting and the recruitment process. Research has most often been undertaken in one location, where a single donation ideology has motivated recruiters. There have been few comparisons of urban v. rural donors, fixed v. mobile sites, or cross-cultural studies. Factors such as the length of time it takes to donate and the donor's perception of how he or she was treated by the staff and peers may be better predictors of donor commitment than attitudes toward moral obligations, etc.

Little attention has been devoted to determining what forces convert a first-time donor into a committed, repeat donor. Recruitment professionals play a key role in garnering first-time donors and in converting them into repeat donors. The personal convictions of the individual recruiter are important factors in motivating donors, and donor recruiters are often active donors themselves (236). Many large blood collection centers have donor recruiters as full-time staff members to organize local media efforts, to encourage and coordinate corporate and institutional drives, and to direct appeals to particular individuals, such as former donors. The conversion of first-time donors into repeat donors is a particularly important aspect, as the retention of past donors may be considerably more efficient than recruiting new donors (382).

Risks for Donors

The risks of whole blood donation are minor and rarely result in serious complications. For virtually all blood donors the loss of 450 ml of blood (up to 13 percent of total volume) is experienced with no untoward effects. Potential risks include local injuries such as bruises or reactions to antiseptics and dressings. The phlebotomy (needle stick) can result in arterial puncture or air embolism. Infections also occur on occasion, but they are usually infrequent and localized (577). The low level of risk to blood donors is evidenced not only by the medical literature and statistics kept by blood donation centers, but also by the dearth of activity in the courts. In contrast to the number of lawsuits brought on behalf of recipients of contaminated blood products, there have been very few court cases involving injuries to donors.

Vasovagal syncope (a transient reaction marked by pallor, nausea, slow heartbeat, and a rapid fall in arterial blood pressure which sometimes results in fainting) is a risk for a small percentage of donors. Although it is impossible to predict with certainty which donors are at risk, certain factors, such as age, weight, a history of fainting and inexperience in donating, may be predisposing.

Along with loss of blood volume from donating, other factors can influence the amount of blood circulating to the brain. Vasovagal activity tends to pool blood in the skeletal muscles and gravity tends to pool blood in the distal veins; this is exacerbated if sitting erect. Eating and drinking pools blood in the stomach and intestines. Vasovagal reactions can, on occasion, include a blocked airway or cardiac arrythmia. Blood donor centers are advised to keep resuscitation equipment on hand. Donors are observed for impending signs of fainting and are usually accompanied to a lounge for a brief period following donation. Obviously, part of the danger in fainting is from resulting bruises, lacerations, or other injuries. Yet, fainting following blood donation is uncommon; an acceptable level of such incidents is 0.3 percent, according to the Red Cross (44).

Plasmapheresis donors undergo some of the same risks as whole blood donors—for example, those associated with phlebotomy (e.g., arterial puncture or air embolism). Unlike conventional blood donation, plasmapheresis involves the removal of whole blood, separation by centrifuge into its constituent parts and reinfusion of cellular components into the donor. Thus, the plasmapheresis procedure entails the additional risk of reinfusion of cells from another donor, which could occasion a hemolytic reaction; Federal regulations specifically require that this risk be disclosed as part of the informed consent process (21 CFR pt. 640.61).

Labeling requirements have been adopted by plasmapheresis centers to decrease the likelihood of such an occurrence, and some centers use portable centrifuges by the donor's chair, which further reduces the chance of a mixup. New technologies being developed to speed up the plasmapheresis process and make it more efficient would remove this risk, as these generally involve membrane or centrifugal separation of blood components in a self-contained system to which the donor is attached continuously.

The greatest controversy regarding risk to plasmapheresis donors has involved limitations on the volume and frequency of donation. The average adult male of 175 lbs has a plasma volume of 3,000 ml. Under Federal regulations donors in the United States can give 1,000 ml of plasma per 48-hour period up to twice a week. (Donors weighing more than 175 lbs can give 1,200 ml per donation (21 CFR 640.65 (4-6).) The regulations allow plasmapheresis donors to give up to 50 or 60 liters of plasma each year; this contrasts markedly with limits set by other industrialized nations—generally 10 to 25 liters annually. Regulations require that plasmapheresis donors undergo a serum protein electropheresis and a measurement of immunoglobulin every 4 months to determine whether they are in normal range.

The effects of plasmapheresis on short- and long-term levels of plasma proteins and other blood components have been vigorously contested. Often the scientific debate has been overshadowed by social, ethical, and political questions concerning commercial plasmapheresis, especially in developing countries. The relative frequency with which U.S. regulations allow plasmapheresis has been decried, especially by European critics (347,348). One critic of U.S. policies regarding commercial plasmapheresis has stated that, "It defies comprehension that the necessary quantities of plasma are not procured by the simple expedient of increasing the number of donors sufficiently to minimize the individual risk" (346).

A group of experts convened by the World Health Organization (WHO) and the League of Red Cross Societies concluded that "no consistent clinical abnormalities have been detected during periods of up to 6 years in donors who have undergone adequately controlled plasmapheresis"

(593). They concluded that plasmapheresis is generally safe when limited to 15 liters per year, and called for retrospective and prospective studies because of "possible effects on lipid transports and deposition, decreased resistance to infections through frequent removal of immunoglobulins and even changes in immune responses toward oncogenic viruses cannot be ruled out .... Disorders might arise out of too frequent plasmapheresis, active immunization and frequent restimulation" (595).

A number of studies have concluded that even frequent plasmapheresis appears safe for both short- and long-term donors who are otherwise healthy and of good nutritional status (150,475). Other studies of plasmapheresis donors over 3 to 4 years have shown small, but statistically insignificant decreases in albumin levels (206,244). In the first 4 to 6 months there is a statistically significant rise in the concentration of α and β globulins and a decrease in the concentration of the immune globulins IgG, IgA and IgM. After a few more months of continued plasmapheresis IgG and IgA concentrations return to normal, while IgM levels continue to be slightly depressed but still within normal limits (206).

Many, including representatives of the plasmapheresis industry, have urged that further studies be conducted "because there are questions about frequency and all the answers are not in" (327).

The studies done to date have been criticized for looking only at donors who are least likely to be at risk, excluding those in poor nutritional status and those who may have stopped donating for health-related reasons (429). Studies have also been difficult to design because of variables such as regularity of donation, volume donated at each session and total cumulative volume (206). Although it is agreed that plasmapheresis can exacerbate problems associated with poor nutritional status and alcoholism, there is still some controversy over whether such individuals continue to form any portion of the donor pool, in spite of the Federal regulations and screening processes at work since the mid-1970s. Because of this uncertainty, it has also been suggested that this screening process should include tests of nutritional status (161).

Other suggestions for long-term studies include assessments of the long-term risks to hyperimmunized donors who supply high-titer antibodies after being immunized with tetanus toxoid or herpes zoster. One group of specially immunized donors produces Rh immune globulin, a product which has saved many lives by dramatically reducing the incidence of erythroblastosis fetalis (hemolytic disease of the newborn). Experts have questioned whether this process is safe for donors over the long term (408a).

PART 4: FEDERAL ACTIVITIES

Introduction

The Federal agencies with primary responsibilities in the blood resources area are the National Institutes of Health (NIH) and the Food and Drug Administration (FDA). NIH supports research and development activities, and FDA is responsible for regulating the efficacy and safety of blood products and the technologies associated with them. Other agencies such as the Centers for Disease Control (CDC) may be involved in specific issues at any given time, such as in AIDS research, where some of CDC's investigations involve blood-transmitted AIDS.

The Medicare program for the elderly (and disabled) also makes the Federal Government a major purchaser of blood products. Escalating costs since Medicare's inception in the mid-1960s have led to a search for methods to restrain cost increases, and in 1983 Congress passed the Social Security Amendments of 1983 (Public Law 98-21), which is based on prospectively paying for inpatient hospital care by diagnosis-related groupings (DRGs), instead of payment on a cost-incurred basis. The Health Care Financing Administration (HCFA), the Federal agency responsible for operating Medicare, began to phase out the cost-based hospital reimbursement system in October 1983, and the DRG system's phase-in is to be completed by October 1986.

The activities of these three Federal agencies, HCFA, NIH, and FDA, are briefly described in the following sections. Payment for hemophiliac care is also briefly described in the first section.

Payment for Blood Products and Services

Health Care Financing Administration

The Medicare program consists of two parts: Part A, the hospital insurance program, and Part B, a supplementary medical insurance plan. Part A is available without charge to those who are eligible, while Part B is optional and requires payment of a monthly premium (about $15/month in mid-1984). Enrollees must choose not to participate in Part B, since premiums are deducted automatically from Social Security checks. In 1982, 99 percent of the elderly and 92 percent of the disabled enrolled in Part A were also enrolled in Part B (544).

The Medicare law has been amended through the years, and various limits have been placed on both hospitals' and physicians' charges; beneficiaries' cost-sharing has also been modified. However, the situation is roughly as follows.

Medicare will pay for the first 90 days of hospitalization, minus a deductible ($356 in 1984). After 60 days, a daily copayment ($89 in 1984) is assessed until the 90th day of care. After the 90th day, a lifetime reserve of 60 days can be drawn upon, but a larger copayment is required ($178 per day in 1984). A copayment of $45 per day is also required for the 21st through the 100th day in a skilled nursing facility.

Under Part B, there is an annual deductible ($75 in 1984) and a coinsurance of 20 percent for the remainder of approved charges (certain limits were placed on the actual level of reimbursement to physicians, although payment is still related to what they charge). Physicians can also accept the level of payment that Medicare will approve on a bill-by-bill basis. If they agree, Medicare will pay them 80 percent of approved charges directly (the patient's coinsurance is 20 percent, which is paid directly by the patient to the physician), but they cannot charge their Medicare patients for the difference between what they charged and what Medicare has determined is the actual level of reimbursement. If they do not agree to accept Medicare's payment as payment in full, Medicare pays the 80 percent to the patient, and the physician has to collect the full amount from the patient—the 80 percent from Medicare, the 20 percent coinsurance which is the patient's responsibility, and the difference between what the physician charged and the amount Medicare determined would be paid.

Part A insurance pays for blood transfusions, drugs, and biologicals when furnished as part of services provided in hospitals or skilled nursing facilities. Part B pays for blood transfusions and drugs and biologicals that cannot be self-administered when provided by physicians or by outpatient hospital services. Part B payments are subject to the deductible and coinsurance payments described earlier.

For both Part A and Part B, the patient is responsible for any nonreplacement fee charged for the first three units of whole blood or packed red cells (the fee applies only to these two blood products). After the first three units, Part A will pay the nonreplacement fee in addition to the processing and transfusion charges, and Part B will do the same subject to the annual deductible and 20 percent coinsurance (568).

Under the diagnosis-related grouping system of prospective payment for Part A, which began to be phased in during October 1983 and which is to be completed by October 1986, 470 diagnosis-related payment categories have been constructed. Hospitals will therefore be paid a single price regardless of how much it costs to provide that care, including the costs of collecting/processing or purchasing blood products. Hospital outpatient services and physicians' services are still based on a charge-based system, and there is no similar limit on the amount of reimbursement that can be made as was legislated for hospital and skilled nursing home care. (Recent and proposed changes in Medicare are discussed in detail in the OTA report on "Medical Technology and Costs of the Medicare Program," July 1984.)

Payment for Hemophilia Care

In 1975, Public Law 94-63 authorized funding for two activities to aid hemophiliacs: comprehensive hemophilia diagnostic and treatment centers, and development and expansion of blood separation centers. Both types of centers were to be administered by public and nonprofit private entities. Funding for blood separation centers was predicated on finding that there was an insufficient supply of coagulation products to meet the needs of hemophiliacs, but it was determined that supplies would be sufficient through 1980 (554). As a consequence, only funds for treatment centers were actually appropriated.

The law required that funds establishing comprehensive hemophilia centers were to be granted in geographic areas with the greatest need for services. However, it also required that programs be established linking geographically designated centers with other, more remote providers of services. Under the law, hemophilia care centers were to provide programs for training of professional and paraprofessional personnel in hemophilia research, diagnosis, and treatment; programs for diagnosis and treatment of hemophiliacs being treated on an outpatient basis; programs of social and vocational counseling for hemophiliacs; and individualized written comprehensive care programs for each individual treated by or associated with the center. Funds for the direct care of patients were never provided. Only $3 million to $4 million were authorized for the establishment of the comprehensive centers for the first 2 years. In 1982, $2.6 million was appropriated (401).

Since 1975, from 22 (504) to 24 (6) major comprehensive care centers, plus many satellites, have been funded, serving about half of the Nation's estimated 15,000 hemophiliacs (6). The centers are funded through the Department of Health and Human Services' Bureau of Community Health Services/Office of Maternal and Child Health.

Unlike the End-Stage Renal Disease Program under Medicare, which recognizes patients with end-stage renal disease as being totally disabled and thus eligible for Medicare coverage for dialysis and transplants, hemophiliacs can receive Medicare coverage only on a case-by-case determination. Self-administered coagulation proteins are also not covered by Medicare. Therefore, in addition to providing for the distribution of coagulation products and establishing a multidisciplinary hemophilia care team, hemophilia care centers have engaged in efforts to establish funding for individual hemophiliacs (504). A variety of State and third-party sources have been used (see, e.g., 400), as, for example, to provide home care coverage (478).

National Institutes of Health

The institute with primary responsibility for blood resources is the National Heart, Lung, and Blood Institute (NHLBI) and its Division of Blood Diseases and Resources (DBDR). In 1948, the National Heart Institute was established under the National Heart Act. In 1969, it was redesignated the National Heart and Lung Institute, when pulmonary diseases were added to its responsibilities. NHLBI was organized in 1976, when its research responsibilities were to include "the use of blood and blood products and the management of blood resources."

The National Heart, Blood Vessel, Lung, and Blood Act of 1972 (Public Law 92-423), however, has most influenced NHLBI. The 1972 legislation established separate funding and renewal periods for the Institute, as had been established for the National Cancer Institute in the previous year. In contrast, other institutes at NIH fall under the general research authority of the Public Health Service Act, which places no specific disease category allocations or time limits on their authorization. The 1972 Act specified the following responsibilities:

- research into the epidemiology, etiology, and prevention of heart, blood vessel, lung, and blood diseases, including the social, environmental, behavioral, nutritional, biological, and genetic determinants and influences;
- research in basic biological processes and mechanisms of the heart, blood vessel, lung, and blood;
- development and evaluation of techniques, drugs, and devices used in diagnosis and treatment of these diseases;
- programs to develop technological devices to assist, replace, or monitor vital organs;

- programs for field studies and large-scale testing, evaluation, and demonstration of approaches to these diseases;
- research in blood diseases and the use of blood resources;
- education and training of scientists, clinicians, and educators in these fields;
- public and professional education in these diseases;
- programs for research of these diseases in children; and
- programs for research, development, demonstration, and evaluation in emergency medical services.

The 1972 legislation also required that: 1) an Interagency Technical Committee (IATC) be established to coordinate Federal health programs and activities in these diseases; 2) no less than 15 percent of appropriated funds be used for programs in lung diseases, and 15 percent in programs for blood diseases and blood resources; and 3) annual reports be issued summarizing that year's accomplishments and plans for the next 5 years from the director of the institute and from NHLBI's National Advisory Council.

The Director of NHLBI chairs the Interagency Technical Committee, which includes representatives from all Federal departments and agencies whose programs involve research in diseases of the heart, blood vessels, lung and blood, and in transfusion medicine. Three reports have been issued, on 1977, 1979 and 1981 activities. The functional arms of the IATC are its working groups, such as those on smoking and blood resources; these meet separately. In 1979, NHLBI provided over $71 million for programs directly related to blood diseases and resources, while other NIH agencies provided nearly $43 million, and other Federal agencies, outside NIH, nearly $21 million (557).

Research program interrelationships between NHLBI and other Federal agencies are the result of activities in similar areas but for different missions. For example, the Department of the Army's 1983 research budget on hemoglobin solutions was approximately equal to NHLBI's (403). The Army is interested in its military applications as a battlefield and other emergency situation resuscitation fluid, and the NHLBI is more interested in its civilian applications and its use in selected circumstances in addition to its use as an emergency resuscitation fluid.

Another example is in research on AIDS. CDC, FDA, and NIH have all been involved in investigations into the cause and treatment of the disease. CDC is conducting various epidemiologic and laboratory studies on AIDS. At FDA, studies of antiviral agents such as interferon and mediators of immunological function such as interleukin-2 were modified to permit interaction with AIDS clinical protocols and to determine in vitro efficacy in correcting immunologic defects. At NIH, work is primarily concentrated in three Institutes—the National Institute for Allergy and Infectious Diseases (NIAID), the National Cancer Institute (NCI), and NHLBI—with AIDS patients also being treated at the NIH Clinical Center (508a). Officials of the various agencies also regularly attend meetings convened by the other agencies; for example, the AIDS Working Group, consisting of non-Federal researchers, which advises NHLBI's Division of Blood Diseases and Resources, has observers/participants from FDA and CDC in attendance.

The Division of Blood Diseases and Resources has four program areas: 1) bleeding and clotting disorders, 2) red blood cell disorders, 3) sickle cell disease, and 4) blood resources.

In 1982, NHLBI conducted a 10-year review of its activities since passage of the landmark 1972 legislation and identified activities that should be undertaken over the next 5-year period (556). Research needs and opportunities were identified in the areas of: 1) blood bank management, 2) cellular elements, 3) plasma and plasma derivatives, 4) safety, 5) apheresis, 6) immunology, 7) blood substitutes, 8) clinical trials, and 9) education. An early 1984 "snapshot" view of the projects which DBDR was supporting in these areas, categorized by the study group's recommendations, is summarized in appendix A. In addition to the laboratory, clinical, and management studies which were being supported, Transfusion Medicine Academic Awards were instituted in 1983 for the integration of educational programs in transfusion medicine into the medical school curriculum, and a study was to be funded in June 1984 to determine future blood data collection, analysis, and reporting activities.

Food and Drug Administration

The Food and Drug Administration's authority to regulate blood products and blood banking technologies derives from several statutory acts (table 4). (The regulations interpreting these statutes are contained in the *Code of Federal Regulations*, ch. 21, pts. 600 et seq.) Regulation is organized in FDA's Center for Drugs and Biologics, with blood products and blood banking technologies under the purview of the Office of Biologics Research and Review. Within the Office of Biologics, the Division of Blood and Blood Products is responsible for all new blood establishment and blood product license applications and amendments, and for approval to market blood products and related technologies, such as products used in typing and compatibility testing and in preserving and storing blood products. The division has five branches: 1) blood products, 2) immunohematology, 3) plasma derivatives, 4) coagulation products, and 5) hepatitis testing (162).

Scientific activities related to the Division of Blood and Blood Products are based at NIH, along with the Office of Biologics Research and Review's other scientific divisions. The Scientific Director of the Center for Drugs and Biologics integrates the scientific and research activities of these divisions with those of the NIH and serves as a member of the NIH's Scientific Directors' Committee.

In 1978, FDA and HCFA signed a Memorandum of Understanding which was approved by the Secretary of the Department of Health and Human Services and published in the *Federal Register* on March 30, 1980 (45 FR 19316). The memorandum provided for HCFA to assume sole responsibility for inspecting all registered blood establishments that did not perform routine collection, processing and transmission of blood and blood products. These facilities were already being inspected by HCFA (including facilities inspected and accredited by the Joint Commission on Accreditation of Hospitals (JCAH) and American Osteopathic Association (AOA) as well as those inspected by the Medicare State survey agencies) for approval to participate in the Medicare program.

As a result of the agreement and its extension, there are approximately 5,000 facilities which are no longer subject to dual inspections (252). HCFA uses the good manufacturing practice regulations and the compliance guidelines and checklists prepared by FDA. FDA inspects blood collection and source plasma establishments biannually, as does HCFA for the establishments for which it has

Table 4.—FDA Statutory Authority to Regulate Blood Products and Blood Banking Technologies

Statutory authority	Group affected	Mechanisms of control
Public Health Service Act and Food, Drug, and Cosmetic Act—1902 and amendments	Blood banks engaged in interstate commerce.	Licensure of establishment, and individual products. Inspection. Labeling review. Amendments to original license applications for nonstandard or new technologies and new blood products.
Public Health Service Act—1902	Manufacturers of biological reagents for blood bank use.	Licensure of establishment and products. Lot release control. Labeling review.
Food, Drug, and Cosmetic Act—1938	Developers of new anticoagulants, collection or storage systems or new blood products.	Investigational New Drug Application.
Medical Device Amendments of the Food, Drug, and Cosmetic Act—1976	Manufacturers of other reagent solutions, supplies and equipment used in blood banking.	Registration. Inspection. Premarket notification or approval. Labeling review.

SOURCES: J. M. Solomon, "Legislation and Regulations in Blood Banking," *Federal Legislation and the Clinical Laboratory*, Morris Schaeffer (ed.) (Boston, MA: G. K. Hall Medical Publishers, 1981); and U.S. Department of Health and Human Services, Public Health Service, Food and Drug Administration, *Working Relationships Agreement Among the Bureaus of Medical Devices, Radiological Health and Biologics*, April 1982.

assumed responsibility. Manufacturers of plasma derivatives and diagnostic reagents used in blood banking are inspected annually by FDA (252).

In regard to medical devices, the Division of Blood and Blood Products performs some of the review functions for blood-related devices for the Office of Medical Devices of the National Center for Devices and Radiological Health. Medical devices are regulated through a three-tiered regulatory structure, with only Class III devices needing to undergo full premarket approval similar to that used in the process of evaluating drugs. Other devices are essentially regulated by manufacturing controls and inspections, and manufacturers need only to notify FDA of their intent to market these devices and to conform to the good manufacturing practices regulations.

The Division of Blood and Blood Products in the Office of Drugs and Biologics, through the interoffice agreement, reviews the notice of intent to market new device products; applications for clinical investigations of Class III devices to gather the information needed to support a premarket approval application; and the application itself for premarket approval of Class III devices that are used in blood banking (162). (The medical devices industry, including its regulation by FDA under the Medical Device Amendments of 1976, is the subject of another OTA report, "Federal Policies and the Medical Devices Industry," published in October 1984.)

Product recalls are voluntary actions and may be taken as a result of FDA findings during inspections, reports from consumers, or new scientific data indicating risks. Although voluntary, a formal procedure is invoked. After FDA is notified, the potential hazard is classified as a market withdrawal (hazard unknown) or Class I, II, or III recall in decreasing severity, and FDA monitors the product recall. FDA may invoke its seizure powers if the health hazard is definable and voluntary recall is not made.

Table 5 summarizes individual recalls between June 1975 and November 1983. Recall actions have been classified since November 1978, and of the 61 recalls since that time, only two (involving whole blood and albumin) have been listed as Class I, considered to be an immediate, serious to deadly hazard. (Reasons for each recall were not tabulated until 1983.)

Table 5.—Blood Product Recalls,[a] June 1975 to November 1983

Product	Number
Diagnostic reagents:	
Reagent red cells	31
Typing antisera	23
Hepatitis test kits	6
Plasma derivatives:	
Normal human albumin	12
Purified protein fraction	2
Immunoglobulin	8
Factor IX Complex	2
Source plasma	11
Recovered plasma	6
Whole blood and components	21
Blood containers and preservative solutions	6

[a]The number of recalls is not indicative of the relative quality of these products. A single unit of red cells would be listed as a recall, while a lot of albumin might represent 20,000 donors, and 10,000 or more units of albumin.

SOURCE: D. Donohue, personal communication, 1984.

Between 1974 and 1984, there were 175 voluntary suspensions and revocations. Fourteen involved establishments providing whole blood and/or components; the rest affected source plasma centers. Most suspensions are temporary, and establishments are reinstated after corrections are verified by reinspections. Deviations in whole blood collections were for hepatitis testing and recordkeeping, particularly in component preparation. Table 6 summarizes the types of actions that led to suspensions of 13 plasma centers in fiscal years 1980-81.

Table 6.—Significant Deviations Leading to Plasma Center Suspensions, Oct. 1, 1979 to Aug. 31, 1981

Deviations[a]	Number of occurrences
Over bleeding (10% or more)	11[b]
Donor suitability inadequately determined	4
Four-month test requirements not met	3
Aseptic technique not used in collection, separation, and/or reinfusion	3
Records incomplete	3
Personnel inadequately trained and/or informed	3
Unsuitable donors drawn	2
Units shipped before receipt of written HBsAG test results	2
Hazards of plasmapheresis not explained	2
Donors drawn after loss of red cells	1
Number of locations suspended	13

[a]More than one deviation may have been incurred by a plasma center.
[b]At least five locations also had inaccurate recordings of whole blood weights.

SOURCE: D. Donohue, personal communication, 1984.

Table 7 summarizes the types and numbers of errors reported to FDA in 1981 and 1982. None of the various errors associated with ABO and Rh typing were reported to have resulted in fatalities. There were 68 reported fatalities in 1981 and 1982. Approximately one-third were due to failure to properly identify the recipient, and six were due to errors in the transfusion service, including improper identification of the patient's blood that was used in crossmatching. Other reported causes included volume overload, hepatitis, and allergic reactions (162).

New products and procedures which have been approved by FDA in the past 2 years are summarized in table 8. Products and related equipment that were in the approval process as of early 1984 are identified in table 9.

Table 7.—Types and Numbers of Blood Processing Errors, 1981-82

Type	Labeling	Testing	Misinterpreted results
ABO	340	73	94
Rh	122	277	194
ABO and Rh	57	6	5
Antibody	95	51	23
STS	21	2	4
HBsAg	30	2	7
Wrong product name	119	—	—
Wrong expiration date	140	—	—

SOURCE: D. Donohue, personal communication, 1984.

Table 8.—New Blood Products and Procedures Approved by FDA in the Past Two Years (approx. 1982-83)

New Products:
Immune globulin intravenous: Provides immediate intravenous immune globulin for patients who cannot receive intramuscular injection.
Lymphocyte immune globulin—anti-thymocyte globulin (Equine): An immunosuppressive agent indicated for the management of renal allograft rejection.
Hepatitis B vaccine: A blood derivative vaccine providing protection against hepatitis B infection.
Hemain for injection: Indicated for the amelioration of recurrent attacks of acute intermittent porphyria (classified as an orphan biologic).

Amendments to existing licensed products:
Streptokinase/urokinase: To include an indication for intracoronary lysis of thrombi obstructing coronary arteries associated with evolving transmural myocardial infarction.
Antihemophilic Factor Human: To include a heat-treated procedure designed to reduce the risk of transmission of hepatitis and other viruses.
49-day dating period for whole blood for transfusion: Previous dating period was 35 days.
5-day dating period for platelets for transfusion: Previous dating period was 73 hours (3 days).

New procedures/equipment:
New plastic materials (CLX, PL-732, PL-1240, DPL-110): Provides for 5-day platelet dating.
New plastic materials (CLX, PL-1240): Eliminates uses of the plasticizer, DEHP.
Closed apheresis kit: Allows 5-day dating for platelets collected by automated pheresis (manual platelet apheresis allows for only a 3-day dating period).
Additive solutions: Allows extended storage of red blood cells without adverse effects on other blood components.

SOURCE: D. Donohue, personal communication, 1984.

Table 9.—Blood Products and Related Technologies in the Approval Process as of Early 1984

Blood products:
Antihemophilic Factor, heated
"Coagulant Complex," heated
Factor IX, heated
Fibronectins
Hepatitis assay systems
Hepatitis vaccines
Immunoglobulins for intravenous administration
(Specific) immune globulins
Interferons
Lymphokines
Monoclonal antibodies
Plasminogen activators
Streptokinases

Blood-related equipment:
Automated cell separators
Automated plasma separators
Staphylococcal-protein A filters
Sterile docking devices
Thrombin-impregnated materials

SOURCE: D. Donohue, personal communication, 1984.

3. The Blood Services Complex

Contents

	Page
Part 1: The Voluntary, Whole Blood, and Blood Components Sector	51
Introduction	51
Blood Collecting Organizations	52
Blood Collections in the Voluntary Sector	57
Costs of Blood and Blood Components	59
Costs and Charges for Blood Products	59
Access	60
Part 2: The Commercial Plasma and Plasma Derivatives Sector	63
Overview	63
Sources of Raw Plasma	65
Finished Products Licensed for Use in the United States	67
Conclusion	73

LIST OF TABLES

Table No.		Page
10.	Whole Blood Collections by Type of Facility and Affiliation, 1980	52
11.	Activities of Three Major Voluntary Blood Service Organizations	53
12.	American Blood Commission Member Organizations and Its Board of Directors, April 1984	56
13.	American Blood Commission Statements of Support, Revenue, and Expenses and Changes in Fund Balances for Years Ended Mar. 31, 1976-83 (thousands of dollars)	57
14.	Blood Center Processing Fees for Blood and Components (1983)	60
15.	American Red Cross Blood Services Statements of Revenue and Expenses and Statement of Assets and Liabilities, 1980-83 (or the year ended June 30) (in thousands)	61
16.	Blood Center Costs and Hospital Charges for Red Cells, 1980	62
17.	Changes in Processing Fees for Red Cells Compared to Changes in Total U.S. Health Care Expenditures	62
18.	Number of Plasma Centers Located in the United States (by owner, fractionator, multi-operator, single operator, and nonprofit)	63
19.	Production and Consumption of Human Serum Albumin and Antihemophilic Factor	65
20.	Albumin and Plasma Protein Fraction Consumption in Selected Countries, 1976	65
21.	Principal Producers of Human Plasma Derivatives for the U.S. Market	66
22.	Manufacturers of Normal Serum Albumin (NSA) and Plasma Protein Fraction (PPF) Licensed for Use in the United States	67
23.	Manufacturers of Coagulation Factors Licensed for Use in the United States	69
24.	Manufacturers of Selected Immune Globulins for Use in the United States	71
25.	Representative Blood Center Prices for Plasma Derivatives	73

LIST OF FIGURES

Figure No.		Page
4.	Relationships Among Blood Collecting Facilities, 1980	52
5.	Increases in Red Cells Available for Transfusion As a Result of Improved Inventory Management and Decreased Outdating	58
6.	Recent Trends in Whole Blood and Components Distributed for Transfusion (Red Cross data only)	58
7.	U.S. Production of Factor VIII (in activity units) and of Albumin/PPF (in 12.5 Gram Equivalents), 1971-82	64
8.	Flow of the Nation's Blood Resources, 1980	74

3.
The Blood Services Complex

PART 1: THE VOLUNTARY, WHOLE BLOOD, AND BLOOD COMPONENTS SECTOR

Introduction

The whole blood sector is called "voluntary" because it collects blood primarily from unpaid donors. In 1980, only 2.2 percent of the 11,880,000 units of whole blood collected was collected from paid donors (518), in contrast to the situation of 10 years ago when over 10 percent of whole blood was collected commercially. Three types of facilities are involved in the voluntary sector: 1) commmunity and regional blood centers which collect and distribute blood to hospitals in circumscribed geographic areas; 2) hospital blood banks which both collect and transfuse whole blood and components; and 3) hospitals which primarily store and transfuse blood, but do not collect it. In addition, the voluntary sector depends on the commercial pharmaceutical firms to fractionate its recovered and salvaged plasma.

Community or regional blood centers generally provide a full range of blood services to a surrounding geographic area. These services may include collection, testing, and labeling of blood, and distribution of blood and blood products to hospitals, physicians, and hemophilia care centers. In addition, blood centers often conduct research and training programs.

Hospital blood banks generally provide a smaller range of services than regional blood centers, usually limited to the collection and storage of whole blood and components. Some common laboratory tests may be available in-house, depending on the size and scope of the blood bank operations, while other tests must be sent out to private laboratories or the regional blood center. Often hospital blood banks orient donor recruitment efforts to the friends and relatives of patients; thus, many of the existing nonreplacement fee programs are associated with hospital blood banks.

The third type of facility involved in the voluntary sector is the hospital transfusion service, which is responsible for the administration of blood and blood components within the hospital. Some hospitals do not collect any blood but obtain their blood and blood products through an outside supplier, either a regional blood center or another hospital blood bank, thus making the transfusion service the primary participant in blood management and use in such noncollecting hospitals. While transfusion services also serve as blood banks, they are called transfusion services to differentiate them from blood banks which collect, as well as store, blood.

Although blood collection began in hospital blood banks, over time they have come to play less of a role in blood collection. In 1971, 69 percent of the blood collected came from regional and community blood centers (555). By 1980, regional and community blood centers collected 88 percent of the total, and comparable, though less reliable figures for 1981 indicate that 91 percent of total whole blood collections were made through blood centers (29). Surgenor & Schnitzer/ABC (518) attribute the predominance of regional centers to the centers' ability to collect blood through constant mobile collections. In 1980, 69.5 percent of whole blood collections was through mobile units. There is some speculation that the dominance of regional blood centers may be reversed in the future as hospitals seek to gain control over costs in the face of such cost containment measures as the prospective payment system—although, as discussed below, there are those who argue that cost containment may accelerate the trend toward more centralized collections (see ch. 5, pt. 3).

Blood Collecting Organizations

As shown in figure 4 and table 10, blood collection and transfusion facilities in the voluntary sector are represented by three organizations with overlapping memberships: the American Red Cross (ARC), the American Association of Blood Banks (AABB), and the Council of Community Blood Centers (CCBC). The American Red Cross has 57 regional centers operating under a single Federal license, and also maintains an affiliation with the New York Blood Center (which is a member of CCBC). The Red Cross regional centers cover about half the geographic area of the United States, and collect about half the Nation's whole blood.

Another 45 percent of the Nation's whole blood is collected by institutional members of the American Association of Blood Banks, including members who belong to CCBC. In 1980, seven ARC regional centers and all but two Council of Community Blood Centers belonged to AABB, as did 1,977 blood collecting hospitals. There were 101 community blood centers that were members only of AABB. Approximately 2 percent of blood collections were through 16 unaffiliated blood centers.

The AABB was formed in 1947 to protect the interests of already existing hospital blood banks in the face of a plan announced by the Red Cross to attempt to collect and organize the Nation's entire blood supply (307). Existing hospital and regional blood banks wanted to maintain their established collection programs. Today, the AABB represents over 2,000 institutional (voting) members, as well as about 7,000 individual members, primarily blood bank personnel (e.g., administrators, medical technologists). Institutional members include blood centers, hospital blood banks, and transfusion services. While blood centers account for two-thirds of the blood collected by AABB members (29), each institutional member has a single vote regardless of its size.

In 1962, the Council of Community Blood Centers was formed by six community blood bank administrators who were dissatisfied with the dominance of the AABB by hospital blood banks.

Table 10.—Whole Blood Collections by Type of Facility and Affiliation, 1980

	Number of facilities	Units collected
Regional and community blood centers:		
AABB only	101	2,163,614
CCBC	41[a]	1,866,586
ARC	57	5,434,783
Unaffiliated.............	16	208,421
Total for blood centers	215	9,673,404
Hospitals:		
AABB affiliated	1,977	1,116,143
Unaffiliated..............	4,455	73,895
Total for hospitals	6,432	1,190,038
Other collections...........		16,637
Total—U.S. collections		10,880,079
Euroblood imported		265,839
Grand total		11,145,918

[a]In 1980 26 CCBC members ran 41 blood collecting facilities.
SOURCE: Surgenor and Schnitzer/ABC, 1983.

Figure 4.—Relationships Among Blood Collecting Facilities, 1980[a]

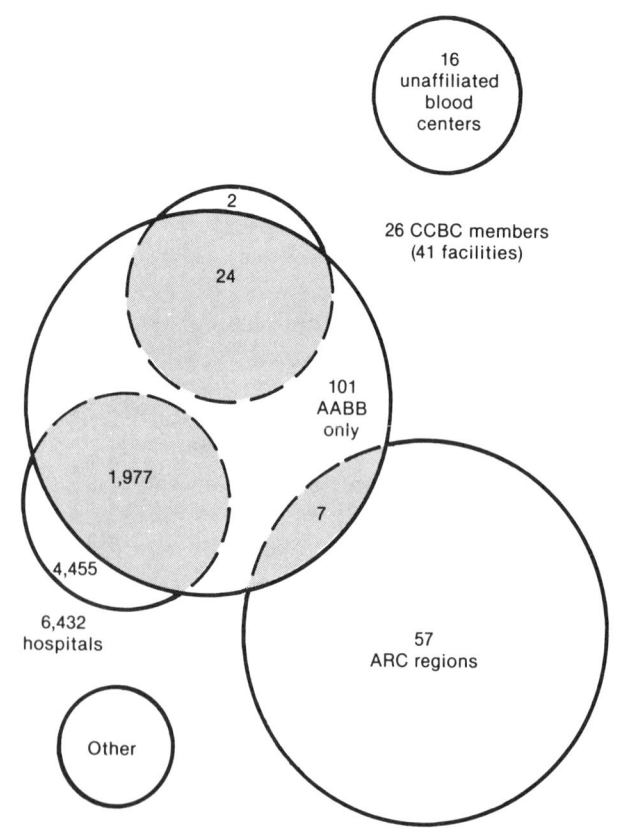

[a]Size of circles represents approximate collection of whole blood in units (see fig. 8).
SOURCE: Surgenor and Schnitzer/ABC, 1983.

CCBC today consists of 27 institutional members, i.e., community or regional blood centers. All but two current CCBC members (New York Blood Center and Puget Sound Blood Center in Seattle) are also members of AABB. CCBC as an organization has played a relatively minor role in the politics of whole blood delivery, which has been dominated by ARC and AABB. CCBC's recent move to the Washington, DC, area, where the Red Cross, the AABB, and the American Blood Commission are headquartered, was a move designed in part to make CCBC more of an active participant in National Blood Policy deliberations.

Thus, three major organizations represent almost all the blood collection organizations in the United States. Although there is some overlap in organizational membership and in function, the three major organizations espouse different philosophies and are designed to serve different functions (see table 11). The AABB and CCBC are organizations which represent individual blood collection facilities. The Red Cross, as a corporation and a blood collector in its own right, provides a Federal license to collect and process blood as well as an organizational framework to its member centers, although each center operates somewhat independently and is required to be more or less self-sufficient.

American Red Cross (ARC) Blood Services

Red Cross chapters choose whether or not to engage in blood services and other services offered by the Red Cross, except disaster services and services to the Armed Forces, which are required to be available from all chapters. In 1982, 1,873 of the 3,011 Red Cross chapters participated in 57 ARC regional blood services. Donor recruitment, blood collection, and processing are performed by volunteers and staff of the regional centers. In addition to blood collection, regional centers also provide diagnostic and other blood-related services. National headquarters provides standards for its 57 regional blood centers and inspects them periodically. Interregional resource sharing is accomplished by the use of a computerized inventory system. ARC national also maintains a Rare Donor Registry, and many of its regions conduct research (50).

Table 11.—Activities of Three Major Voluntary Blood Service Organizations

	ARC	AABB	CCBC
Actual blood services:			
Number of institutional members	57 regions 1,873 chapters	2,176	27
Units of blood collected by organization or members in 1981[a]	5,799,024	3,395,854[b]	2,320,750[c]
Actual blood collection	x	*	*
Formal resource sharing program	x	x	
Other activities or characteristics:			
Management conferences	x	x	x
Government liaison	x	x	x
Organ and tissue procurement	x	**	**
Scientific programs	x	x	
Scientific and educational publications	x	x	
Rare donor registry	x	x	
Blood bank procedures manual	x	x	
Standards published[d]	x	x	
Institutional inspection and accreditation	x	x	
Training for technologies	x		
Incorporation as single entity	x		
Plasma products marketed	x		
Formal ongoing strategic planning activity	x		

*Collected by members.
**Several members of these organizations are engaged in organ and tissue procurement.
[a]Source: AABB, untitled, 1983.
[b]Excludes amount collected by the 24 CCBC members and 7 ARC regions who are also AABB members.
[c]Excludes Euroblood.
[d]AABB publishes standards for the industry. ARC publishes standards which are used internally; however, these have been cited in court cases as the basis for standards of care.
SOURCE: Office of Technology Assessment.

Red Cross Blood Services also maintains a plasma products division operating out of its national headquarters, which is responsible for arranging contracts for fractionation of plasma from Red Cross blood collections and marketing of the products on a competitive basis with the commercial fractionation industry (see below). The Red Cross recently entered into an agreement with Baxter-Travenol which would give it more control over fractionation of the plasma it collects (and the ability to develop new products), but Red Cross does not fractionate its own plasma. In general, 85 percent of the plasma products sold by the Red Cross (primarily albumin and Factor VIII) is marketed by and within Red Cross regions; and the remaining 15 percent is marketed outside the regions (486). Eleven Red Cross regions are also licensed as source plasma centers.

Other fairly new activities of the Red Cross include efforts at strategic planning and management, and involvement in organ and tissue procurement (see ch. 7, pt. 2). In the last year, Red Cross Blood Services has created a Planning, Marketing, and Operations Research Division at National Headquarters. Blood services is one concern of an organization-wide planning group called the President's Council. The Red Cross is concerned that particularly because of technological advances such as genetic engineering, blood services as it exists today may be a declining industry. Currently, Blood Services accounts for almost 60 percent of the Red Cross's gross revenues (see "Costs and Charges for Blood Products" for further discussion of Red Cross Blood Services finances).

The entire ARC organization holds a special position in the national blood services complex. ARC is the only one of the blood service organizations with a congressional charter, although the charter is for disaster relief, not blood collections. (The charter is dated 1905, and Red Cross blood collections were not begun until the 1940s.) The President of the United States is ARC's honorary chair, and other cabinet members serve as honorary counselor and treasurer. The President appoints eight of the ARC's Board of Governors, and by an act of Congress ARC audit reports are reviewed by the Department of Defense. For these reasons, ARC is sometimes described as a quasi-governmental agency.

American Association of Blood Banks (AABB)

The American Association of Blood Banks characterizes itself as the only organization devoted exclusively to blood banking and blood transfusion services (28). As a scientific and administrative association, AABB sets technical standards which are followed by its members (see, e.g., 583), inspects and certifies the operations of its institutional members, and serves as a liaison with the Federal Government and with the other blood collection organizations. A major part of AABB's operation is its National and Regional Clearinghouse (see "Coordination of Blood Resources" in ch. 5), which accounted for two-thirds of its assets at the end of 1982 ($1.3 million of AABB's $2 million total) (20).

The basic standards in blood banking were first formalized and published by the AABB. The Red Cross and AABB have agreed to keep their standards essentially identical and even jointly publish the "Circular of Information" which must be included with shipments of blood components as required by the Food and Drug Administration (FDA). The AABB also initiated the first formal nongovernment inspection and accreditation system. All institutional members of AABB are inspected on a regular basis and are dropped from membership if they are not in compliance. AABB also conducts inspections of approved schools for training specialists in blood banking to ensure that the required educational standards are maintained.

Council of Community Blood Centers (CCBC)

The primary audience for CCBC activities is blood center managers. (The AABB has recently become more actively concerned about blood center administration; to date, the AABB has oriented itself primarily to hospital blood banks and to the day-to-day technological aspects of blood services.) CCBC describes itself as serving as a forum for blood center administrators, medical directors and senior management. It publishes no technical or procedures manuals, and does not operate a formal resource exchange system, but holds two meetings a year to discuss management issues. CCBC is a relatively small organization which has struggled financially in the past. It derived almost all of its $207,000 income in 1983 from membership dues (136).

Each of the three organizations described above also serves its members or chapters by representing them on the American Blood Commission's Board of Directors.

American Blood Commission (ABC)

The American Blood Commission is the one formal mechanism enabling the AABB, ARC, and CCBC to work together, along with other health care providers (e.g., American Hospital Association, American Medical Association), consumer groups (e.g., National Hemophilia Foundation, National Kidney Foundation, American Legion), and representatives from the commercial plasmapheresis industry (e.g., Pharmaceutical Manufacturers Association of America). A list of ABC's members and governing board is shown in table 12.

Given its unique position as a private voluntary association charged with implementing public policy, ABC has been forced to influence blood policy through nonregulatory channels. Its potential effectiveness was limited by its lack of enforcement powers. In addition, philosophical differences persist among ABC's member blood collecting organizations, both voluntary and commercial, and the organizations fear losing control over their operations to the ABC. Many early attempts by the commission to mediate a compromise between the major blood collection organizations failed. For example, while ABC's Board adopted the recommendation of its 1977 Task Force on Donor Recruitment that the nonreplacement fee be abolished, it was never acted upon by the full commission because of AABB's opposition.

Some of ABC's progams and initiatives are widely credited for catalyzing change in the blood industry—or at the very least, for maintaining constructive dialog conducive to problem-solving. It has been suggested that ABC may have succeeded in its role as conscience of the blood industry (270) by providing a public forum for discussion of blood policy issues. ABC has established standing committees on donor recruitment, and regionalization, for example; both are issues in which the exchange of information, and an eventual consensus, are of value both to the industry and to those served by it.

ABC, and many others, see its regionalization recognition program as having been fairly successful, with 44 regions, representing over 50 percent of the Nation's blood supply, having achieved full recognition status. ABC's attempt at a more far-reaching effort at resource sharing (which would have overcome the discontinuities between the AABB Clearinghouse and the ARC system) was delayed when the commercial sector objected to limiting resource sharing to noncommercial blood, and the Red Cross withdrew in fear that a civil suit would be filed. The Red Cross has substantial assets which it fears could be attached if such a suit were filed and won.

In an attempt to get an agreement about resource sharing signed, the ABC Board contemplated, but never enacted, a motion to seek Federal legislation that would, in effect, exempt participation in resource sharing from antitrust action. The strategy now is to see whether the move of the AABB National Clearinghouse operation to the Washington, DC, area will make resource sharing seem more feasible. The continuing failure of the blood collectors to agree on a means of coordination has been frustrating to the consumer representatives on the ABC Board, but it is not clear that such coordination would contribute significantly to the efficiency of blood collection (see ch. 5, pt. 2).

ABC's effort at coordinating an ongoing system of data collection and analysis was a mixed success. While the 1979 and 1980 data collected for the ABC's National Blood Data Center represent the only systematic national data collection since 1972, ABC was unable to maintain data collection on an ongoing basis, or to make it commercially viable, as had been hoped. The effort was marked initially by heated debates among the participating organizations (e.g., on the collection of information on outdated blood, which was defined differently by different organizations (270; see also 547). Further, National Blood Data Center data do not include information on the com-

Table 12.—American Blood Commission Member Organizations and Its Board of Directors, April 1984

Member organizations:
American Association of Blood Banks
American Association for Clinical Histocompatibility Testing
American Association of Donor Recruitment Professionals
American Association of Retired Persons
American Association of Tissue Banks
American College of Physicians
American College of Surgeons
American Federation of Labor—Congress of Industrial Organizations
American Heart Association
American Hospital Association
American Legion
American Medical Association
American Nurses' Association, Inc.
American Osteopathic Association
American Red Cross
American Society of Anesthesiologists
American Society for Apheresis
American Society of Clinical Pathologists
American Surgical Association
College of American Pathologists
Communications Workers of America
Cooley's Anemia Foundation
Council of Community Blood Centers
Health Insurance Association of America
Leukemia Society of America
National Association for Sickle Cell Disease, Inc.
National Association of Patients on Hemodialysis and Transplantation, Inc.
The National Hemophilia Foundation
Pharmaceutical Manufacturers Association
United Way of America
Veterans Administration

Board of Directors:
Ray Andrus
  American Federation of Labor—Congress of Industrial Organizations
J. Newton Ashworth, Ph.D.
  Pharmaceutical Manufacturers Association
Fred A. Barnette, at-large
  Ortho Diagnostics, Inc.
Carl G. Becker, M.D.
  American Heart Association
Hamp Coley
  United Way of America
Margaret M. Diener, MPH
  National Association of Patients on Hemodialysis and Transplantation, Inc.
Suellyn Ellerbe, R.N., M.N.
  American Nurses' Association, Inc.
Ralph G. Golden, Ph.D.
  American Association of Retired Persons
Charles R. Goulet
  Blue Cross/Blue Shield Association
David Guri, at-large
  Alpha Therapeutic Corp.
Douglas Holloway, at-large
James B. Hubbard, Vice President
  American Legion
Alfred J. Katz, M.D.
  American Red Cross
Roland H. Lange
  American Red Cross
Paul McCurdy, M.D.
  American Society of Hematology
Franklin D. McDonald, M.D., Secretary
  National Kidney Foundation
Mary L. Mays
  Communications Workers of America
Harold T. Meryman, M.D.
  American Association of Tissue Banks
John D. Milam, M.D.
  American Association of Blood Banks
William V. Miller, M.D., President, at-large
Gerald S. Moss, M.D., FACS
  American College of Surgeons
Victor H. Muller, M.D.
  American Society of Clinical Pathologists
Richard E. Palmer, M.D.
  American Medical Association
Peter J. Quesenberry, M.D.
  Leukemia Society of America
Randall H. Rolfe
  American Hospital Association
Dale A. Smith, at-large
  Baxter-Travenol Laboratories, Inc.
James M. Stengle, M.D.
  The National Hemophilia Foundation
Bill T. Teague, B.S., M.T. (A.S.C.P.), S.B.B., Treasurer
  American Association of Blood Banks
John L. Thornton, M.D., Vice President
  Council of Community Blood Centers
Martin J. Valaske, M.D.
  College of American Pathologists
Edward L. Wampold, at-large
  Cooper Diagnostics
Charles F. Whitten, M.D.
  National Association for Sickle Cell Disease, Inc.
Edward C. Zaino, M.D.
  Cooley's Anemia Foundation

SOURCE: American Blood Commission.

mercial plasmapheresis industry, which was collected and published separately by the American Blood Resources Association.

Government support for ABC has diminished over the years, necessitating increases from private funding (see table 13). ABC now receives no Federal funding. A great blow was the withdrawal of the American Cancer Society, the American College of Emergency Physicians, the American Osteopathic College of Pathologists, and the National Medical Association in 1983. Although members are often delinquent in their dues, collections of membership dues for fiscal year 1984

Ch. 3—The Blood Services Complex • 57

Table 13.—American Blood Commission Statements of Support, Revenue, and Expenses and Changes in Fund Balances for Years Ended Mar. 31, 1976-83 (thousands of dollars)

	1983	1982	1981	1980	1979	1978	1977	1976
Public support:								
U.S. Government contracts	$ 56	$296	$467	$337	$348	$526	$389	$129
Private grants					12	42		100
Contributions	126	123	46	51	61	46	7	
Total public support	$182	$419	$513	$389	$420	$614	$395	$229
Revenue:								
Membership dues	$166	$169	$179	$179	$159	$144	$144	$141
Investment income	20	19	9	8	3		1	4
Conference fees	10	8	23	10				
Publications and miscellaneous	9	22	6	3	2	2		
Loss on sale of equipment	(3)							
Total revenue	$202	$219	$217	$200	$163	$147	$144	$145
Total support and revenue	$384	$638	$730	$589	$583	$761	$540	$374
Expenses:								
Program services:								
Technical advisory panel	3	3	16					
Resource sharing		12	8					
Policy operations	93	137	142	173	149	139	169	
National Blood Data Center	73	240	277	191	165	237	106	29
Regionalization	57	84	103	70	87	88	72	36
Management and Logistics Conference			8	3				
Plasma study			2	4				
Utilization					5	7	4	
Long range planning					1			
Commonality						46	107	39
Clearinghouse						5	5	
Donor recruitment						44	63	20
Planning and implementation								35
Total program service expenses	$225	$475	$555	$440	$407	$565	$525	$158
Supporting services:								
Management and general	$110	$157	$178	$141	$119	$172	$ 85	$ 40
Financial development	7	4	13	2	21			
Total supporting services	$117	$161	$190	$143	$139	$172	$ 85	$ 40
Total expenses	$342	$636	$746	$583	$547	$737	$609	$199
Excess (deficiency) of public support and revenue over expenses	$ 42	$ 2	$ (16)	$ 6	$ 37	$ 24	$ (69)	$175
Fund balances, beginning of year	157	156	172	166	129	106	175	
Fund balances, end of year	$199	$157	$156	$172	$166	$129	$106	$175

SOURCE: American Blood Commission, 1983.

exceeded ABC's goal. Nevertheless, as a consequence of corporate contributions not meeting ABC's goal, ABC now projects a $20,000 shortfall in fiscal year 1985. Some believe that the decline in support indicates that there is no longer a need for such an organization to resolve differences among blood collectors.

Blood Collections in the Voluntary Sector

Whole blood collections have been able to keep up with increasing demand at the same time that paid whole blood donations have decreased significantly (fig. 1 in ch. 1). This increase has occurred through increased recruitment, improved inventory management, and a large increase in the use of blood components instead of whole blood.

The most recent comprehensive data on whole blood collections and transfusions are for 1979 and 1980 (518). Partial data are available from blood collection centers (but not transfusion services) represented by ARC, AABB, and CCBC for 1981 (29) and from the American Red Cross through June 1983. In 1980, out of 11.15 million units of whole blood collected, 14.8 million units of blood components were transfused, exclusive of blood that was outdated or lost (see fig. 2 in ch. 1). Between 1971 and 1980, whole blood collections increased from 8.8 million to 11.15 million units, while whole blood and red cell losses decreased from 2.44 million to 1.15 million units, an improvement in losses from 28 to 10 percent of blood collected (see fig. 5). (Solutions increasing the storage life of blood from 21 to 35 days were introduced in 1980, and this effect is only partially reflected in the 1980 data. Recent approval of a solution that allows a 49-day shelf life for packed red cells should result in further improvement, although the additional cost of such solutions may limit their widespread acceptance.)

Losses in Red Cross centers have remained fairly stable in the years since 1980 but these data do not include reports from hospitals and other blood banks to which blood is shipped. Red Cross data shown in figure 6 for products distributed for transfusion (but not necessarily transfused) indicate that trends toward component therapy and the use of blood components have continued.

Figure 5.—Increases in Red Cells Available for Transfusion As a Result of Improved Inventory Management and Decreased Outdating

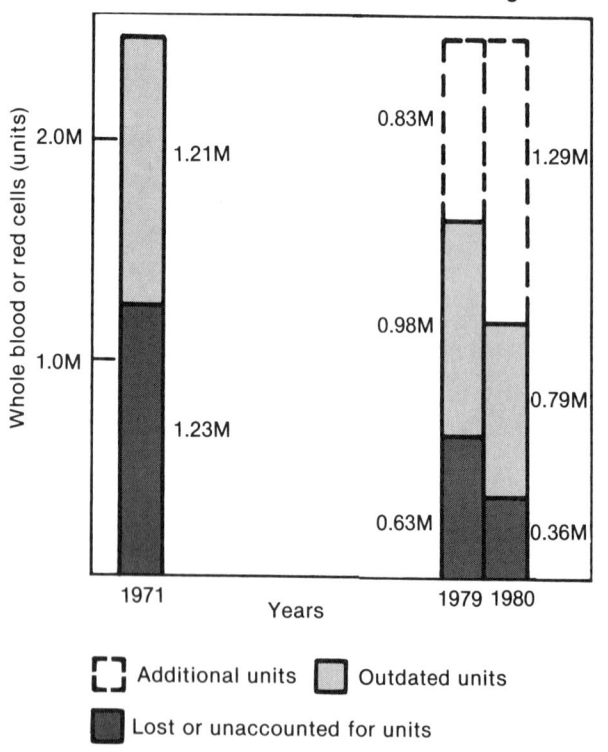

SOURCE: Surgenor and Schnitzer/ABC, 1983.

Figure 6.—Recent Trends in Whole Blood and Components Distributed for Transfusion (Red Cross data only)

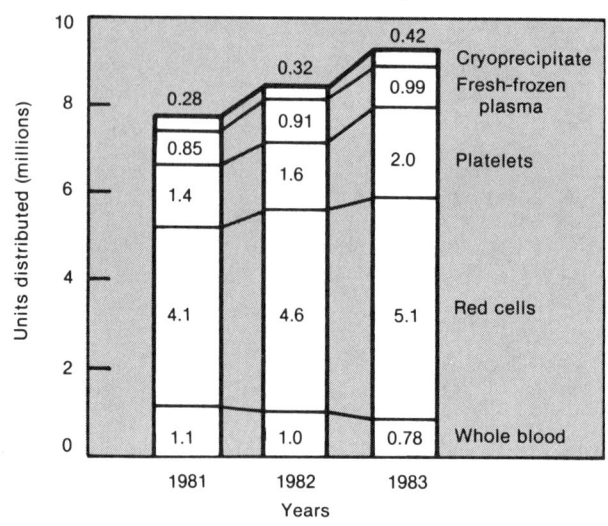

SOURCE: American Red Cross, *Blood Services Operations Reports: 1981-1983.*

Red blood cells (including whole blood) continue to dominate use and are the driving force behind collection efforts in the voluntary sector. Platelet use rose from 0.41 million units in 1971 to 2.86 million units in 1980. (Approval in 1982 of platelet storage bags that extend the storage period from 3 to 5 days is expected to increase the availability and use of platelets, as well as to decrease outdating, which is substantial.) Most platelet concentrates are made from whole blood, but platelets are also collected directly (plateletpheresis). Plateletpheresis collections have increased steadily in Red Cross regions since 1979 (45,46,47,48). The reported nationwide drop in plateletpheresis collections between 1979 and 1980 (518) may be misleading because of a simultaneous increase in combined leukaplateletpheresis procedures (470).

Fresh-frozen plasma (FFP) production has also increased, although indications for its use are limited and have become the topic of private and Federal scrutiny (see ch 5, pt. 4). In the Red Cross alone, 3.2 million units of FFP were produced in 1983, a 27.2-percent increase over the previous year. However, only 30 percent of the fresh-frozen plasma produced was distributed for transfusions. Two-thirds was used for fractionation.

Use of the final product from voluntary whole blood collections, cryoprecipitate, which contains antihemophilic factor (AHF) and other coagulation proteins, remained constant from 1972 to 1980, primarily because of availability of a more effective and stable way to inject concentrates of AHF derived from pooled plasma. However, in light of the AIDS crisis, and because new uses have been found for the substance (see ch. 5, pt. 4), cryoprecipitate production has increased recently (23,48).

Costs of Blood and Blood Components

On the whole, the cost of blood and blood products has not been a major factor in discussions of health care expenditures, probably because it has been estimated that the total valuation of collected and transfused blood and blood products (including plasma derivatives) is only about 1 percent of total health care expenditures (31a). However, the National Blood Policy (NBP) pointed out that costs could have an impact on access to health care. Another issue addressed by the NBP was the need for public confidence in the reasonableness of service charges to encourage voluntary donors. To this end, the National Blood Policy encouraged development of accounting and reporting systems to identify relationships between the costs and charges for all services and materials associated with transfusion therapy (180; see table 2 in ch. 2).

In 1979, the U.S. General Accounting Office recommended that the Health Care Financing Administration (HCFA) investigate the relationship between costs and charges for blood products to determine if Medicare was being overcharged by hospitals (546). Concern had also been raised about whether nonreplacement fees constituted "profiteering," especially when patients were charged for nonreplaced blood that was originally obtained from unremunerated donors (e.g., see 511). The nonreplacement fee was also viewed as causing problems of access to health care for Medicare patients, who are responsible for paying a three-unit deductible if they cannot arrange to replace the blood transfused in hospitals charging a nonreplacement fee.

Costs and Charges for Blood Products

The costs associated with voluntarily donated blood derive from donor recruitment, equipment (hardware and software) and labor, testing, inventory management and distribution, and transfusion. When donors are paid, the costs of remuneration must be added. Blood collecting and transfusing facilities in the voluntary sector have not developed a uniform industrywide system for allocating costs to each step in the collecting and transfusing process. The American Red Cross and some larger independent blood centers (e.g., the New York Blood Center) have developed cost accounting systems for internal use.

There is wide variation in the fees charged to hospitals and patients by blood collectors and by hospitals to patients. As shown in table 14, 1983 processing fees for whole blood charged by American Red Cross regions ranged from $28 (in San Juan, PR) to $59 (in San Jose, CA). Charges in some community blood centers can be higher, e.g., $67 for whole blood in San Mateo, CA (including a replacement fee); $75 at the Irwin Memorial Blood Bank in San Francisco. Similar variations are found for other components. Production and sale of the several blood components means that an average Red Cross blood center could collect up to $105.54 from a single unit of whole blood donated in 1983, not including revenues from recovered plasma (higher if red cells are frozen or washed).

Increases in processing fees for blood components, as well as better inventory management, have meant that blood suppliers have been able to accumulate substantial fund balances. For example, as shown in table 15, Red Cross net assets at year-end increased by 18 percent from 1980 to 1981, by 30 percent from 1981 to 1982 and by 32 percent from 1982 to 1983. Although apparently substantial on a cumulative basis, Red Cross net assets of $36,053,000 for the year ended June 30, 1983, amounted to only 8.5 percent of that year's entire blood services revenues, representing fewer than 36 days of operating expenses, according to the Red Cross (43). Some blood centers (e.g., Puget Sound Blood Center, Hoxworth Blood Center) have deliberately accumulated revenues over

Table 14.—Blood Center Processing Fees for Blood and Components (1983)

Blood components	Average processing fees ARC	CCBC	Range[a]
Whole blood	$ 41.83	$42.59	$28.00 (San Juan)—$ 59.00 (San Jose)
Red blood cells	41.17	40.41	28.00 (San Juan)— 59.00 (San Jose)
Red blood cells deglycerolized	131.55	—	91.00 (Portland) — 225.00 (Atlanta)
Red blood cells washed	86.00	NA	60.25 (Roanoke) — 160.00 (Atlanta)
Fresh-frozen plasma	25.08	24.49	17.00 (Waco) — 38.00 (San Jose)
Cryoprecipitated AHF	12.28	12.68	8.00 (Great Falls, Daytona) — 18.00 (4 centers)
Platelets	26.41	25.31	17.00 (Waco) — 40.00 (Boston)

[a]Red Cross data only.
NA = not available.
SOURCES: ARC—American Red Cross (1983), fees shown are as of June 30, 1983, and do not include the NYBC; CCBC—Huitt, letter to OTA, 1984; fees shown are as of July 1983.

those required for operating expenses in order to provide for capital expansion (221,242). Red Cross headquarters usually does not exercise direct control over blood services assets; such assets are used at the discretion of individual blood services regions (141). A small portion of Red Cross revenues is devoted to research—less than 2 percent.

The difference between community blood center processing costs and hospitals' charges to patients is shown in table 16. In table 17, the processing fee for red cells charged by blood centers to hospitals is compared to hospital charges to patients. In 1980 the average community blood center red cell processing fee to hospitals was about $32. (The average cost of $45.91 for collecting and processing a unit of whole blood is offset by sales of remaining blood components.) The average total hospital charge for a unit of red cells was $88.97. In addition to a processing fee, hospital charges might include an additional processing fee, a replacement charge, a laboratory charge, an infusion charge and other charges (table 16). Data for processing fees for hospitals include hospitals which also collect their own blood. Wallace & Wallace/ABC (576) found that total charges are higher at collecting than at noncollecting hospitals, and that higher processing fees and replacement fees accounted for the higher total charges. As might be expected, there is substantial variation in hospital charges for red cells (the only component for which hospital data are available), with standard deviations from a quarter to a third of the mean.

Increases in blood costs have not exceeded increases in total health care costs. As shown in table 17, national health expenditures have increased on an average of 15 percent per year (for 1980 to 1982), while blood center processing fees have increased 7 percent (CCBC members) and 12 percent (Red Cross regions). Increases in hospital charges for blood appear closer to increased hospital charges in general, although it is difficult to draw conclusions with information from only 2 consecutive years.

Access

Issues of access are more difficult to sort out than issues of cost/charge relationships. It is currently unlikely that individuals will be denied hospital care because they cannot afford the cost of blood to be transfused during their hospital stay, but the issue may become more complicated as prospective payment systems are phased in (see ch. 5, pt. 4). At present the only real threat to access posed by the cost of blood products seems to be that uninsured hemophiliacs may receive less Factor VIII than is optimal.

At present, there is wide variation in the way third-party payers cover the costs of blood products. Since 1968, Blue Cross/Blue Shield national policy has been to encourage voluntary donation and replacement, and blood assurance programs (79). Like Medicare, then, most Blue Cross/Blue Shield policies have a three-unit deductible for nonreplacement fees when they are charged. For Federal employees covered by Blue Cross/Blue Shield, however, replacement fees are partially covered by the supplemental portion of the policy (i.e., 80 percent coverage for high option; 75 percent coverage for low option). Policies more costly to patients are followed in at least one State.

Table 15.—American Red Cross Blood Services Statements of Revenue and Expenses and Statement of Assets and Liabilities, 1980-83 (for the year ended June 30) (in thousands)

	1983	1982	1981	1980
Revenues:				
Blood Services processing	$418,962	$371,901	$301,685	$241,155
Investment income	5,389	3,695	2,252	1,213
Contributions	177	200	—	—
Government and private foundation grants	73	101	66	209
Other income	1,292	1,371	2,016	1,021
Total revenues	425,893	377,268	306,019	243,598
Expenses:				
Blood Services expenses	379,091	342,813	292,281	233,684
Less—expenses incurred by chapters funded from non-Blood Services support and revenue	(9,821)	(9,469)	(9,673)	(10,633)
Net Blood Services expenses	369,270	333,344	282,608	223,051
Excess of revenue over expenses before property and equipment acquisitions	56,623	43,924	23,411	20,547
Property and equipment acquisitions—net of proceeds from sales of property	(20,570)	(17,927)	(10,130)	(9,577)
Net Excess of Revenues Over Expenses and Property Acquisitions:				
Increase in designated balances approved by Board action for:				
Replace and improvement of buildings and equipment	9,271	—	—	—
Other specific purposes	6,193	—	—	—
Net operating assets required	20,589	—	—	—
	36,053	25,997	13,281	10,970
Designated Net Assets, Beginning of Year	111,364	85,367	72,086	61,116
Designated Net Assets, End of Year	$147,417	$111,364	$ 85,367	$ 72,086
Assets:				
Cash and time deposits	$ 14,392	$ 6,425	$ 5,982	$ 6,658
Investments	46,415	29,350	15,181	9,365
Receivables	47,745	47,073	41,458	31,129
Inventories	55,116	47,268	51,975	52,351
Other assets	1,084	799	541	353
Due from undesignated funds	8,172	4,015	—	—
Total assets	172,924	134,930	115,137	99,856
Liabilities:				
Accounts payable and accrued liabilities	25,480	23,132	20,018	15,136
Notes payable	27	434	494	602
Due to undesignated funds	—	—	9,258	12,032
Total liabilities	25,507	23,566	29,770	27,770
Net Assets	$147,417	$111,364	$ 85,367	$ 72,086
Net assets—as follows:				
Replacement and improvements of building and equipment	$ 20,511	$ 11,240	$ 6,577	$ —
Other specific purposes	16,405	—	—	—
Net assets required for operations	110,501	100,124	78,790	—
Net assets—as above	$147,417	$111,364	$ 85,367	—
Notes: Compared to:				
*Total ARC Public Support and Revenue	$722,159	$637,059	$556,911	$484,300
**Total Net Assets of ARC	628,658	559,949	231,298	214,647

SOURCE: American Red Cross Annual Report, 1980-83.

Table 16.—Blood Center Costs and Hospital Charges for Red Cells, 1980

Average community blood center cost per unit whole blood collected....	$45.91 (15.34)[a]
Average total hospital charge for unit of red cells	88.97
Charges may include:[b]	
Processing fee (average)	37.94
Replacement fee (average)	27.54
Laboratory fee (average)	40.51
Infusion fee (average)............	20.41
Other (e.g., blood delivery, general administration)..........	17.32

[a]Figure in parenthesis is standard deviation.
[b]Charges do not add to total average hospital charge because not all hospitals charge all types of fees. Of the 2,441 respondents to the survey conducted by Wallace and Wallace/ABC, 2,250 charged a laboratory fee, 1,756 charged a processing fee, 1,656 charged an infusion fee, 351 charged a replacement fee, and 60 charged a fee related to some other service.

SOURCE: Wallace and Wallace/ABC, 1982.

Mississippi Blue Cross/Blue Shield has a three-unit deductible for all costs associated with blood transfusions, including processing charges and administration charges.

Some blood centers offer coverage incentives to donors in addition to replacement credits. The Gulf Coast Regional Blood Center in Houston has two blood assurance plans. "Life Plan I," for families and individuals covers the donor (and certain selected others) for all Gulf Coast Regional Blood Center service fees for blood and blood components transfused in the gulf coast region served by the blood center. Hospital charges for typing and crossmatching etc. are not covered, and, as in most insurance plans, preexisting conditions are not covered. "Life Plan II" is a group plan which fully covers participating donors and their immediate families and also provides partial coverage (equal to one replacement donation) for nondonors in the group, if there is 25 percent participation. Gulf Coast also charges and covers replacement fees.

Mississippi Blood Services (MBS) has probably the most generous coverage plan for donors. Its "donor protection program" covers any out-of-pocket blood charges (including any hospital replacement fees) up to $10,000 for any MBS donor, without geographic restrictions. MBS itself does not charge a replacement deposit fee. In 1983, MBS paid out-of-pocket blood charges amounting to $51,163 for 393 patients. The largest single payment for one patient was $3,759. MBS acknowledges that such a system would not be feasible for blood centers on a large-scale basis because insurance companies might increase their deductibles if such a plan were adopted nationwide, or even in entire regions.

Table 17.—Changes in Processing Fees for Red Cells Compared to Changes in Total U.S. Health Care Expenditures

Processing fees charged by community blood centers	ARC	CCBC[3]	Percent change from previous year ARC	CCBC	Percent change in national health expenditures[4]
1976-77	22.19[1]	n/a	—	—	11.9
1979	n/a	32.30	—	—	13.5
1980	30.23[2]	34.14	8.04	5.7	15.8
1981	38.30[2]	36.98	26.7	7.7	15.1
1982	38.80[2]	39.72	1.3	7.4	12.5
1983	41.47[2]	40.41	6.9	1.7	n/a

Hospital charges[5]	Total	Processing Fee	Replacement	Laboratory	Infusion	Other
1979.........................	79.06	32.07	28.31	33.94	19.94	13.60
1980.........................	88.97	37.94	27.54	40.51	20.41	17.32
Percent change 1979-80........	13%	18%	−3%	19%	2%	27%

n/a = not available.
SOURCES: [1]Wallace and Wallace/ABC, 1982.
[2]American Red Cross Operations Reports; data as of June 30.
[3]Huitt, personal communication, 1984; data for 1983 is as of July.
[4]Gibson, R. M., Waldo, D. R. and Levit, K. R., *National Health Expenditures, 1982*.
[5]Wallace and Wallace/ABC, 1982.

PART 2: THE COMMERCIAL PLASMA AND PLASMA DERIVATIVES SECTOR

Overview

Demand for large amounts of plasma, principally for production of albumin, antihemophilic factor (AHF, or Factor VIII), and immune serum globulins, has led to what is known as the "source plasma" industry, in which donors provide plasma, not whole blood.

The source plasma sector is largely commercial and has three main components: collectors, or plasmapheresis centers; fractionators; and brokers, all of whom operate on a for-profit basis. Not-for-profit blood banks and blood centers also play a part in the commercial plasma industry when they sell recovered or salvaged plasma (i.e., plasma recovered after components have been removed from whole blood, or after whole blood has outdated) to fractionators, or when they contract with commercial firms to fractionate plasma into derivatives which they then market themselves.

Forty-five percent of the Red Cross' recovered plasma is fractionated by commercial fractionation companies (486). It is estimated that from 17 to 20 percent of the plasma derivatives sold in the United States is sold by the voluntary sector (i.e., by the Red Cross and the New York Blood Center). These sales put the not-for-profit industry in direct competition with the commercial plasmapheresis industry.

As shown in table 18, at present there are approximately 336 source plasma centers licensed by the FDA: 317 U.S. centers are commercially operated, and 19 are community or Red Cross blood centers—i.e., they are not operated for profit. The largest portion (90 percent) of source plasma centers is owned by independently operated multi-location companies. These multi-location centers are owned by 30 companies marketing biological products. Some of these biologicals companies are subsidiaries of larger corporations (e.g., Sera-Tec Biologicals, owned by the Rite-Aid Corp. in New York, operates nine centers in the East and Midwest, most of which are near college campuses). The plasma collected by commercial plasmapheresis centers is either sold to U.S. fractionators who separate it into a number of products, primarily albumin, Factor VIII (antihemophilic factor) and immune globulins, or exported to fractionators in Europe, Japan, or South America.

The way plasma is provided from plasmapheresis centers to fractionators varies. Four fractionation companies "self-source"; i.e., they run their own source plasma centers. According to the latest figures, 98 (30 percent) of the U.S. source plasma centers are owned by fractionation companies. Most centers contract annually with fractionators to provide a certain amount of plasma, although there is some "spot buying." Recovered plasma (from whole blood) is not contracted for, but is marketed through the efforts of nine major brokers. Both the brokers and the for-profit source plasma centers are members of the American Blood Resources Association (ABRA), a nonprofit trade association organized in 1972 to represent the interests of businesses engaged in the collection, manufacturing or distribution of certain biological products—in particular, plasma for further manufacturing (437).

Table 18.—Number of Plasma Centers Located in the United States
(by owner, fractionator, multi-operator, single operator, and nonprofit)

	Nov. 1979	July 1980	Mar. 1981	Apr. 1984	Percent change
Fractionator owned	121	123	107	92	− 24%
Multi-operator	171	167	213	177	+ 4%
Single operator	98	104	50	48	− 51%
Non-profit	9	9	11	19	+110%
Total	399	403	381	336	− 16%

SOURCE: *Plasma Quarterly*, summer 1984.

The market for source plasma is largely controlled by four pharmaceutical companies (Hyland Therapeutics, Cutter Laboratories, Alpha Therapeutics, and Armour), which are in turn subsidiaries of major corporations (Travenol, Bayer, Green Cross of Japan, and Revlon, respectively). Each commercial fractionator accounts for about 1 million of the 4 million liters of plasma fractionated in the United States annually (459). In addition, the nonprofit New York Blood Center operates its own 300,000-liter-capacity plant for fractionating plasma recovered from its own donors and from a portion of Red Cross donors. (The States of Michigan and Massachusetts each have small [approximately 50,000 liters each] fractionation capacities, with derivatives distributed primarily in each State.)

The U.S. source plasma collection industry is the most important contributor to worldwide plasma fractionation. The approximate disposition of both source and recovered plasma collected in the United States at the present time is shown in figure 3 in chapter 1. About 1.3 million of the 6 million liters of source plasma are exported, in addition to the exportation of plasma derivatives manufactured in the United States. About 5.5 million of the 12.5-million-liter worldwide manufacturing **capacity** in 1978 was in the United States. Of the 7-million-liter capacity outside the United States, about 5 million liters were in the commercial sector, and about 2 million liters were in the voluntary sector. But there were only about 77 plasma fractionation firms worldwide (439), and commercial plants outside the United States operate at about 68 percent capacity, compared to about 85 to 90 percent of capacity in the United States (459). As shown in figure 7, domestic production of AHF and albumin have increased steadily. In 1971, 110 million activity units of Factor VIII were sold; in 1982 the figure was 528 million. Comparable increases have occurred for albumin. Albumin accounts for the largest share of total sales (see table 1 in ch. 1). It is estimated that in 1984, approximately one-third of the albumin and one-half of the Factor VIII produced will be used in foreign countries (see table 19).

Figure 7.—U.S. Production of Factor VIII (in activity units) and of Albumin/PPF (in 12.5 Gram Equivalents), 1971-82

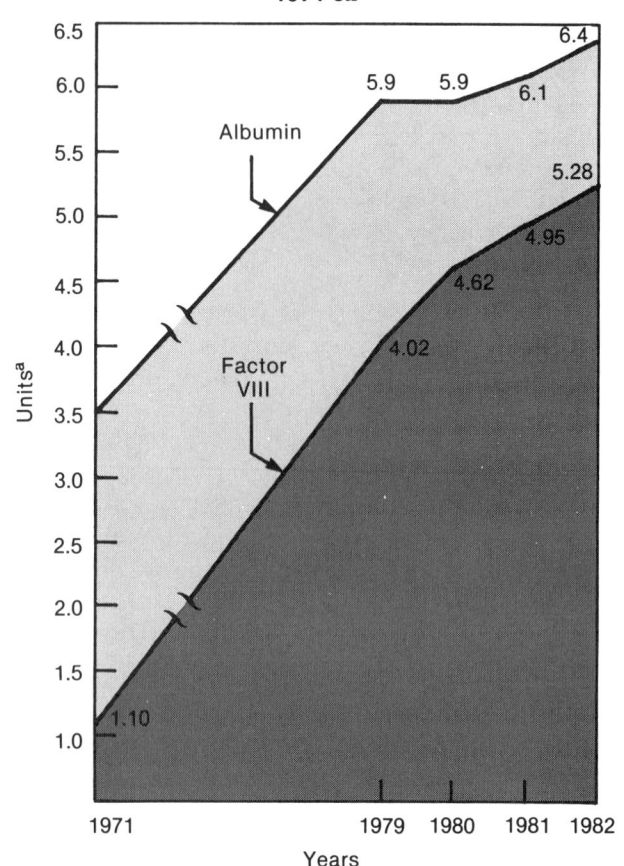

[a]Albumin/PPF in millions of 12.5 gram equivalents; Factor VIII in hundreds of millions of activity units.

SOURCE: Rodell, personal communication, 1983.

Thus, much of the plasma and plasma derivatives used worldwide comes from U.S. sources.

The principal products of the source plasma industry that are used in this country are albumin, AHF, and plasma protein fraction (PPF), which is used much as is albumin. Other products include intravenous gamma globulin (IVGG), immune serum globulin and hyperimmune globulins. Worldwide use differs from use in the United States. For example, in 1978, at a time when IVGG was not licensed in the United States, it accounted for 23 percent of worldwide demand for

Table 19.—Production and Consumption of Human Serum Albumin and Antihemophilic Factor

	1971	1976	1979	Forecast 1984
Plasma processed in the United States (thousands of liters)	1,950	2,910	3,950	6,920
HSA production in the United States (millions of grams)	39	67	91	159
HSA consumption:				
Domestic (millions of units)	2.9	4.6	5.8	8.5
Foreign (millions of units)	0.3	0.7	1.5	4.2
Total (millions of units)	3.2	5.3	7.3	12.7
Domestic	94%	87%	80%	67%
Foreign	6%	13%	20%	33%
HSA revenues:				
Domestic (millions of dollars)	$58	$133.4	$168.2	$300
Foreign (millions of dollars)	4	20.3	43.5	148
Total (millions of dollars)	62	153.7	211.7	448
Plasma processed globally for AHF (thousands of liters)	365	1,600	2,750	5,320
AHF units processed (millions)	80	400	688	1,330
Domestic consumption:				
Millions of units	72	300	412	648
Average price (cents/units)	15	10	10	14
Sales (millions of dollars)	10.8	30	41.2	91
Foreign consumption:				
Millions of units	8	100	275	682
Average price (cents/units)	40	30	30	27
Sales (millions of dollars)	3.2	30	82.5	184
Total AHF sales (millions of dollars)	14	60	123.9	275

SOURCE: Office of Technology Assessment, based on data and estimates in M. M. Le Coney, "Who Needs Plasma?" *Plasma Quarterly* 2:68-93, September 1980.

plasma fractions (see table 1). Table 20 summarizes differences in albumin/PPF consumption between selected countries in 1976.

Sources of Raw Plasma

In the 1960s, the introduction of plastic bags for collection of whole blood enabled component separation to increase, and blood centers began to address the need to more effectively utilize plasma from whole blood. Today, plasma in excess of a region's needs is supplied by blood centers to plasma derivative manufacturers for further processing. Plasma is supplied as fresh-frozen plasma or liquid recovered plasma to licensed processors (253).

Table 20.—Albumin and Plasma Protein Fraction Consumption in Selected Countries, 1976

Country	Consumption in kilograms/ 1 million population
West Germany	499 kg
United States	301
Austria	259
Finland	213
France	59
Japan	50
Brazil	14

SOURCE: Adapted from T. Drees, *Plasma Forum*, 1979.

The American Red Cross, which has been involved in providing plasma for fractionation since the pioneering work of E. J. Cohn, does not operate any facilities for production of plasma derivatives. One regional blood center, the New York Blood Center (NYBC), has its own plasma fractionation facility. The Red Cross maintains a number of contracts with domestic and foreign plasma fractionation facilities to process Red Cross plasma in accordance with Red Cross specifications, and the products are returned to Red Cross regional blood centers for distribution to hospitals and other users (319). Through its system of regional blood centers, the Red Cross collects more plasma for fractionation than any other single entity in the world. As described earlier, however, the vast majority of the plasma required to meet the needs of the United States and other parts of the world is provided by commercial plasmapheresis centers. While some of the major manufacturers operate their own plasma collection centers, many are operated by independent multi-location companies.

Plasmapheresis has several advantages over recovery of plasma from a single unit of whole blood. First, the volume of plasma recovered per donation is greater with plasmapheresis. Up to 600 ml of plasma can be taken per donation, versus an average recovery of 200 to 250 ml per donation of whole blood. Second, under current FDA guidelines, a donor can be plasmapheresed twice each 7 days, while a whole-blood donor can contribute only once every 8 weeks and a maximum of five times per year. Third, because plasmapheresis collections are specifically for fractionation into derivatives, the plasma is frozen immediately upon collection, thereby preserving more of the labile protein fractions whose functional loss is proportional to delays in freezing.

Finished plasma derivatives for the U.S. market are produced and supplied by several companies. Most manufacturing facilities that produce human plasma derivatives are located in the United States, but some are located in Europe and Canada. The principal producers of human plasma derivatives for the U.S. market are identified in table 21. None of these licensed manufacturers produce all of the plasma derivatives approved for distribution in the United States. In addition to those listed, numerous other manufacturers produce plasma derivatives for use in other parts of the world (319).

The cost of plasma is generally determined by the number of products that can be made from the plasma and the anticipated protein yield. Frozen source plasma, collected by plasmapheresis, and fresh-frozen plasma obtained from whole blood but frozen shortly after processing, have traditionally provided the highest product and protein yield. Although all plasma processing is based on the basic Cohn process (described in ch. 4), modifications and improvements in methods or equipment enable some fractionators to process plasma more cost effectively than do their competitors.

The time from collection to processing into licensed, finished products takes as much as 4 to 6 months, depending on the products produced and the manufacturer. Temporary shortages and surpluses can occur, with parallel increases and decreases in price. In addition, such factors as price variances between nations, due to prices governments and insurance plans pay for a particular plasma derivative, affect where products are distributed. Many manufacturers have distribution networks in numerous countries and direct their products to the markets where demand is great and prices are higher.

Barriers to entry into the plasma fractionation business are substantial, due to the need to develop cost-effective production techniques, construction of a capital-intensive facility, and stringent licensing requirements for biological products. For these reasons and the volatile and competitive nature of the plasma derivatives market, no new production facilities have been constructed in the past 12 years by firms not already in the business. In the recent past, except for continued marketing of some immune globulins, several firms have left the plasma derivatives market, including large pharmaceutical firms such as Parke-Davis, Squibb, Upjohn, and Merck Sharp & Dohme.

Table 21.—Principal Producers of Human Plasma Derivatives for the U.S. Market

Company	Manufacturing location	Ownership
Alpha Therapeutics	California	Green Cross/Japan
Armour	Illinois	Revlon/USA
Connaught	Canada	Connaught/Canada
Cutter	North Carolina	Bayer/Germany
Hyland	California	Baxter Travenol/USA
Immuno	Michigan/Austria	Immuno/Austria
Massachusetts State Laboratory	Massachusetts	State of Massachusetts
Michigan State Laboratory	Michigan	State of Michigan
New York Blood Center	New York	New York Blood Center
Swiss Red Cross	Switzerland	Swiss Red Cross
Netherlands Red Cross	Netherlands	Netherlands Red Cross

SOURCE: Grossman & Schmitt, 1984

Finished Products Licensed for Use in the United States

Normal Serum Albumin and Plasma Protein Fraction

Normal serum albumin (NSA) and its close relative, plasma protein fraction (PPF), are produced from Cohn Fraction V, with PPF also containing proteins from Cohn Fraction IV-4. Under FDA standards, greater than 96 percent of the protein in NSA must be albumin, while for PPF the requirement is that only greater than 85 percent of the protein in the solution must be albumin. The production of PPF instead of NSA is economically advantageous to plasma fractionators due to the allowed differential in albumin concentration in the final product.

Normal serum albumin is available in 5 and 25 percent concentrations in various vial sizes. PPF is available in 5 percent concentrations in various vial sizes. NSA and PPF are generally regarded as generic products by users, and distributors and hospitals often obtain these products from several sources (319).

Many of the major manufacturers of NSA and PPF often contract to deliver their products to users on a direct basis. The need for these products and the size of the market requires that numerous outlets be made available. Users include hospitals, nursing homes, dialysis centers and pheresis centers, as well as the local physician who requires an occasional vial to treat a patient in his office.

NSA and PPF account for approximately one-half of the total dollar volumes of plasma derivatives distributed in the United States. In the last 5 years, there has been a steady decrease in the use of PPF, with increasing use of 5 percent NSA displacing PPF (486).

One liter of plasma processed into NSA will yield approximately 25 grams of protein. Based on market prices in mid-1984, the value of the product would be between $2.50 and $2.80 per gram, or between $62.50 and $70.00 per liter of plasma. The manufacturers that operate FDA-licensed facilities for the processing of plasma into NSA and PPF for the U.S. market are listed in table 22.

Table 22.—Manufacturers of Normal Serum Albumin (NSA) and Plasma Protein Fraction (PPF) Licensed for Use in the United States

Alpha Therapeutics
Armour Pharmaceutical
Connaught Laboratories
Cutter Biological
Hyland Laboratories
Immuno
Massachusetts State Laboratory
Michigan State Laboratory
New York Blood Center
Netherlands Red Cross
Swiss Red Cross

SOURCE: Grossman & Schmitt, 1984.

Although there are numerous distribution outlets, the vast majority of these products are supplied by the manufacturers and the Red Cross directly to hospitals. Distributors are used to service the specialized needs and regional requirements of other users.

Every institution that uses NSA and PPF independently determines the purchasing method that provides it the most benefits. The various purchasing alternatives currently available are: 1) arranging an independent purchase contract with a manufacturer, 2) participating in group purchasing contracts, 3) purchasing from local American Red Cross centers, and 4) purchasing from a community blood center or distributor. Institutions that have special requirements, in addition to negotiating prices, make these needs known to their suppliers. Some of these special requirements often preclude delivery of products in large shipments to one central warehouse facility. When this occurs, the cost of servicing an account is greatly increased, and manufacturers may lose the contract to smaller distributors or regional blood centers.

One of the most common ways of pricing NSA and PPF is by annual bidding from the various manufacturers and suppliers. Some hospitals negotiate annual prices with a local blood center or distributor that can provide supplies in quantities that meet the hospital's special needs.

Many not-for-profit hospitals have joined together to form joint purchasing groups. The concept of a joint purchasing program is that a supplier will bid a lower price if it can more easily obtain a substantial and reliable quantity of business. Member hospitals provide the joint purchasing programs with projected use figures. The information is consolidated, and bids are solicited from approved manufacturers and suppliers.

Most purchasing groups operate as clearinghouses for information between their respective members and potential vendors, and never actually take delivery of the products. Orders are placed by each member institution directly with the supplier. Delivery and supply arrangements are coordinated between the hospital and the supplier. The purchasing group receives a rebate directly from the supplier, based on the actual volume of business, and manufacturers supply monthly reports to the purchasing groups.

Some purchasing groups or shared service corporations actually take ownership of the products. These purchasing groups provide warehousing and delivery services for its members as required. Shared service warehouses offer the hospitals numerous advantages, such as ordering all supplies, not only PPF and NSA, from one source. The manufacturer benefits by reducing costs for shipping and billing, since an order will only have to be sent to one location and billed to one account.

One of the problems arising from purchasing group programs is that manufacturers or distributors who are awarded supply contracts are required to rebate a specified percentage of the revenue to the purchasing group to offset its costs. Since these costs are paid by the supplier, they must be factored into the bid price and are ultimately paid by the hospital. The issue is often debated as to whether or not direct purchases could be made for less, especially by the larger hospital members.

The large chains of proprietary hospitals also solicit annual bids from the major producers. In many cases each hospital is given the opportunity to negotiate a more favorable supply arrangement with a local supplier. If a more favorable pricing arrangement cannot be made, the hospital can purchase from the vendor who has been awarded the national supply agreement for the chain. Dialysis centers and nursing homes requiring NSA and PPF usually negotiate with local sources at spot market prices because their requirements are often very sporadic.

In all cases, however, supply is a major factor. Reliability is often more important than saving a few cents per vial. When an organization can avoid having to carry a large dollar item in inventory, such as NSA and PPF, it often offsets these costs by purchasing from local sources rather than purchasing in large quantities from one of the manufacturers.

Supply and availability of all plasma derivatives are dependent on both the availability of the raw material (human plasma) and the prices obtainable for manufactured products. Prices as well as supplies have traditionally had very large "peaks and valleys." To offset price volatility, suppliers and manufacturers often resort to product transfer from one country to another.

Competition for business among the manufacturers and suppliers of NSA and PPF is very fierce. Traditional emphasis has been for pricing to act as the main element for differentiation. Purchasing groups which control a substantial volume of the NSA and PPF market tend to treat these products as commodities. The market is sensitive to price changes and thus maintains a high level of price-competitiveness. Margins earned by manufacturers on the sale of NSA and PPF are substantially below those characteristically earned on the sale of pharmaceutical products.

The second major determinant of consumer preference in the purchase of NSA and PPF is confidence in the suppliers's ability to fulfill its purchase obligation. Long production lead time, as well as sudden pricing shifts, make it difficult for suppliers to plan for and rapidly provide additional material. Some hospitals have encountered supply problems with a particular vendor and are often reluctant to purchase from that firm again, even if the price offered is lower than that of a competitor.

Other less significant determinants of purchaser preference are items such as packaging, which does affect sales to some accounts. Package size, type of intravenous hanger, cap or stopper, as well as the administration set used, have become competitive opportunities.

Differentiations between NSA and PPF products have become more related to the source of service, packaging, and availability than to the product itself.

Coagulation Factors

Approximately one-quarter of the total dollar volume of plasma derivatives distributed in the United States are represented by coagulation factors, which are used for treatment of individuals with congenital deficiencies of Factor VIII or Factor IX. Antihemophilic factor, or concentrates of Factor VIII, is distributed and prescribed by the number of "activity units" desired. An "activity unit" is defined as that amount of Factor VIII present in 1 ml of normal plasma. The protein is very unstable and is therefore prepared as a lyophilized powder, which is reconstituted with sterile water prior to injection. AHF is available in reconstituted volumes of 10 to 40 ml, with associated activity unit ranges from 250 or 400 to 1,250 or 1,500. Manufacturers licensed by the FDA for Factor VIII and Factor IX sales in the United States are listed in table 23.

All major plasma fractionators in the United States produce AHF (see table 23). Unlike other plasma derivatives, coagulation factors are produced only from plasma frozen within 24 hours of collection. The activity of these factors decreases rapidly unless the plasma is frozen and stored at $-18°$ C or colder until used by a plasma fractionator. Economics dictate that plasma be frozen as quickly as possible after collection in order to maximize product yields.

One of the major disadvantages of use of AHF has been the inability to treat the product in a manner that would reduce or eliminate the potential for disease transmission. Recently all four commercial manufacturers received approval from FDA to begin marketing of heat-treated AHF. Although some manufacturers have data which indicate the process may reduce the transmission of viral diseases, there is no AHF product which has yet been proven to be entirely free of risk.

One liter of frozen plasma processed for AHF will yield approximately 200 AHF activity units. Based on market prices in mid-1984, the value of this product would be between $0.07 and $0.10 per activity unit, or between $14.00 and $20.00 per liter for non-heat-treated product. The heat-treated product sold during the same period for $0.11 to $0.16 per activity unit, or approximately $22.00 to $32.00 for the yield from 1 liter of frozen plasma. (It has been reported that the yield of heat-treated Factor VIII is slightly less than the yield of non-heat-treated Factor VIII from 1 liter of frozen plasma.)

The second major coagulation factor is Factor IX Complex, which is a product consisting of coagulation factors II, VII, IX, and X. Factor IX Complex is used in treatment of hemophilia B, as well as in treatment of some patients with inhibitors to Factor VIII. As with AHF, Factor IX Complex is measured in activity units and is prepared as a lyophilized powder which is reconstituted prior to injection.

Most of the U.S. market for Factor IX Complex is shared by two plasma fractionators, Cutter and Hyland. The total U.S. consumption of Factor IX Complex is estimated at approximately 130 million activity units per year. Based on a yield of approximately 400 activity units per liter, it takes 325,000 liters of plasma to meet this need. Based on market prices in early 1984, the value of Factor IX Complex was between $7.8 million and $13 million.

The other coagulation factor product is "activated" Factor IX, or anti-inhibitor coagulant complex, for treatment of patients with inhibitors to Factor VIII. This part of the market is serviced by two companies, Hyland and Immuno.

In addition to the manufacturers listed above, who distribute the products manufactured in their own processing facilities, the American Red Cross

Table 23.—Manufacturers of Coagulation Factors Licensed for Use in the United States

Manufacturer	Factor VIII	Factor IX Complex	Anti-Inhibitor Complex
Alpha	X	X	
Armour	X	X	
Cutter	X	X	
Hyland	X	X	X
Immuno			X
New York Blood Center	X		

SOURCE: Grossman & Schmitt, 1984.

has plasma fractionated into the various clotting factors by selected manufacturers. These plasma derivatives are returned to the Red Cross regional blood centers for distribution to hospitals and hemophilia treatment centers. Numerous suppliers and regional blood centers also purchase products for distribution to their local hospitals and hemophilia treatment centers.

Distribution channels for the coagulation proteins vary from region to region. Availability is often dependent on whether there is a hospital or hemophilia treatment center in a particular region. Most large urban areas have at least one major hemophilia treatment center that routinely stocks the various clotting factors.

Depending on the size of the region, patient requirements, and product preferences, numerous purchasing channels can be encountered. The hospital may solicit bids for the various factors required through its Purchasing Office in conjunction with the Pharmacy or Blood Bank, but there does not appear to be a standard as to which department should take responsibility for purchasing, inventory control, or distribution of coagulation factors within a hospital.

Depending on the institution, it could be assigned to the Blood Bank, Pharmacy, Purchasing Office, or Hemophilia Treatment Center. It is not uncommon for one company to receive the entire award for a 1-year period for a particular product at a hospital or hemophilia treatment center. When numerous patients are treated at a hospital, the treating institution may require products manufactured by several manufacturers. To assist hospitals and reduce their inventory requirements, many institutions utilize the services of a local distributor or regional blood center, which maintains adequate supplies of each of the needed clotting factors.

In recent years, home care treatment of hemophiliacs has increased. At least one manufacturer, numerous distributors and pharmacies, and several regional blood centers have begun to supply these products directly to the patient at home. Orders are filled in response to instructions from the treating physician, and home care treatment has lifted the burden from the patient of having to visit the hospital each time a treatment is required. The regional blood centers, manufacturers, distributors, and pharmacies that distribute clotting factors to home care patients often provide the supplies needed to administer the clotting factors—which saves time, money, and effort in having to secure them from another source.

Some manufacturers will only supply end-users, such as hospitals or blood centers, or directly to patients. Other suppliers provide products to end-users, distributors, and other suppliers. Suppliers of coagulation factors vary from region to region, as does the availability of these products. Purchase and selection of a specific brand is often left to the patient, unless the physician specifies a particular brand.

Packaging, supplies, and availability, as well as price contribute to the numerous differences in the supply and use of the various clotting factors. Brand awareness of the product on the part of physicians, nurses, and patients often plays an important role in sales of various coagulation factors.

Brand loyalty is encouraged by manufacturers by supplying information at educational seminars and through direct communication with the physician and hemophilia nurse-clinician. Information is also provided directly to the patient by company representatives at many of the various national and local hemophilia meetings. Manufacturers provide a wide array of product sizes, and product preferences and loyalty are often based on the successful response a patient has had with the product in past treatment episodes, not on what manufacturers tell patients.

Immune Globulins

Immune serum globulins (ISG) account for approximately 10 percent of the total dollar volume of plasma derivatives distributed in the United States. A typical preparation of ISG will contain multiple antibodies to a wide variety of infectious agents.

ISG is available in either "normal" or "hyperimmune" preparations. The "normal" product is produced from the plasma of donors who have not been stimulated to produce elevated levels of specific antibodies. "Hyperimmune" ISG products are obtained from donors with elevated levels of a specific antibody. This elevation may occur naturally, as with antibodies to the Rh blood type (Rho(D)) or hepatitis B, as a result of the donor's prior medical experience, or may be obtained by injection of materials designed to produce an immune response in the form of antibody formation (319).

Specific types of ISG which are presently available in the United States include normal immune serum globulin, and hyperimmune globulins against hepatitis B, measles, mumps, pertussis, tetanus, rabies, varicella zoster, and RHo(D). All of these ISG products are available for intramuscular, not intravenous, injections. ISG is prepared as a 16.5 percent protein solution and distributed in vials ranging from 2 to 10 ml each.

In the United States, varicella zoster immune globulin (VZIG) is manufactured only by the Massachusetts Biologics Laboratory and is distributed primarily by the American Red Cross and other regional blood centers. Since this limited market drug was licensed, no other manufacturer has begun to produce it for distribution within the United States.

Intravenous gamma globulin is indicated for maintenance treatment of patients who are unable to produce sufficient amounts of IgG antibodies. Use of this product may be preferred to that of the intramuscular immunoglobulin preparations, especially in patients who require an immediate increase in intravascular immunoglobulin levels, in patients with small muscle mass, and in patients with bleeding tendencies in whom intramuscular injections are contraindicated.

Intravenous gamma globulin (IVGG) is currently produced only by Cutter, and is available directly from Cutter, regional blood centers, or distributors for purchase by prescribing hospitals and physicians. Immuno and Sandoz have applied for licensing of their IVGG products. The products under review by FDA are prepared in a lyophilized form, whereas Cutter's IVGG is prepared in solution. Manufacturers of some of these products are listed in table 24.

Manufacturers of the various immune globulins distribute their products through many channels.

Table 24.—Manufacturers of Selected Immune Globulins for Use in the United States

Manufacturer	ISG	IVGG	RHoD	HBIG	VZIG
Abbott			X	X	
Armour	X		X		
Connaught/BCA			X		
Cutter	X	X	X	X	
Hyland	X				
Immuno		X[a]			
KABI				X	
Massachusetts Biologics Laboratory					X
Merck Sharp & Dohme				X	
New York Blood Center	X				
Ortho			X		
Sandoz		X[a]			

[a]Application for licensing pending before FDA as of May 1984.
KEY: ISG: immune serum globulin; IVGG: intravenous gamma globulin; RHoD: anti-RH antigen immune globulin; HBIG: hepatitis B immune globulin; VZIG: varicella zoster immune globulin.
SOURCE: Grossman & Schmitt, 1984.

While almost every hospital utilizes some or all of the immune globulins, there is usually no central distribution or supply network as is available for normal serum albumin or coagulation factors. Some manufacturers, such as Ortho, have a large share of a specific market such as for RHo(D), but they do not sell other plasma derivatives in the United States.

Immune globulin products are routinely delivered by pharmaceutical distributors, hospital supply companies and blood centers, as well as directly by manufacturers to the numerous hospitals, nursing homes, physicians, and clinics that prescribe these preparations.

Many manufacturers have their own sales representatives, who contact individual physicians to encourage the ordering of brand-specific products. Within the hospital, these products may be ordered by the Pharmacy, Purchasing Office, Blood Bank, or by a special user department. The department requesting the product often specifies which supplier or manufacturer should be used, based on services and product results in the past.

Annual bidding for each immune globulin product is not as prevalent as for other human plasma derivatives, but is gaining. Usually, an award is made for one company's product, and supply has not been a factor since all manufacturers usually have adequate inventories.

Many other manufacturers of immune globulins offer various products and numerous customer advantages, including low prices, well-located distribution outlets, and ease of ordering. The two most important advantages are availability at the time the product is needed and pricing.

Reagent Products

Plasma not suitable for further manufacture into injectables is available for use by reagent manufacturers. Plasma for this market is available from a variety of sources, including regional blood centers, hospital blood banks, plasmapheresis collection centers, and plasma fractionators.

The number of manufacturers within the United States requiring plasma for reagents is quite large, and each one has strict requirements for the plasma that it obtains. Usually, human plasma destined for reagent use is sold to plasma dealers who routinely supply laboratory reagent manufacturers and are familiar with the necessary specifications. Many of these dealers also provide a wide array of animal proteins to the same laboratory reagent manufacturers.

Each manufacturer of reagent products provides its sources of human plasma with the requirements that must be followed in the preparation of the material. These strict manufacturing specifications often limit the sources of plasma to a highly select group of hospitals, plasma collection centers, and bulk product manufacturers. Plasma suppliers that specialize in meeting the reagent manufacturer's specifications usually maintain a long-term relationship with these manufacturers. Some collection centers specialize in preparation and segregation of plasma from donors with special or rare characteristics for use by selected reagent manufactures.

Other Plasma Derivatives

At the present time, many proteins found in human plasma are being evaluated and studied for their therapeutic value. Proteins such as Alpha I Antitrypsin, Antithrombin III, Factor XIII, Fibronectin, Tissue Plasminogen Activator, von Willebrand Factor, and Interleukin-2, as well as new immune globulin preparations, are being evaluated by numerous commercial and nonprofit research facilities. The American Red Cross and the Michigan Department of Public Health are jointly evaluating as a new plasma derivative a Factor IX Concentrate depleted of Factors II, VII, and X; and a concentrate of C1 Inactivator (373).

Several new plasma derivatives have been licensed for use in other countries and will, after passing the necessary testing, be licensed in the United States. Some of these products are: 1) Antithrombin III, currently marketed in Europe by Behring (Germany) and Kabi (Sweden); 2) Factor XIII, currently available in Europe by Behring (Germany); and 3) Fibrin Tissue Sealant (Tissell), currently marketed in Europe by Immuno (Austria) and projected to be available in the United States in 1985.

Costs of Major Plasma Derivatives

As already discussed, the market structure for plasma derivatives differs substantially from that for whole blood. However, the voluntary collectors compete with the commercial sector when marketing plasma products. Prices charged by selected not-for-profit blood centers are shown in table 25. Current retail prices for Factor VIII in the not-for-profit centers range from $0.10 to $0.147 a unit for non-heat-treated Factor VIII and higher for heat-treated Factor VIII. Prices charged by hospitals to patients are reported to range from $0.09 to $0.26 per unit in the United States (99; 464). Assuming an average consumption of 50,000 units per year (293), Factor VIII could cost the average hemophiliac from $4,500 to $13,000 per year, although "average" consumption can be a misleading figure.

Hemophiliacs can require a large infusion of Factor VIII for surgery, including minor surgery. Needs also vary for mild, moderate, and severe hemophiliacs. In addition, from 10 (99) to 15 (76) percent of hemophiliacs have inhibitors to Factor VIII and require anti-inhibitor coagulant complex, which can cost from $0.70 to $1.00 per unit (99).

Federal activities in support of hemophiliacs were discussed in chapter 2. While provisions for hemophilic care have improved in the last decade, coverage for coagulation proteins on an out-

Ch. 3—The Blood Services Complex • 73

Table 25.—Representative Blood Center Prices for Plasma Derivatives

Major blood derivatives		Goldman (Okla.)	S.E. La.	Sacramento	Central (Pittsb.)	NYBC[a] List	Actual
Serum Albumin 5%	250 ml	34.10F			28.00	41.00	31.00
Serum Albumin 5%	500 ml	67.65F			55.65	82.00	62.00
Serum Albumin 25%	20 ml				20.00		
Serum Albumin 25%	50 ml	35.20F	31.00		28.00	41.00	31.00
Serum Albumin 25%	100 ml			75.00	55.65	82.00	62.00
Plasma Protein F.	250 ml			36.00	27.35	41.00	31.00
Plasma Protein F.	500 ml				54.35	82.00	62.00
Factor VIII		0.132iu C			0.10iu	0.11 N	0.11
						0.147A1	0.147
						0.11Ar	0.11
						0.104C	0.104
						0.108H	0.108
Factor VIII, (Heat-treated)		0.165iu H				0.187A1[b]	0.187
						0.145Ar	0.145
						0.142C	0.142
						0.129—	0.129—
						0.153H	0.153H
Factor VIII Anti-Inhibitor Complex 200-600 FECU		0.77iu FB				0.75FB	.75
Factor VIII Inhibitor Complex 200-600 FECU		1.22H				1.01H	1.01
Factor II, VII, IX, X complex 500 u vial		57.20C		62.50	0.12iu	0.066A1	0.066
						0.057Ar	0.057
						0.065C	0.065
						0.113H	0.113

Legend: Al = Alpha Therapeutics product; Ar = Armour product; C = Cutter product; F = Fenwal product; FB = FEIBA product; H = Hyland product; N = New York Blood Center product.
Where no letter is given, product name was not specified.
[a] Through June 30, 1984. Price includes New York Blood Center service fee for development and maintenance of data management and hemophilia research project, and hemophilia home care service.
[b] Prices may be unrealistic because NYBC does low volume in this product. Prices range from 0.11 iu (Cutter) to 0.165 (Alpha).
SOURCE: Grossman & Schmitt, 1984.

patient basis varies widely, and they are often not covered because they are regarded as drugs rather than biologics. When they are covered, copayment provisions can burden patients. Pharmaceutical companies that distribute Factor VIII sometimes ignore the copayment requirement for individual hemophilic patients.

The price of albumin has not been challenged per se, but some have encouraged the use of less expensive alternatives for volume restoration (see ch. 5, pt. 4). A 12.5 gram dose of albumin, prepared by a commercial fractionator and purchased from a blood center, cost approximately $32.00 in 1984. In 1982, the cost from commercial manufacturers was $27.40 (464).

CONCLUSION

U.S. blood resources consist of two distinct sectors, a voluntary whole blood system and a commercial source plasma industry (fig. 8). Human blood is the common denominator, but there are distinct differences between the two sectors in donor populations, recruitment policies, type of blood collected, markets (domestic v. international), indications for use, and Federal policy attention and directives. Even the acquisition and use of the products of these two sectors differ. Whole blood and its components are ordered and monitored through blood banks and transfusion

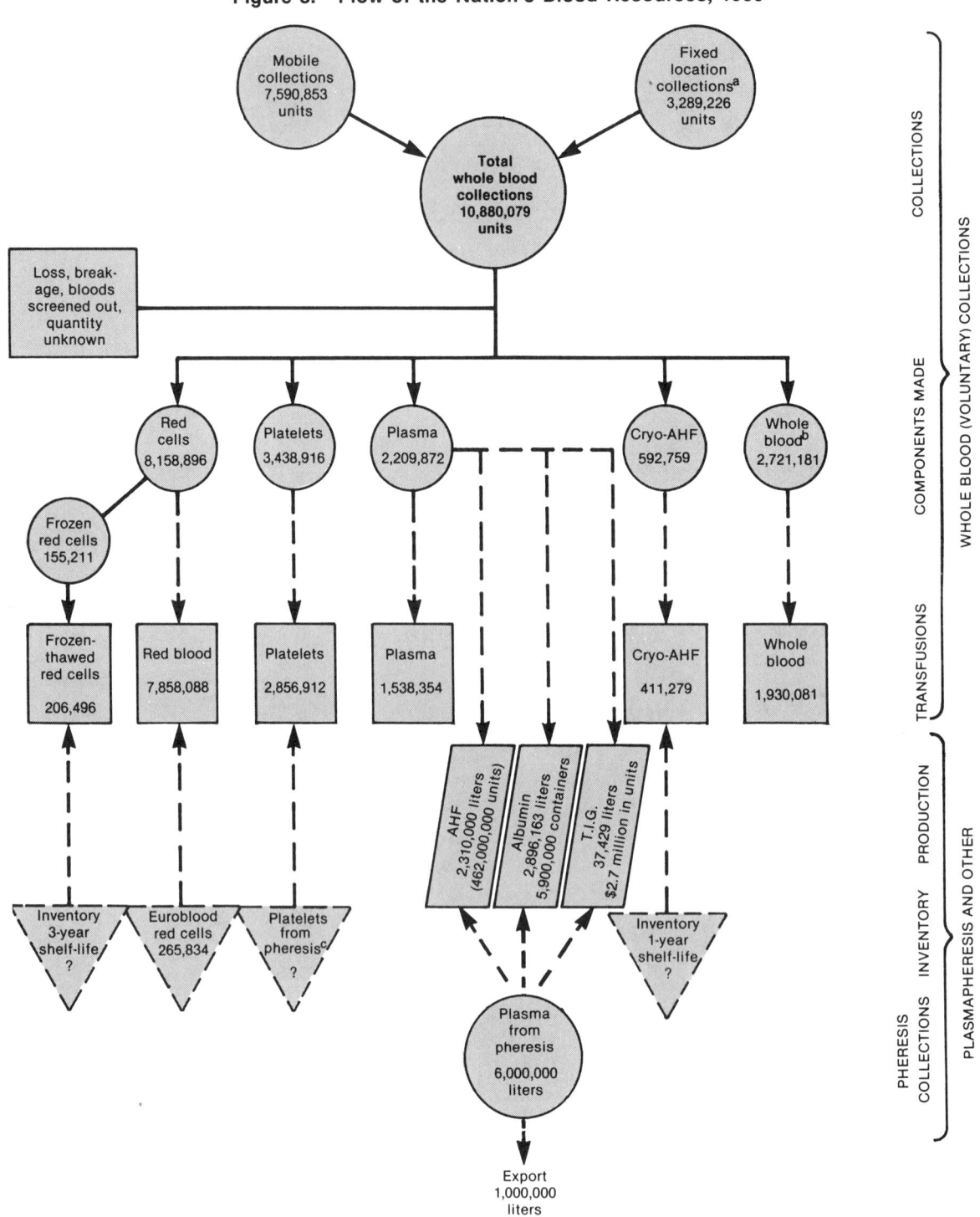

Figure 8.—Flow of the Nation's Blood Resources, 1980

[a] No question on the ABC National Blood Data Center Survey for this value. Number shown is the difference between total collections and mobile collections.
[b] No question on the survey for this value. An unknown quantity of whole blood, not made into components, was screened out (because of hepatitis B or other complications) or lost/broken during handling.
[c] Units of platelets were derived from plateletpheresis procedures. Platelets transfused include apheresis figures.

SOURCES: Figure adapted from Surgenor and Schnitzer/ABC (1983). *Whole blood figures:* Surgenor and Schnitzer/ABC (1983).
  Plasmapheresis figures: Reilly, personal communication, 1983; Rodell personal communication, 1983.

services, while plasma derivatives are usually ordered through the pharmacy and monitored through pharmaceutical committees.

Growing use of specific blood components has contributed to the continuation of this dual blood supply system, because different demands for each component or derivative make it unlikely that whole blood collections could meet and balance the demand for all blood products. In addition, the use of components has led to excess plasma in the voluntary sector, and this excess contributes to a significant extent to plasma used for fractionation and in providing additional revenues to voluntary blood banks.

An interesting contrast with the voluntary system in the United States are the voluntary systems in Switzerland, West Germany, Belgium, and the Netherlands. These countries collect more whole blood than they can use in an attempt to meet their needs for both blood and plasma products, but they still import plasma derivatives. This emphasis on whole blood collections results in excess red cells in these countries, and a small portion of these red cells are imported into the United States as "Euroblood." In 1980, there were 10,880,079 units of whole blood collected in the United States, with an additional 265,839 units of red cell "Euroblood" imported (518). The plasma derivatives market is even more international in scope, with even the Swiss and Dutch Red Cross selling some plasma derivatives in the U.S. market.

In the United States, the commercial sector's involvement in blood resources began with fractionation technologies arising from World War II needs, and there will continue to be markets for their products at home and abroad as long as human blood continues to be the principal source of these products, and as long as the United States and other countries are not able to meet their total needs for blood products (plasma derivatives as well as blood components) with blood supplied from their own citizens on a voluntary basis.

4.
Blood Technologies

Contents

	Page
Part 1: Technologies for Blood Collection and Processing	79
Introduction	79
Blood Collection	80
Blood Component Preparation	84
Testing and Labeling of Blood From Donors	85
Pre-Transfusion Testing Techniques	90
Conclusions	91
Part 2: Plasma Fractionation Technologies	91
Introduction	91
Plasma Collection	91
Fractionation Methods and Products	93
New and Emerging Technologies	95

LIST OF TABLES

Table No.	Page
26. Standard Blood Collection Container Systems	82
27. Plateletapheresis Technologies	83
28. Testing of Blood Donor Samples	86
29. Determination of ABO Blood Group	86
30. Comparison of Manual Technologies for Red Cell Serological Testing of Blood Donors	87
31. Automated ABO/Rh Test Technologies in the United States, 1983	88
32. Traditional Automated Technologies v. Automated Microplate Systems (AMS)	89
33. Current Technologies for HBsAG Testing	90

LIST OF FIGURES

Figure No.	Page
9. Uniform Labeling Format for Blood Products	81
10. Derivation of Blood Components	84
11. The Crossmatch	90

4.
Blood Technologies

PART 1: TECHNOLOGIES FOR BLOOD COLLECTION AND PROCESSING

Introduction

Modern blood bank technology began less than 100 years ago, when several technological obstacles were overcome. First, it was necessary to arrest the blood clotting mechanisms which normally convert liquid blood into a gel in a matter of minutes. Second, physicians needed tools by which blood could be collected from one individual and infused into another with minimum risk to donor and recipient. Third, there was a lack of understanding of the immune system and the potential for incompatibility between donor red blood cells and red blood cell antibodies produced by recipients.

The coagulation problem was solved by the addition of citrate into freshly collected blood (344); citrate compounds are still the basis for stored blood anticoagulants today. Preservatives such as glucose were soon added to extend the shelf life of stored red cells from several days to several weeks.

Devices used in collecting, storing, and administering blood have ranged from quill and tubing contraptions to syringes (used currently for newborn exchange transfusions), to reusable vacuum glass bottles, still the standard in parts of the world today. In the United States, glass bottles have been replaced by flexible plastic containers with attached satellite bags to hold separate blood components.

Landsteiner's description of ABO blood groups in the early 1900s and other researchers' elucidation of antigen/antibody relationships led to simple laboratory tests for compatibility between donors and recipients, but 15 percent of transfusion recipients remained at risk until the Rhesus or Rh blood types were discovered (331,342). From that time to the present, determination of the donor and recipient ABO and Rh blood types has been the most important procedure in preventing potentially fatal hemolytic transfusion reactions.

In 1945, a new test was described (Coombs) which made possible the recognition of previously undetectable antigens and led to the identification of more than 400 new red blood cell types over the subsequent 30 years (284). However, probably fewer than 30 of these types are of clinical concern in routine transfusion practice (220).

As the demand for blood increased, the larger blood banks began to consider adaptations of clinical chemistry analyzers which could perform multiple tests on a single blood sample to remove some of the tedium and manual labor from mass blood-typing. These systems have evolved into computerized testing devices which deliver samples, interpret results, and flag any spurious findings for further investigation.

In the beginning, donor blood collection and testing were conducted in the same setting as blood transfusion; each hospital would screen donors on the basis of specific patient needs, and donors were often a patient's family and friends. World War II resulted in the creation of donor centers across the United States to collect large amounts of plasma for use in treating combat casualties, and intensive research into improving the storage life and function of red blood cells. When the war ended, community blood centers began to appear under the auspices of American Red Cross chapters, community service clubs, and local medical societies. These centers acted as staging areas from which mobile operations could be sent for blood collections, after which the blood was returned to the center for processing and subsequent distribution to hospitals.

Blood collection and processing in a community blood center can function as an assembly-line operation because of the need for repeating the same battery of tests on a number of donor samples, ranging from 200 per day in medium-size centers to over 1,000 per day in large centers. On the other hand, transfusion services repeat the entire workflow upon receipt of physician orders which, except in cases of standing orders for elective surgeries, are unpredictable and often urgent. Therefore, batch or assembly-line processing is not as feasible, except for verification of donors' blood types and elective surgery workups.

Blood is inherently variable, with each collected unit representing a unique "lot." Because it is impossible to test each unit for effectiveness before transfusion, the use of scientifically proven protocols and regular checks on representative products are important.

The use of computers for donor resources and inventory management at the community blood center, and standard policies for surgical blood needs at the transfusion service have improved blood utilization, decreased outdating, reduced charges to the patient, and improved management of donor resources. Computer management of discrete functions has been accomplished at many U.S. blood centers, but often lack coordination among donor recruitment, collection, laboratory, inventory, and financial management departments. One comprehensive information system has been designed as a joint venture between two community blood centers (Blood Center of Southeastern Wisconsin and the South Florida Blood Service) and Arthur Andersen & Co. The goals of all such systems are to minimize manual documentation and subjective analysis, and provide useful statistics for operational management and planning.

A number of automated data management systems throughout the world utilize uniform bar coding technology for the identification of donor units and samples for production and inventory management. This uniformity, which has the advantage of standardized machine-readable as well as simplified eye-readable features, is the result of a special task force of the American Blood Commission, whose efforts were funded by the National Heart, Lung, and Blood Institute and endorsed by the International Society for Blood Transfusion.

Figure 9 shows an example of this labeling format. The labeling scheme has been endorsed by FDA (182) and appears on 60 to 70 percent of products distributed by U.S. blood banks. However, not all blood centers who label their products with bar codes have the equipment to make use of the machine-readable information, and few transfusion services have the capability. Nevertheless, eye-readable uniformity and simplicity are universally appreciated aspects of the commonality label, given a history of multiple color-coded label schemes and superfluous information on earlier blood product label formats. The uniform label has allowed developers of automated testing systems and management information systems to design equipment and software around a single machine-readable format for use in the United States and several countries in Europe and the Far East.

As yet untapped, but applicable, technologies include: recruiting by computerized telecommunications linkages, donor and physician education via cable health networks, and robotics laboratories to perform certain repetitive tasks (209). The feasibility of these alternatives is unproven, but studies are under way.

Blood Collection

Technologies involved with collection of blood from donors address three basic functions: 1) accurate identification of donors, 2) determination of donor suitability, and 3) collection of blood.

Donor identification is accomplished in most blood banks by the use of a cardboard or plastic card embossed with name, address, permanent identification number, and blood type. Most blood banks also have rosters of "special" donors against which the donor's identification is compared. "Special" donors include individuals whose blood is extraordinarily rare (for special needs), as well as those whose blood is unacceptable for transfusion due to laboratory findings on previous donations.

Donor suitability is determined by an assessment of current health status (temperature, blood pressure, screening test for anemia, etc.) and an

Figure 9.—Uniform Labeling Format for Blood Products

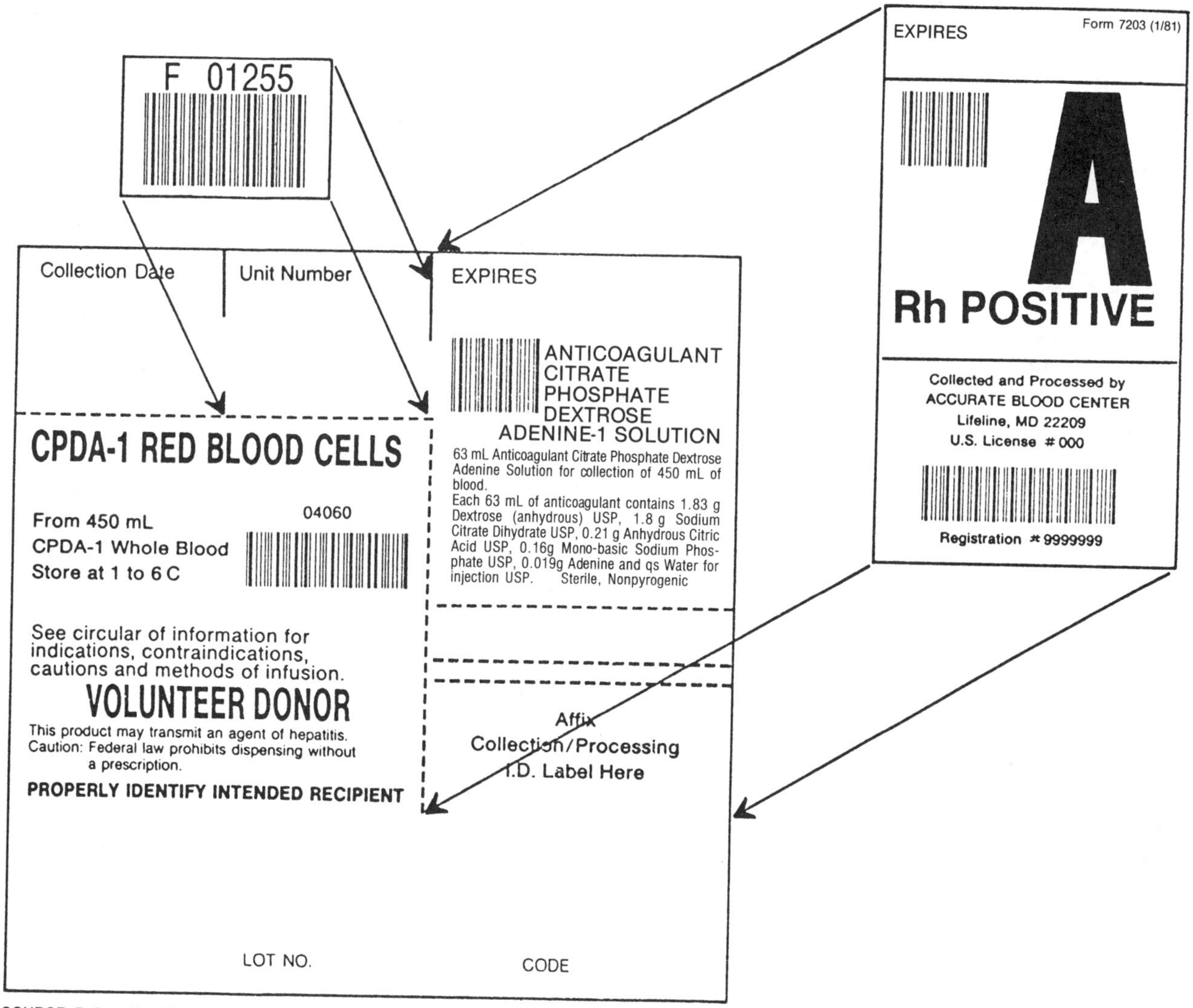

SOURCE: E. Rossiter, "Technologies for Blood Collection," 1984.

interview covering past and present illnesses, immunizations, hospital procedures, or other conditions (including travel outside the United States, lifestyle, and exposure to other individuals) which could make donating blood unsafe for the donor or transfusion unsafe for the recipient. While some of the donor acceptability criteria are straightforward, most are subject to varying degrees of interpretation at the time of screening. In the absence of factual information to support all the decisions that affect donor suitability, intuition is often used (598). There are also concerns among blood bank physicians about the adequacy of current donor criteria when used for frequent, long-term donors (562).

Pre-donation cell counts or hemoglobin measurements generally assure that donating will not be unduly risky for the donor and that an adequate number or volume of the desired component can be collected. Findings of diminished platelet effectiveness in individuals taking aspirin has led to deferral of such donors in plateletapheresis programs (565). (See ch. 2, pt. 3, for a discussion of the risks to donors.)

One measure of the safety of the collection process is the frequency of moderate to severe reactions in which donors faint or lose consciousness during or after donation. A rate of 0.3 percent or less is regarded as acceptable (44).

Collection of whole blood is accomplished by the use of pre-sterilized collection sets which consist of a needle, tubing and container pre-filled with anticoagulant/preservative solution. The main collection bag may have one or more smaller, satellite bags attached to it by tubing. After venipuncture, blood flows by gravity into the main container, mixes with the anticoagulant/preservative and remains there until an internal closure is opened to the satellite containers for component preparation. Table 26 lists the usual types of components that can be made from each container configuration.

Underutilization of the multiple bag set can result when changes in blood orders or incidents during the collection process necessitate preparation of fewer or different components than the ones for which the configuration was designed. For example, a bad (traumatic) venipuncture results in decreased platelet and cryoprecipitate yields; therefore, if a triple pack is assigned to a donor who subsequently has a traumatic venipuncture in the collecting process, only red blood cells and plasma may be prepared. The empty, extra satellite container, which represents a cost of $4.52 (based on differences in the price of double and triple packs with a 5-day platelet storage container in 1984) is lost. The extent of this problem has been estimated by some to affect 7 to 10 percent of collected units (472).

Successful adaptation of sterile docking devices to routine component production operations could eliminate the need for multiple bag configurations; all blood could be collected into single packs (at $3.18 each in 1984) and those units needed for component production could be coupled with separate transfer packs (at $2.25 each in 1984) via sterile docking technology (projected cost of $0.50 per component) (3). Savings of $0.50 to $1.00 per component would be possible. Further savings could be realized on less expensive storage containers for products designated for further manufacturing (e.g., plasma fractionation).

During the last 10 years, a new technology originating in the United States called "apheresis" has become popular for the collection of large amounts of a specific component from a single donor. (The therapeutic use of this technology was reviewed in a July 1983 OTA case study, *The Safety, Efficacy, and Cost Effectiveness of Therapeutic Apheresis*.)

Plasmapheresis can be accomplished by manual techniques, which involve collection containers and techniques similar to those for whole blood collection. After centrifugation and separation of the plasma, the red cells, white cells, and platelets are reinfused into the donor. The entire process is then repeated, resulting in two final plasma products and involving a second reinfusion of the donor's residual cells. The procedure takes approximately 90 minutes. Plasmapheresis is a relatively uncommon procedure in community blood centers and transfusion services; for example, less than 0.1 percent of the total plasma collections in the Red Cross in 1983 were by plasmapheresis (48).

Plasma may be collected as a byproduct of automated cytapheresis (cells) procedures for platelets or white blood cells. Current automated

Table 26.—Standard Blood Collection Container Systems

Bag configuration	Components prepared[a]	Cost per pack[b]
Single pack	Whole blood	$ 3.18
Double pack	Red blood cells Plasma	$ 6.52
Triple pack	Red blood cells Cryoprecipitate or platelets Plasma	$11.04[c]
Quadruple pack	Red blood cells Platelets Cryoprecipitate Plasma	$14.55[c]
Quintuple pack	Pediatric doses of red blood cells and plasma	$17.78

[a]Products listed do not include modified whole blood and resulting byproducts, or components prepared by breaking original (sterile) seals.
[b]List prices for CPDA-1 systems from Fenwal Division, Baxter-Travenol, Deerfield, IL.
[c]Price is for 5-day platelet product; 3-day platelet or cryoprecipitate container price is reduced by $1.44.
SOURCE: E. Rossiter, "Technologies for Blood Collection," 1984.

technologies are not cost effective compared to manual methods for routine plasmapheresis (2), but are useful nonetheless in collecting large amounts of antibody-rich plasma from specially immunized donors for reagent use or further manufacturing into injectable products, such as hyperimmune anti-Rh(D) for prevention of hemolytic disease in the newborn.

Membrane filtration technology under development may provide a cost-effective alternative to automated plasmapheresis. One developer projects a 20- to 35-minute procedure in which operator intervention is minimized by microprocessor control.

All automated apheresis devices work on the principle of centrifuging whole blood to enable the separation of components, transfer of the desired component to a storage container, and reinfusion of the remaining components. The first apheresis devices were largely mechanical processors, but later machines are microprocessor-controlled with multiple modes for different component schemes. Operator experience and technique have been shown to substantially affect equipment performance.

Collection techniques for plateletapheresis are fairly new. Effectiveness and safety data show some variation in end-products, mainly in platelet yield and undesirable contamination by extraneous white blood cells and red blood cells (198).

Current plateletapheresis technologies are summarized in table 27. The costs of all systems are comparable (1984 prices); hardware is approximately $30,000 and collection container systems $65-85, except for the 5-day container system.

Platelets collected by apheresis (single-donor platelets) have been proven to be as safe and effective as platelets prepared from whole blood (random-donor platelets) (301,501), but there is controversy surrounding the extent to which plateletapheresis products should be used in lieu of platelets from whole blood collections. Critics of "routine" plateletapheresis cite economic reasons (pheresis platelets costs ranged from $200 to $350 per dose; manually collected platelets, from $125 to $200 in 1984), the higher prevalence of donor complications, and lack of clinical data to support widespread and indiscriminate use of plateletapheresis technology (483). Nevertheless, few blood bankers doubt that apheresis technologies could someday replace manual platelet collections.

The 24-hour shelf life of apheresis platelets (compared to the 3- or 5-day shelf life of platelets separated from whole blood collections, because the collection system in apheresis is opened in the separation and reinfusion of the donor's cells) has been a major problem in inventory management with these products. But one company, Fenwal, is now marketing a closed system for the production of apheresis platelets with a 5-day shelf life.

Table 27.—Plateletapheresis Technologies[a]

Technology	Manufacturer/model	Year developed	Product dating period	Comments
Intermittent-flow centrifuge............	Haemonetics 30	1973	24 hrs.	First system approved by FDA. Requires extra step to remove extraneous cell contamination.
	Haemonetics V-50	1983	24 hrs.	Produces platelet-rich plasma.
Continuous-flow centrifuge................	Fenwal CS 3000	1979	24 hrs.	Fewer extraneous red blood cells. Lower extracorporeal volume.
		1983	5 days	Sterile docking device technology and a different type of storage container add $40 to collection container costs.
Dual stage continuous-flow centrifuge............	IBM 2997	1977	24 hrs.	Manufacturer plans no further development of product line.[b]

[a]These devices can also be used to collect white blood cells.
[b]Letter to customers from IBM, Jan. 24, 1984.
SOURCE: OTA, 1983, Poindexter, 1984, and Fenwal Division of Travenol Laboratories, Inc.

Leukapheresis (for collection of white blood cells) can also be performed (independent of or concomitant with platelet collection) with the same technology; costs and techniques are similar to those for plateletapheresis. Although the safety, effectiveness and efficiency of leukapheresis technologies, and leukocytes as a transfusion product have been under study for over a decade, use of the technology remains controversial (90,405,468). Clinical data to support the use of white blood cell transfusions are extremely difficult to obtain because of the morbidity of the recipients; white blood cells have generally been used for individuals with overwhelming infections unresponsive to antibiotics.

Blood Component Preparation

The proportion of whole blood donations that are separated into components varies among blood centers from around 50 to more than 99 percent, reflecting local medical preferences and practices. The minimum yield from one unit of whole blood is one unit of red cells and one unit of plasma. Additional components which are commonly separated are platelets and cryoprecipitate.

The plasma and cellular components of collected whole blood will separate by gravity over a period of about 24 hours. The most dense cells, red blood cells, settle out to fill the bottom half of a container. Less dense white cells settle in a thin, visible layer on top of the red cell mass. Platelets are distributed among the white blood cells, with some platelets remaining suspended in the plasma layer.

This separation process can be accomplished in a matter of minutes using high-speed centrifuges. The flexibility of the plastic collection container allows removal of the top layer into a sterile attached satellite bag.

The original collection container configuration dictates the number and type of components which can be prepared from whole blood (see table 26). Through a scheme of primary and secondary processing steps, a variety of end-products can be produced, either for direct transfusion or for further manufacturing into other products (fig. 10). Secondary processing adds to product cost and is generally limited to special applications.

On average, 80 percent of whole blood collections are processed into two or more components, most commonly red blood cells and frozen or liquid plasma. Platelets are also prepared from over 30 percent of collections and have become the "driving force" behind scheduling and planning of component production. Platelet shelf life is the

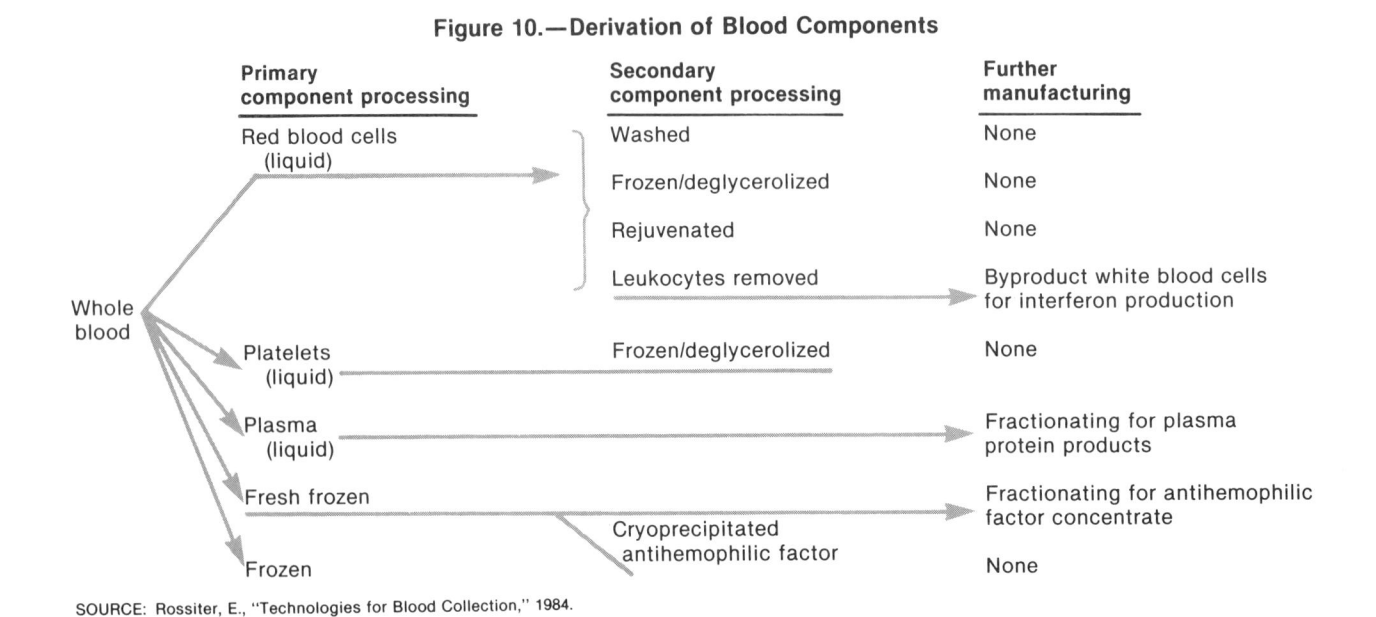

Figure 10.—Derivation of Blood Components

Whole blood	Primary component processing	Secondary component processing	Further manufacturing
	Red blood cells (liquid)	Washed	None
		Frozen/deglycerolized	None
		Rejuvenated	None
		Leukocytes removed	Byproduct white blood cells for interferon production
	Platelets (liquid)	Frozen/deglycerolized	None
	Plasma (liquid)		Fractionating for plasma protein products
	Fresh frozen	Cryoprecipitated antihemophilic factor	Fractionating for antihemophilic factor concentrate
	Frozen		None

SOURCE: Rossiter, E., "Technologies for Blood Collection," 1984.

shortest of all whole blood components, except for granulocytes; the product must be prepared within several hours of blood collection to preserve platelet function and survival. Because over 60 percent of blood collection operations are offsite periodic shuttles back to the blood center are necessary throughout the day. Special collection operations are scheduled over weekends and holidays to avoid shortages.

The development in 1981 of new plastics for storing platelets increased shelf life from 3 to 5 days and has alleviated some of the production constraints. Initial studies show improved efficiency by an increase in product availability and decrease in outdating (414b). Longer shelf life has also allowed a reduction in the number of shuttles and weekend operations, further improving component production efficiency. Notable increases in platelet demand and utilization were experienced in 1983 in the Red Cross, where 75 percent of the platelet production was in the 5-day plastic containers (48,351).

The extended shelf life of platelets is possible because of two different new plastics which allow better exchange of oxygen and carbon dioxide through the walls of the platelet storage container, thereby preventing the buildup of acid (as metabolic processes continue in the stored product) that is toxic to platelets. The new plastics have an additional advantage over previous formulations in that they lack DEHP, a common plasticizer used in construction, home furnishings, clothing, etc., which is known to leach into blood during storage and therefore has caused concern over potential toxicity (562).

The storage life of liquid-stored red blood cells and whole blood was extended from 21 to 35 days by the addition of adenine to the basic preservative solution in 1978. The improved efficiencies from this change have resulted in 50 percent reduction in outdating, now at approximately 5 percent (48). Further extension of red blood cell shelf life to 49 days is now possible. Red blood cells are first suspended in CPD anticoagulant (one of the standard preservatives), then an additive nutrient solution (AS-1, or ADSOL™, from the Fenwal Division of Travenol Laboratories) is added after other components are separated. It is not known whether the additive system approach (still in the introductory phase in 1984) will allow appreciable further reduction in red blood cell outdating, but there are other advantages to additive systems recognized from years of use in Sweden and Australia (267,345). They include increased plasma recovery (the additive solution replaces the buffering function of plasma during storage), better red cell survival in the recipient, and transfusion viscosity similar to that of whole blood.

Potential disadvantages include the additional cost of the collection container (approximately 13 percent more), extra manipulation during component preparation, and the potential need to remove excess solution in patients subject to circulatory overload (392). Nevertheless, the additive solution approach represents a technology designed to make possible specific preservative solutions tailor-made for each blood component (315).

Future component storage research is aimed at further increases in platelet shelf life and the use of ascorbate (vitamin C) to improve maintenance of certain red blood cell functions.

Recent advances and commercial successes in extending the shelf life of platelets are likely to spawn further improvements in dating periods. Use of additive solution systems, if widely accepted in the blood banking community, will facilitate research into component-specific preservatives. There also is interest in automating component production by the adaptation of robotics systems used in the U.S. automobile industry. Such a system has been designed, and its feasibility and potential impact are under study (209).

Testing and Labeling of Blood From Donors

With every donation, blood samples are tested for selected red blood cell antigens and antibodies and certain transmissible diseases (table 28). Test methods, their scientific bases, and potential clinical relevance vary greatly.

Table 28.—Testing of Blood Donor Samples

Test	Test detects	Reason performed	Clinical significance
Red cell antigens and antibodies:			
ABO group	A and/or B antigens on red blood cells. Presence of antibodies to A or B in plasma.	Assure ABO compatibility of donor and recipient; prevent hemolytic transfusion reaction.	Hemolytic transfusion reaction could occur in 97% of recipients due to natural antibodies to A and B red cell antigens.
Rh type	D antigens on red blood cells.	a. Prevent immunization of an Rh negative recipient.	a. 15% U.S. population is Rh negative; one-half of these would be immunized by an Rh positive transfusion.
D^u	Weak variant of D antigen.	b. Prevent hemolytic transfusion in a recipient already immunized.	b. 1% of Rh negative patients already immunized to D from transfusion or pregnancy.
Antibody screen	Unexpected antibodies (other than A or B).	a. Prevent passive transfer of antibody to recipient. b. Prevent antigen/antibody reaction in recipient. c. Identify rare donors or those with reagent-grade plasma.	a. Confusing results in subsequent blood bank testing. b. Rarely notable. c. Less than 0.5% of donor population has any antibody; reagent-grade or rare types much rarer.
Screens for transmissible disease:			
Syphilis screening (STS)	Reagin, an antibody-like substance present in people who have syphilis and a number of other acute and chronic conditions.	a. Originally, prevention of the transmission of syphilis by transfusion. b. Control of syphilis in donor population. c. Detection of biological false positive donors.	a. No longer a problem. b. Of doubtful effectiveness. c. Unclear; accounts for 70-90% positive STS tests.
Serum or Type B hepatitis	Hepatitis B surface antigen (HBsAg).	Prevention of transmission of type B or serum hepatitis.	7-10% of blood recipients at risk for some type of hepatitis; HBsAg test has significantly reduced posttransfusion type B, but has had no effect on other types—1-3% mortality for hepatitis B.

SOURCE: U.S. Department of Health and Human Services, FDA Panel, 1979.

Red blood cell tests determine the donor's ABO and Rh type. Mild incompatibility can result in an ineffective transfusion due to reduced red blood cell survival. Major ABO group incompatibility can result in fatal hemolytic transfusion reactions. Because of this danger, the donor ABO and Rh type are confirmed by the transfusion service, and ABO compatibility may be verified by crossmatching.

Standard tests for red cell antigens and antibodies are based on the principle of hemagglutination; i.e., the clumping of red blood cells that can occur as a result of specific antigen-antibody reactions. When a red cell antibody comes into contact with its target antigen on the surface of red blood cells, it combines with the antigen, forming antibody "bridges" between cells, which lead to visible clumps. Some antibodies (e.g., A and B) are very effective in bridge formation; others need antiglobulin (Coombs) reagent to form visible antibody bridges.

Table 29 demonstrates the serological basis for determining the ABO group of an individual. Because A and B antibodies are naturally produced by individuals who lack one or both of the antigens, it is possible to determine the ABO group by testing for either antigens or antibodies. Common practice is to perform both tests and check for agreement.

Rh type is determined by testing for D antigen on red cells; there is no naturally occurring an-

Table 29.—Determination of ABO Blood Group

Donor blood group	Antigens on donor's red blood cells A	B	Antibodies in donor plasma A	B
O	No	No	Yes	Yes
A	Yes	No	No	Yes
B	No	Yes	Yes	No
AB	Yes	Yes	No	No

SOURCE: E. Rossiter, "Technologies for Blood Collection," 1984.

tibody to D as with A and B antigens. Some blood banks perform two different tests for D antigen to provide an internal check. Blood banks also perform additional, more sensitive antiglobulin (Coombs) testing on samples giving negative results for D antigen. This technique will detect weak or suppressed D antigen, but its clinical significance is unclear.

ABO and Rh types are genetically determined and do not change. For this reason, some European blood centers do not repeat ABO and Rh determinations on donors who have been previously tested (sometimes multiple testing will be conducted before subsequent testing is discontinued). This practice would significantly reduce the testing workload in the United States, because approximately 80 percent of blood donors have donated before (48). However, Federal regulations currently require ABO and Rh testing on every donation. On the other hand, some blood banks in Canada and Europe do more elaborate Rh typing than is done in the United States, testing for C and/or E antigens (of the same family as D). This practice has been discontinued in most U.S. blood banks with no increased risk to recipients (562).

ABO and Rh testing can be performed by manual or automated methods. Table 30 summarizes the different manual techniques used for detecting red cell antigens and antibodies. All manual techniques involve mixing of sera-containing antibodies and red blood cell suspensions, and visual examination for clumping. Tube and microplate techniques allow centrifugation of the test mixture for easier reading of the test reaction. The predominant manual test technique is the tube method, although use of microplates (actually a miniaturization of the tube technique) has been increasing since the late 1970s. In 1984, within the Red Cross alone, 14 centers used manual microplate techniques as their primary method, and another 7 used microplates as a backup to automated methods.

The Technicon AutoAnalyzer, introduced in 1967, was the first attempt to automate routine donor testing. It used continuous flow technology already proven in clinical chemistry analysis. It automatically samples and performs ABO, Rh, and STS (serological test for syphilis) tests, but relies on the operator to identify samples, read reactions, and interpret and record results. Nevertheless, the AutoAnalyzer was widely used (still about 200,000 worldwide), easy to repair and maintain, and, at about $30,000, within the price range of a number of medium to large blood centers; the largest of them often had two. The AutoAnalyzer is no longer produced but is still used in a number of centers.

Table 31 lists the fully automated testing technologies used in the United States in 1984. All identify samples via bar-coded label, sample automatically, perform tests, read results by a photometer, and interpret results via dedicated computer. All systems also have some capability to perform antibody screening and STS, but are not generally used for these purposes in the United States. Costs per donor sample range from $0.83 to $1.23 v. $0.53 for the AutoAnalyzer (208). These systems are much more difficult to maintain and repair. Overall costs of the fully automated

Table 30.—Comparison of Manual Technologies for Red Cell Serological Testing of Blood Donors

Type	Advantages	Disadvantages
Slide/tile testing	Simple, fast, inexpensive.	Less sensitive. Not adaptable to automation. Difficult to use in batch testing. Coombs testing impossible without supplemental use of tubes.
Tube testing	Allows the use of more sensitive techniques than slide. Adaptable to batch testing up to approximately 200 samples.	Requires labeling and manipulation of tubes. Uses larger amount of reagent and sample than slide or microplate.
Microplate	More sensitive than tube or slide. Uses less sample, reagent and space. Easily adaptable to large batch testing.	More dexterity required for sampling and plate handling. May require new reaction interpretation techniques.

SOURCE: E. Rossiter, "Technologies for Blood Collection," 1984.

Table 31.—Automated ABO/Rh Test Technologies in the United States, 1983

System name	Manufacturer	Principle	Number of centers	Price (×1,000)
AutoGrouper	Technicon[a]	Continuous flow analysis	11	$184
MiniGroupamatic	Kontron[b]	Discrete analysis	5	$115
G-2000	Kontron	Discrete analysis	8	$260
G-360	Kontron	Discrete analysis	8	$460

[a]Tarrytown, NY.
[b]Everett, MA.
SOURCE: L. Friedman, "Status of Automated ABO/Rh Testing in the U.S." ARC Internal Report, 1983.

systems are beyond the grasp of most community blood centers (only 32 of 213 U.S. community blood centers were using them in 1984).

The testing of blood donor samples for unexpected antibodies involves the use of reagent red blood cells selected on the basis of antigenic content. The test was originally designed to detect antibodies in recipient plasma that might cause difficulty in crossmatching, but it has become a standard test for every sample entering the blood bank. Tube or microplate testing is necessary to detect clinically significant antibodies that react only with Coombs reagent. Microplate techniques are more efficient and more sensitive for this purpose (487).

Although traditional screening techniques have included multi-phase testing with various enhancers and potentiators, there is little justification for elaborate procedures on donor samples. Regular blood donors who have not been transfused or pregnant since the last negative antibody screen could be excluded from subsequent testing, but the effort required to selectively exclude these donors may negate the benefits of decreased testing.

A new and abundant source of antibody production was developed in the 1970s and is being applied commercially in the 1980s. Monoclonal antibody technology (see ch. 6, pt. 2) allows large-scale production of antibodies with selected specificity and potency (575). Production of antibodies in this manner should eventually become less expensive and have the added advantage of reducing variability in test results that is inherent in using naturally produced human or animal serum. Monoclonal antibodies also can be easily labeled with indicator substances (radioactive, fluorescent, etc.) (436). Only a few monoclonal reagents have been approved for blood bank products, but many are under development.

Recent increases in the use of microplates for manual ABO/Rh testing have led to renewed interest in automating that technique. Initial developmental work from at least three companies indicates that "ELISA" readers, photometers currently used for reading enzyme-linked immunosorbent assays (an immunologic test) can be adapted for reading hemagglutination reactions. Coupled with dedicated computers for data analysis and interpretation, market projections indicate that these devices could be a more economical alternative for automated ABO/Rh testing (table 32). The automated microplate system prototypes require more manipulation of test samples than the current automated technologies, but the techniques for manual and automated microplate testing are the same, allowing easy conversion from one technology to the other.

Still another technology under development for several years by Gamma Biologicals, Inc. (Houston, TX) involves modified microplate technology (Microtear™), which offers visual or automated interpretation of hemagglutination by the "streaming" of red blood cells after centrifugation.

All of the testing technologies described thus far are liquid-phase tests; i.e., they involve the mixing of sera-containing antibodies with red blood cells in suspension, and the qualitative reading of the presence or absence of agglutination. A solid-phase immunoadsorbance technique has been patented by Rosenfield and Kochwa (U.S. patent # 4,275,053, June 23, 1981), and similar developmental work has been presented by Plapp and associates (1983), which offer quantitative evaluation of antigen-antibody interactions. Greatly increased sensitivity results from

Table 32.—Traditional Automated Technologies v. Automated Microplate Systems (AMS)

	Traditional[a]	AMS[b]
Machine costs	$115K-$420K	$25K-$60K
Cost per sample ABO/Rh	$0.83-$1.23	$0.68
Operator intervention	Minimal	Centrifugation, resuspension, and loading of microplates required.
Backup technology	Second machine, manual tube, or microplate.	Standard manual microplate technology is inherent alternative.

[a] Figures are based on actual operations.
[b] Developers include Dynatech Laboratories, Alexandria, VA; Flow Laboratories, McLean, VA; and Kontron International, France. Figures are based on estimates from developers.
SOURCE: Friedman, personal communication, 1983.

affixing the reaction components to a solid surface (usually a microplate well), but the utility of this technique in routine donor processing has not been proven.

Except for the semiautomated AutoAnalyzer techniques developed in the late 1960s, screening technologies for syphilis have been unchanged for the past 15 to 20 years. The tests are not specific; approximately 90 percent of positive reactions are due to causes other than syphilis. Questions have been raised about the health status of false positive reactors; some scientists believe the test may be indicative of pre-disease states, the infectivity of which is unknown (562). However, the overwhelming opinion of FDA expert panels, AABB, and ARC is that the STS test need not be required for donor samples. Federal regulations and most State health departments currently require STS testing, in spite of the lack of scientific evidence to support its continued use.

Hepatitis testing technologies have undergone rapid evolution since the discovery of Australia antigen (80). The antigen so discovered was a marker of hepatitis B virus and led to development of a succession of increasingly more sensitive tests for hepatitis B surface antigen (HBsAg). Like other tests on donor blood, it is repeated on every donation, regardless of the donation frequency and history, and once a donor has had a confirmed positive test, he or she is permanently disqualified as a donor. No confirmation of the (negative) test is performed by the transfusion service.

Current "third generation" technologies for HBsAg testing are compared in table 33. Enzyme immunoassays (EIA) are of equal sensitivity as radioimmunoassay (RIA) techniques, but are increasingly preferred over RIA due to cumbersome monitoring, licensing and waste disposal requirements for the radioisotopes used in RIA testing. Both EIA and RIA have automatic reading of reactions and interpretation of results. Abbott Laboratories, the leading company in the field of HBsAg testing, is developing a more complete automated system which identifies samples by bar code and can interface with other blood center computers.

Once all testing is completed on donor samples, blood components with unsatisfactory test results must be disposed of and satisfactory units labeled according to ABO, Rh and a statement of satisfactory test results (e.g., for HBsAg), and released for distribution. This is a most crucial procedure, since the mistaken release of a unit reactive to HBsAg would go undetected, and blood labeled incorrectly for ABO group could be transfused into an incompatible recipient.

Labeling and release of blood components are tedious and laborious tasks. They are usually performed in batches by a team of two or more persons, with one individual applying adhesive labels and the other checking laboratory and donor records. To minimize human error and facilitate the process, computers storing laboratory and donor suitability data can be used to print appropriate labels or to verify that a correct bar-coded label has been applied, and that all testing on a blood component has been satisfactory. Such systems, fully integrated with automated testing sys-

Table 33.—Current Technologies for HBsAG[a] Testing

Test surface	Agglutination test type		Immunoassay test type	
	Latex	Red blood cell	Radio-plastic	Enzyme-plastic
	Slide/tile	Microplate	Bead or tube	Bead or tube
Sensitivity	Good	Good	Excellent	Excellent
Specificity	Fair	Good	Excellent	Excellent
Interpretation of results	Subjective	Subjective	Objective	Objective
Positive results indicated by	Clumping of particles	Clumping of red blood cells	"Radioactive"[b] bead	Colored solution
Automated reading	No	Under development	Yes	Yes

[a]Hepatitis B surface antigen.
[b]Higher than levels of background radioactivity.
SOURCE: Huestis, Bove, and Busch: *Practical Blood Transfusion*, 1981.

tems, are operational in probably not more than 10 community blood centers, and no onsite printers approved by the American Blood Commission are being used, but they are the ultimate goal of any facility introducing computers into the laboratory.

Pre-Transfusion Testing Techniques

The purpose of test procedures in the transfusion service is to minimize risk of major serologic incompatibility. The ABO/Rh type of the donor unit is rechecked, the ABO/Rh type of the recipient determined, and a crossmatch performed between the recipient sample and selected donor samples. Though not required by Federal regulations, AABB accredited transfusion services must also perform a recipient antibody screen. Recipient antibody screening yields much the same information as the crossmatch, and there has been increasing questioning of the need for both tests since the antibody screen was required for accreditation by AABB in 1970. The next revision of the AABB standards is likely to allow some options in choosing between the tests.

The first crossmatch was a simple mixing of two blood samples and observing for hemagglutination. The test eventually evolved into two distinct procedures—mixing of recipient plasma with donor red blood cells, and mixing of donor plasma with recipient red blood cells (fig. 11). The former is now regarded as the "major" crossmatch, because it is of prime importance in predicting the likelihood of a hemolytic transfusion reaction (recipient's antibodies would destroy the infused red cells). The latter, "minor" crossmatch, is no longer required by Federal or voluntary standards.

Figure 11.—The Crossmatch

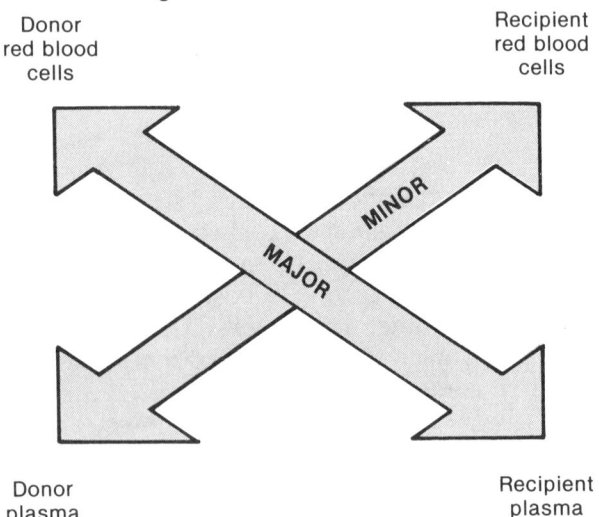

Donor red blood cells — Recipient red blood cells
MAJOR   MINOR
Donor plasma — Recipient plasma

SOURCE: Rossiter, E., "Technologies for Blood Collection," 1984.

In spite of the diversity of approaches taken in testing, decisions about when to crossmatch and how many units to hold available have become increasingly standardized. Eighty-three percent of responders to a recent survey (588) used a type-and-screen (T&S) procedure in which preliminary testing (ABO, Rh, and antibody screen) is performed on low-risk surgical patients, and blood is made available (though not crossmatched). The T&S policy is implemented after each blood bank reviews its own transfusion statistics across "surgery-related" groups and determines which elective surgical procedures seldom result in transfusion. In the rare instances in which blood is needed during or after these surgeries, blood will be released for transfusion with an abbreviated crossmatch.

Studies of the safety of T&S practices indicate that they are both safe (408b) and economical (203). T&S and similar policies which establish a standard number of crossmatched units for surgeries that usually require transfusion, improve blood resources management through lower inventory needs, improved utilization, and decreased outdating.

Conclusions

Technologies developed and put into use during the last 10 years have made blood products more effective, and have increased their safety. The biggest improvements have been in efficiency, with increased availability and better utilization of products.

Trends for the next 5 to 10 years in the use of technologies will be continued increases in automation and computerization, and further improvements in blood preservation. These changes are a natural result of technological changes made since the late 1970s and reflect the dynamic climate in which U.S. blood banks operate.

PART 2: PLASMA FRACTIONATION TECHNOLOGIES

Introduction

Plasma fractionation began in this country during World War II. At the onset of the war, liquid human plasma was in use in the battlefields of Europe, but there was a need for a blood substitute that was easy to transport and which could be administered on the battlefield under widely varying climatic conditions.

At the request of the Medical Advisory Committee of the Red Cross and the National Research Council's Committee on Blood Transfusions, Edwin J. Cohn, head of the Department of Physical Chemistry at Harvard University, agreed to undertake an investigation to determine whether or not the plasma of animals could be made safe for transfusion. By mid-1940, Cohn notified the Red Cross of the development of a system which would yield not only albumin but other protein components of plasma as well, but said he felt that dependence should be placed on the use of human plasma rather than that of animals. The Red Cross then opened a blood donor facility at Peter Bent Brigham Hospital in Boston to provide plasma to support Cohn's work. In April 1941, the first human serum albumin produced by Cohn was released for clinical trials, and by July 1941, pilot production facilities had been expanded.

In December 1941, clinical studies had not yet been concluded, but human derivatives from Harvard were rushed to Pearl Harbor for use in treatment of injured servicemen. By 1942, the Armed Forces had authorized regular use of normal serum albumin (NSA) and issued production contracts to several pharmaceutical firms. Training of technical personnel from these firms was conducted by Cohn and his staff. Cutter began to supply the product in late 1942, and by 1943 seven U.S. companies were involved in fractionation and supply of human plasma products. Following World War II, these companies continued to process plasma to meet the demand for various plasma proteins for civilian use.

During the beginning of plasma fractionation in the 1940s, albumin production and sale provided the economic support for the industry. Later in the 1950s, the need for gamma globulin for prophylaxis against poliomyelitis, infectious hepatitis, and childhood viral diseases provided financial security for the industy. Subsequently, prevalance of these diseases was markedly decreased, and at about the same time methods for recovering Factor VIII were greatly improved, leading to increased treatment of hemophiliacs in the United States and abroad. As a result, sales of Factor VIII have been a significant source of revenues from the mid-1960s to the present.

Plasma Collection

Three types of plasma are used to produce plasma derivatives; liquid single-donor plasma, fresh-frozen, single-donor plasma, and "source" plasma, which is collected by plasmapheresis. Liquid and fresh-frozen, single-donor plasma are primarily obtained through volunteer agencies as "recovered" plasma from whole blood donations. "Recovered" plasma is either fresh frozen within 6 to 24 hours of collection or is salvaged from outdated whole blood at the time the red cells are discarded. Only fresh-frozen plasma is suitable for Factor VIII fractionation. Increased use of components has resulted in an increasing proportion of recovered plasma being frozen within a few hours of collection to protect the labile coagulation factors. Single units of fresh-frozen plasma are then shipped directly to the fractionators.

In plasmapheresis, 500 ml of whole blood is drawn into a sterile container in which there is anticoagulant solution (either ACD Formula A, CPD, or Trisodium Citrate). The container is then detached and the blood centrifuged in order to separate the red cells from the plasma. During this time the phelebotomy needle is kept open with an infusion of isotonic salt (NaCl) solution. The red cells are then reinfused into the donor, and the process is repeated a second time. The 0.5 to 0.6 liters of collected plasma are then frozen. The average elapsed time for such plasmapheresis is 90 minutes. Each donor is permitted to undergo a double-bleeding of this type twice per week.

At least three systems for the automation of plasmapheresis are currently undergoing research and development: membrane filtration, continuous flow centrifugation, and intermittent flow (batch) centrifugation. As yet, none is able to compete economically with the traditional manual technique. Although the manual system is labor-intensive, the total cost of a double pack of plasma is in the range of $22 to $25 (277), including $7 to $10 for the donor fee, $8 for the blood bag set and saline solution, $2 for donor screening and testing, and $5 for labor. In the case of automated centrifugal systems, the disposable plastic bowls alone cost more than this; Haemonetics $55, Fenwal $60, and IBM $65. However, these costs could plummet if simplified to be used for source plasma alone. The state of the art of the automated centrifugal system has been developed far beyond the needs for plasma collection because the same basic hardware (with costs of approximately $20,000) and disposable plastic bowls can be used to prepare platelet concentrates, buffy coats (leukocytes), and washed red cells.

On a theoretical basis, filtration through membranes of appropriate pore size should be the simplest way to separate liquid plasma from the cells in whole blood. Earlier development of this technology has been hampered by the fact that filtration does not simultaneously yield cellular components such as platelets to help amortize the development costs. However, its potential value in therapeutic plasmapheresis may catalyze its evaluation in the collection of normal (source) plasma. Membrane filtration at low temperatures has also been attempted experimentally to isolate Factor VIII-rich cryoprecipitate. Large-scale application of this new technology has not been attempted.

The estimated time required for a centrifugal plasmapheresis separation is 30 to 40 minutes, and for continuous flow membrane filtration, 50 to 60 minutes. When donor preparation time is added in, the overall plasmapheresis time is slightly longer than 1 hour. This compares with approximately 90 minutes for the traditional manual system (2). The interrupted flow centrifugal system also requires only a single venipuncture, as opposed to the two needles or large, double lumen needle necessary for continuous flow. The principal advantages of automated plasmapheresis are: 1) the donor is always attached to his/her own red cells or whole blood, thus preventing accidental administration of mismatched cells; and 2) the potential population of plasma donors may be able to be expanded significantly throughout the world. Automation also raises the possibility of decentralized plasmapheresis, and, by shortening the overall procedure time, also enhances the possibility of inclusion of volunteer donors for source plasma. The remaining unanswered question is whether or not increased volumes of plastic disposables will lower costs sufficiently to compete with a manual system in which labor costs are only 20 percent of final production costs.

There are two types of plasmapheresis donors: standard donors and specialized donors. High-titer antibody preparations (hyperimmune globulins) are made from the plasma of specialized donors. Successful passive immunization is greatly improved by use of gamma globulin fractions high in specific antibody content against the individual diseases. The hyperimmunization of selected (specialized) donors through repeated stimulation of their immune systems with specific antigens (noninfectious products made from the inactivated protein of the underlying virus or bacteria) can provide a pool of high-titer antisera. This technique has provided specific globulins for the management of such diverse disorders as rabies, herpes zoster, and hepatitis B.

In a similar manner, individuals who inadvertently have been immunized through prior blood transfusions or pregnancy, or who elect to become donors of blood group antibody sera, can have their titers restimulated over a period of years and maintain their role as specialized plasmapheresis donors for the production of anti-A, anti-B, or anti-Rh immune globulin for blood group typing, or, in the case of anti-Rh, for the prevention of Rh hemolytic disease of the newborn (erythroblastosis fetalis).

Some overlap occurs between standard and specialized plasmapheresis donors. Immunization against tetanus, for example, is so commonly practiced and easily accomplished that it is common for standard donors to receive occasional booster doses, making possible the recovery of a high titer of tetanus antibodies from routine gamma globulin fractionation.

Fractionation Methods and Products

The principal method used for the isolation of the different plasma proteins continues to be the cold-ethanol precipitation technique of Cohn and collaborators (127). This method employs a four-variable system of temperature, ionic strength, ethanol concentration, and pH to precipitate:

- Fraction I—chiefly Factor VIII and fibrinogen,
- Fraction II—the gamma globulins,
- Fractions III and IV—other coagulation proteins and trace components such as ceruloplasmin and iron-binding globulin, and
- Fraction V—the albumins.

Fraction VI, the residue remaining, is currently discarded due to lack of known therapeutic usefulness.

Method XII, the final technique evolved by the Cohn group (128), gave promise of considerable simplification by using metallic precipitation of the globulins with zinc diglycinate, but this method was never commercially adopted due to preliminary evidence of contamination of the albumin fraction with hepatitis virus. It also was impractical in its requirement for decalcified plasma (through ion-exchange treatment) rather than the usual citrated plasma.

Due to a shortage of industrial sources of alcohol in England following World War II, the principal fractionation facilities which were constructed at the Lister Institute were modified to permit use of ether rather than ethanol. The basic principle of the four-variable Cohn system was nonetheless used, and this method was continued for a period of approximately 20 years, following which the ethanol system was again employed. Nevertheless, many minor modifications of the basic alcohol precipitation technique have been introduced successfully with improvement in yield, cost effectiveness, and stability of individual products.

Factor VIII

In the original alcohol fractionation method, Factor VIII precipitated with fibrinogen in Fraction I-$_0$. The yield of Factor VIII by this method was similar to that developed by cryoprecipitation, but contamination of the final product with other proteins was considerably higher with the original alcohol fractionation method. These concentrates were used to treat hemophilia during the 1940s and 1950s, and were marketed primarily for their fibrinogen content. After the development of the cryoprecipitate technique by Pool, et al. (442), Fraction I-$_0$ was abandoned as too crude a preparation to use for its Factor VIII content. The fibrinogen, which the recipient received as a side effect of the Factor VIII replacement, led to problems in red cell crossmatching. Contamination with hepatitis virus was also so prevalent as to no longer justify its commercial preparation, and approval of Fraction I-0 (fibrinogen) as a plasma product was withdrawn by FDA in the late 1970s.

"Cryoprecipitate" was discovered by Pool and associates (442,443) to trap a significant portion of Factor VIII, and thus provided a simple physical step to harvest it. Currently, cryoprecipitate is either prepared as a single unit in a plastic bag during the routine collection and processing of a single unit of plasma in a blood bank, or the plasma is frozen and shipped to the fractionation industry.

The concentration of Factor VIII in cryoprecipitates varies widely, depending on such factors as the size of the ice crystals which form and the local salt concentrations left behind when water crystallizes into ice (419). Federal regulations require that the average Factor VIII potency of a single unit of cryoprecipitate be greater than 80 units as determined on four representative containers each month (21 CFR pt. 640.56). (The Factor VIII content of any single unit that is being used therapeutically cannot, of course, be measured.) For example, the average content of a bag of cryoprecipitate as determined by one Red Cross blood bank was assayed as containing: 1) 120 units of Factor VIII (range of 105 to 130), 2) 46.6 mgm of fibronectin, 3) 326 mgm of fibrinogen, and 4) present but not quantified amounts of von Willebrand factor (420).

With commercial preparations of Factor VIII concentrates, a higher concentration of Factor VIII can be achieved with less volume of infusion needed to administer it, and an exact Factor VIII content of each preparation can be assayed rather than assumed. Moreover, the stability and packaging of the concentrates is more suitable for home therapy.

When large pools of frozen material are processed, thawing is carefully controlled to improve yield and stability. The best yields of Factor VIII from cryoprecipitate are approximately 25 percent of the starting material. (As mentioned in ch. 3, heat-treated Factor VIII concentrates are now available.)

Gamma Globulins

Essentially all gamma globulins are recovered from Cohn Fraction II using the classic cold-ethanol technique. Immune serum globulin (ISG) is dispensed as a 16 percent protein solution for intramuscular injection in amounts up to 10 ml, or as a solution for intravenous injection (Intravenous gamma globulin, or IVGG).

Albumin

The production of albumin from fraction V_0 utilizes pH, ionic strength, and ethanol concentration to precipitate a highly purified concentrate of this principal oncotic agent of plasma. The powdered albumin is then resolubilized as either a 5 percent solution, with the same oncotic pressure as normal plasma, or as a 25 percent concentrate of salt-poor albumin. The 25 percent concentrate is marketed as a hyperoncotic concentrate which draws water from the extravascular tissues to restore blood volume and circulatory competence in a recipient suffering from hypovolemic shock.

An alternative method of albumin production is the elimination of the subfractionation steps which precipitate Fractions IV and V and reconstitution of these pooled fractions as an albumin solution. This material, plasma protein fraction (PPF), contains 83 to 90 percent albumin, no more than 17 percent of the total protein as alpha or beta globulin, and no more than 1 percent as gamma globulin. Currently, after the preceding fractions are removed, 30 percent of all fractionated plasma goes into PPF production and 70 percent into albumin production.

Albumin (and gamma globulin) can also be prepared from human placentas. Such processing is different from plasma because of the large amount of connective tissue, free supernatant hemoglobin, and other extraneous material which must be removed by filtration, adsorption, and centrifugation, but the final products are of high purity. The average yield of albumin by this technique is 5 gm/kg of placenta.

Factor IX Complex

Other modifications of the basic cold-ethanol technique have been developed for the preparation of specific concentrates. Among these is a product which contains the coagulation proteins of the prothrombin complex, (i.e., Factors II, VII, IX, and X). Like Factor VIII, Factor IX Complex is capable of transmitting viral diseases. For the past decade, its principal use has been: 1) in the treatment of hemophilia B (Christmas disease), and 2) in cases of hemophilia A patients with circulating inhibitors and who are unresponsive to Factor VIII treatment. Recent heat-treatment of the coagulation concentrates and the simultaneous reevaluation of viracidal agents such as ultraviolet irradiation give promise of increasing Factor IX Complex use significantly if sterilization proves possible without major loss of coagulant activity.

In the original cold-ethanol method of fractionation, Factor IX was concentrated in Fraction IV. Currently, most Factor IX Complex is produced by ion exchange chromatography (53). Protein absorbants such as tricalcium phosphate or aluminum hydroxide are also used at the beginning of the fractionation process to remove Factors II, VII, IX, and X prior to the standard cold-ethanol precipitation steps.

New and Emerging Technologies

Despite development over the past 40 years of new technologies for separation of proteins, they have remained largely confined to laboratory use or to the production of reagent and research products. Among the technologies are the separation of proteins on the basis of: 1) their differing electrical charges (electrophoresis), 2) their physical size and shape by passage through inert columns of different porosity (filtration), 3) their molecular weight (ultracentrifugation), and 4) different inert substances such as cellulose and resins, from which plasma proteins can then be recovered by elution.

Modifications of the cold-ethanol system have nonetheless been applied. One foreign producer, for example, uses ultrafiltration to separate hemoglobin from the alcohol solution of albumin, and ion exchange chromatography to absorb pigments, pyrogens, and residual reagents. Unfortunately, chromatography is difficult to adapt to systems which handle greater than 500 liters/week, which is only one-tenth of the standard volume deemed commercially necessary.

Failure to exploit these different technologies into manufacturing techniques for plasma derivatives is due to the market for plasma products not being large enough to warrant such developmental expenses, and the extensive retooling that would be required for major changes in technology. Still another reason new developments have been inhibited is that the whole field of plasma fractionation as it is known today may have a finite life span. Application of revolutionary new synthetic techniques such as recombinant DNA makes the same products potentially possible without relying on plasma as an organic source.

5.
Current Issues

Contents

	Page
Part 1: Impact of Aids on Blood Collection and Use	99
Part 2: Coordination of Blood Resources	107
Regionalization	108
Resource Sharing	111
American Association of Blood Banks	112
American Red Cross	114
Volume of Sharing	115
Conclusion	116
Part 3: Impact of Health Care Cost Containment	117
Part 4: Appropriate Use of Blood Products	121
Introduction	121
Whole Blood	121
Red Cell Concentrates	122
Platelets	124
Granulocytes	125
Cryoprecipitate	125
Fresh-Frozen and Single-Donor Plasma	126
Albumin and Plasma Protein Fraction	126
Factor VIII	127
Methods to Change Usage Patterns	127
Conclusion	129

LIST OF TABLES

Table No.	Page
34. Centers for Disease Control's Characterization of Groups at Increased Risk for AIDS in the United States (percent of total reported AIDS cases as of Dec. 19, 1983)	99
35. Resource Sharing Inventory Shipment Fees	114
36. AABB Clearinghouse Transactions by Type	114
37. Utilization of AABB Clearinghouse, 1973-83	115
38. Blood and Blood Components Moved by American Red Cross Regional Blood Centers in 1982 and 1983	116
39. Movement of Blood and Components Through the American Red Cross, 1979-83	116
40. Total Movement of Blood and Blood Components in the United States, 1979-83 (including both the AABB and the American Red Cross)	117
41. Blood Utilization by Major Disease Categories Ranked by Total Units Transfused and Percent of Units Transfused: Operated Males, Nonoperated Males, Operated Females, Nonoperated Females, and All Patients in Each Category	123

5.
Current Issues

PART 1: IMPACT OF AIDS ON BLOOD COLLECTION AND USE

Acquired immunodeficiency syndrome (AIDS) is a disease now shown almost conclusively to be of viral origin, with a high mortality rate (>40 percent of all diagnosed cases), and which is apparently transmitted through body fluids (e.g., semen, blood) through such means as sexual contact and intravenous drug abuse.

The disease is characterized by a profound disturbance of the immune system, with death usually due to extreme susceptibility to infections by organisms which rarely cause disease in persons with normal immunity (e.g., *pneumocystis carinii* pneumonia) and/or the development of a type of cancer (Kaposi's sarcoma) that is usually seen only in elderly or severely immunocompromised individuals.

The probable agent for AIDS attacks a type of white blood cell, T lymphocytes, which help to mediate the body's immune system through helping or suppressing the production of antibodies. It appears related to another virus which has been recently identified as the cause of human T-cell leukemia. The probable agent for AIDS apparently selectively infects and kills T-lymphocyte "helper" cells, whereas the T-cell leukemia virus infects T cells and, instead of killing them, turns them into cancerous leukemia cells (211,444, 476,488). (AIDS is examined in an OTA Technical Memorandum, "A Review of the Public Health Service's Response to AIDS" (in press).)

In the United States, the early AIDS cases were concentrated among homosexual and bisexual men, intravenous drug abusers, and persons of Haitian origin. As time passed, however, cases began to show up in hemophiliacs, and investigations of cases of unknown origin appeared to show a relationship between blood transfusions and subsequent development of AIDS (143). There was initial skepticism toward the conclusion that some AIDS cases were due to blood transfusions, but at a February 1984 meeting of blood banking representatives convened by the Centers for Disease Control (CDC), there was agreement that the evidence was conclusive enough that AIDS could be and had been transmitted through blood products, that no further studies need be conducted to prove/disprove the association, and that studies to quantify and clarify the risks were needed.

Table 34 summarizes the percent of AIDS cases according to groups at risk as of January 1984. The "other" category includes some cases of apparent transfusion-related AIDS in infants, whose immune status is sufficiently different from adults so that CDC has classified these infant cases separately from adult cases. Some of these infants, however, either had transfusions or were children of known AIDS patients.

In an April 1984 telephone conference call with representatives of blood banking organizations, CDC reported that there were: 1) 43 adult cases of AIDS associated with blood transfusions, with an additional 10 cases in children; and 2) 33 cases of AIDS in hemophiliacs. CDC had completed its investigations of 13 adult and 7 pediatric transfusion cases. In 12 of the 13 adult cases, at least one donor was identified who was either in a high-risk AIDS group (e.g., homosexual or bisexual

Table 34.—Centers for Disease Control's Characterization of Groups at Increased Risk for AIDS in the United States (percent of total reported AIDS cases as of Dec. 19, 1983)

	Percent of total reported AIDS cases
Homosexual and bisexual men	71
Intravenous drug abusers	17
Haitians living in the United States	5
Heterosexual contacts of persons at increased risk for acquiring AIDS	1
Hemophiliacs	1
Recipients of blood transfusions	1
Other (unknown)	4
Total	100% (3,000 cases)

SOURCE: CDC, *Morbidity and Mortality Weekly Review*, Jan. 6, 1984.

men) or who had an abnormal T-lymphocyte helper:suppressor ratio. At least one high-risk donor was identified in five of the seven pediatric cases with completed investigations.

The incidence of transfusion-related cases of AIDS is difficult to estimate because CDC traced blood donations as far back as 5 years in their search for a possible cause. CDC's first report of an association of transfusions with AIDS, for example, stated that the first 18 cases they reported on were diagnosed during approximately a 12-month period (to August 1983), when over 3 million persons in the United States received transfusions. But most of these cases were transfused between 1979 and 1982, when the prevalence of AIDS was much lower than during late 1982 and early 1983 (143). An incidence rate based on the time of diagnosis would be 18 per 3 million persons transfused, or 6 cases for every million persons transfused. At a rate of approximately 10 million units of blood components transfused per year (518), there would have been approximately 2 cases of AIDS for every million units transfused.

Cases in hemophiliacs have occurred at a much higher rate. Estimates are that there are 15,000 moderate to severe hemophiliacs in the United States (6), and 5,000 more mild hemophiliacs (173), or a rate of about 1/500 for the 37 AIDS cases diagnosed as of June 1984.

Hemophiliacs have been at highest risk of all blood group recipients, probably through the use of Factor VIII (and Factor IX) concentrates. If AIDS is indeed a virus, and based on the histories of the transfusion-related AIDS cases (143), all blood components—whole blood, red cells, platelets, cryoprecipitate, and plasma—are also capable of transmitting the agent.

Several methods have been employed to screen out AIDS from the blood supply. These include: 1) donor screening in addition to those methods which were already employed, 2) laboratory tests to identify donors at risks for AIDS, 3) product recalls, and 4) attempts to inactivate the AIDS agent.

FDA, in consultation with the major blood banking and plasma derivative organizations, the National Hemophilia Foundation, the National Gay Task Force, the Centers for Disease Control, and the National Institutes of Health, issued a recommendation in March 1983 to initiate the following procedures (566):

1. Educational programs to inform persons at increased risk of AIDS to refrain from blood or plasma donation. Persons at increased risk of AIDS were defined as follows: persons with symptoms and signs suggestive of AIDS, sexually active homosexual or bisexual men with multiple partners, Haitian entrants to the United States, present or past abusers of intravenous drugs (such intravenous drug abusers were already excluded by prior regulations), and sexual partners of persons at increased risk of AIDS.
2. Expanded medical screening of blood and plasma donors to identify individuals with early signs or symptoms of AIDS, with revision of standard operating procedures to include questions to elicit a history of night sweats, unexplained fevers, unexpected weight loss or signs of lymph node enlargement or Kaposi's sarcoma.
3. Examination of source plasma donors for lymph node enlargement by a physician (initially and annually), and by an adequately trained individual at each donation.
4. Measurement of body weight of source plasma donors prior to each donation to detect unexplained weight loss. If loss was detected, a physician's examination was recommended prior to continued plasma collection.

The sensitivities involved in screening high-risk donors are obvious; homosexual or other sexual activities and the use of injectable drugs are activities associated with a high degree of social stigma and illegal in many States. In negotiations surrounding the adoption of screening policies, spokespersons for the gay community have expressed fears about what the "stigma of bad blood" would do to a group already vulnerable socially, politically, and economically (66,322). To compound matters, it appears that the risk of contracting and transmitting AIDS is linked to the degree of sexual activity and number of sexual partners. Leaders of the gay community have objected to the use of the value-laden term, "promiscuity" (368). Gay physicians have cooperated and urged the adoption of a more restrictive definition of what constitutes a degree of sexual activity sufficient to contraindicate blood donation.

It has also been recognized that, while AIDS has been linked with male homosexual practices, women contracting the disease have been in other risk categories—e.g., sexual partners of bisexual men, intravenous drug users, or recent Haitian immigrants. Thus, gay women have continued to be safe prospective donors, and the blood banking community has continued to include them in appeals for blood donations.

As part of generalized public information campaigns about the risk of AIDS, the Public Health Service has included warnings about who should refrain from donating blood. Blood banking organizations such as the American Association of Blood Banks (AABB) have also waged their own public information efforts, aimed at both increasing awareness of high-risk donors and allaying groundless fears that AIDS could be contracted by simply donating blood (which involves a sterile needle that is disposed of after a single use).

In addition, many blood banks have introduced procedures which allow donors to privately indicate whether or not their blood donations should be used for transfusions, because such individuals may be especially reluctant to acknowledge their homosexuality or use of injectable drugs before their peers at school, business, or community blood drives. The New York Blood Center, for example, initiated a confidential form in February 1983 on which donors could indicate whether their blood could be used for transfusions or only for laboratory studies. A more common mechanism is to inform donors that they can call the blood bank after donating to indicate whether or not their blood should be used for transfusions. The Red Cross formally adopted such a mechanism on January 1, 1984.

For source plasma collectors, an additional recommendation from FDA was that plasma collected in geographic areas at high risk should not be used to manufacture the coagulation proteins. Manufacturers have ceased to accept plasma for Factor VIII and Factor IX products from prisons and the cities of New York, San Francisco, and Los Angeles (Hollywood area) (162).

A number of commentators have expressed concerns that any system aimed at screening high-risk donors, rather than the blood itself, will be imperfect. In the early debates over whether potential benefits from screening questions outweighed the dangers of invasion of privacy, an AABB Transfusion Transmitted Diseases Task Force resolution stated, "In fact there is evidence that such questions, no matter how well-intentioned, are ineffective in eliminating those donors who may carry AIDS."

While it may be too early to gauge the success of the screening procedures, some tentative initial assessments indicate that there has been a drop-off in donations by males between the ages of 18 and 35. Spokespersons for the New York Blood Center, for example, have reported a high degree of cooperation from the gay community, with whom they initially forged ties during the years of studies concerning transfusion associated hepatitis, when thousands of gay men were recruited as subjects (230). Blood bank recruiters have said that the same sense of civic responsibility that led to donating in the first place has convinced gay men to refrain from donating or allowing their blood to be used in transfusions (144).

On the user side, the National Hemophilia Foundation (NHF) (399) recommended that cryoprecipitate be used to treat newborn infants and children under age 4, newly identified patients never treated with Factor VIII, and patients with clinically mild hemophilia who require infrequent treatment. Similar recommendations have been made for Factor IX deficient patients when fresh-frozen plasma can be used instead of Factor IX Complex. No specific recommendations have been made between cryoprecipitate and Factor VIII for the treatment of severe hemophiliacs because of controversy over their advantages and disadvantages. Thus, the NHF recommends the continuation of early and appropriately intensive replacement of Factor VIII or Factor IX in the form of Factor VIII or Factor IX Complex at each hemorrhagic episode, for the approximately 90 percent of severe and moderately severe hemophiliacs now so treated in this country.

These recommendations came in the wake of a number of anecdotal reports that hemophiliacs were reducing the amount and frequency of administration of coagulation concentrates, foregoing treatment when indicated, or using smaller doses for bleeding crises. Such practices risk increasing the long-term morbidity associated with the disease, especially the orthopedic problems occasioned by bleeding into the joints, one of the most vexing problems of hemophilia. There have also been accounts of hemophiliacs declining necessary dental treatments or elective surgery, procedures which can require massive doses of coagulation products as a precautionary measure (5).

Plasma from a few donors subsequently diagnosed as having AIDS, or even from a single donor, has led to uncertainty over the safety of all the Factor VIII (and IX) concentrates derived from the thousands of plasma units containing the plasma from donor(s) with AIDS. All four commercial manufacturers of coagulation proteins, as well as the Red Cross and the New York Blood Center, have voluntarily withdrawn lots of Factor VIII or Factor IX upon learning that an AIDS victim had donated plasma used in their preparation.

The potential dimensions of this problem are enormous. Because of the preclinical, asymptomatic phase of AIDS, donors could give many times before becoming aware of having contracted the disease. In one recall case, an Austin, TX, man had sold plasma to a commercial center 50 times before being diagnosed as having AIDS. The process of pooling thousands of products also contributes to the need to quarantine a great deal of the product; the largest of the voluntary withdrawals involved enough Factor VIII to represent 500 patient-years of treatment (434).

All four manufacturers of coagulation factors have also recently received FDA approval to market heat-treated Factor VIII. These preparations have been shown to reduce the infectivity of hepatitis viruses and a variety of marker viruses added prior to the treatment process, with the hope that viruses from other heat-sensitive classes such as the retroviruses (in which the proposed AIDS organism belongs) may be similarly affected. The heat treatment is also estimated to decrease potency of these preparations by about 10 to 20 percent (162).

While donor screening has been most controversial among the affected donor groups, the methods that have raised the most controversy among blood bankers have been attempts to screen out AIDS from the blood supply through the use of laboratory tests. No specific test for AIDS is available, although one may become available in the relatively near future if the tentative identification of an AIDS virus is confirmed and tests can be devised to be used on a mass scale as promised (256). In the absence of a specific test for AIDS, attempts have focused on "surrogate" tests. These are of two types: 1) detection of abnormalities associated with AIDS or the preclinical stages of the disease, and 2) evidence of past infections with diseases that have a high incidence in the same population groups that are at increased risk for AIDS. Both of these types of surrogate tests will be positive in a much higher number of people than actually have the AIDS agent.

The total costs associated with surrogate tests include the cost of testing each individual unit, the loss of blood which tests positively, and higher recruitment costs associated with seeking donors to replace those excluded. Moreover, tests purporting to reveal abnormalities implicated in the preclinical stages of the disease raise questions about what kind of information to share with those who test positively. Conditions other than AIDS can lead to abnormal test results in tests of the first type. For example, the Stanford University Blood Bank now tests all whole blood donations for the T-lymphocyte helper:suppressor ratio. About 1 to 2 percent of collections are positive and discarded, but donors are not deferred permanently, since short-term virus infections can also cause an abnormal ratio (445).

In the second type of surrogate test that tests for past infections with other diseases, the diseases tested for have much higher incidences than known for AIDS. For example, in May 1984 Irwin Memorial Blood Bank in San Francisco initiated the test for antibodies against hepatitis B core antigen (anti-HBc)(indicating past infections with hepatitis B) and expects that deferrals will increase by 5 to 7 percent because of positive tests (445). (Irwin expects that the test will also help to prevent non-A, non-B hepatitis transmission, another infectious agent that so far has not been identified specifically, although current research indicates it is a virus(es).) Cutter, one of the four fractionators of plasma, also announced at approximately the same time that it also would use the anti-HBc test and expects that approximately 15 percent of its donors will have positive tests. Cutter plans to use their plasma only in producing albumin and immune globulins, which have not been implicated in AIDS (137).

A study group of the Food and Drug Administration's (FDA) Blood Products Advisory Committee has also been studying whether surrogate tests, specifically, the anti-HBc test, should be instituted for all whole blood and plasma collections, with the majority believing that the test was not appropriate as a means of identifying AIDS high-risk group members. This group also recommended in March 1984 that another surrogate test be studied in pilot tests. This test would be for beta-2 microglobulin, a cell surface protein component of the immune system that has been found to be elevated in patients with AIDS. Finally, the study group also recommended that a pilot study be conducted to measure the effectiveness of procedures by which plasma donors could privately indicate that their plasma should not be used in the manufacture of coagulation products.

Pressure to adopt some type of surrogate test may have been temporarily alleviated by the announcement on April 23, 1984, by the Department of Health and Human Services of its claim to identifying the AIDS virus, and its promise that a blood test would become "widely available within about 6 months," which should "identify AIDS victims with essentially 100 percent certainty" (256). Whether or not this expectation will be realized should be known soon.

Pressure to institute some type of laboratory screening test reflects the preoccupation with safety with blood resources, with costs a secondary consideration. This is manifest in the decision by some blood banks and plasma fractionators to use surrogate tests, despite their high "false positive" rates for AIDS, loss of donors, and the increased recruitment effort needed to replace excluded donors. Blood bankers have also noted that costs and benefits must be weighed in the balance and that, moreover, the potential costs of not performing surrogate tests include those associated with the treatment of additional AIDS cases and the potential for lawsuits arising from transfusion associated AIDS.

Assurances of safety from surrogate tests, whatever their validity, can also become factors in competition for patients. For example, an additional reason for San Francisco's Irwin Memorial Blood Bank's adopting the anti-HBc surrogate test was Stanford University Blood Bank's use of another surrogate test, the T-lymphocyte helper: suppressor ratio test. Apparently, the use of a surrogate test by Stanford and not by Irwin was perceived by some patients and doctors as reflecting a "safer" blood source at Stanford (445).

For the longer term, costs may become a more prominent factor in decisions to adopt additional safety measures because of prospective payment systems that are currently being implemented (discussed in a subsequent section of this chapter). Even if a "guaranteed" screening test for AIDS becomes available, the question still remains whether it should be required of every whole blood and plasma collector, or limited to high-risk whole blood collection areas and to plasma supplies, the latter because of the pooling of thousands of units prior to fractionation into coagulation products.

The impact of AIDS has had other effects on the blood supply besides the search for good methods to screen out AIDS. Interest in autologous donations, where a patient banks his/her own blood prior to elective surgery, has increased dramatically. Autologous donations have long been supported by the blood banking community as the safest method of transfusion, and indeed, a substantial portion of requests for autologous transfusions probably originate with physicians rather than patients, since in many institutions physicians must give their written permission for such a request and in many cases must point out to the patient that it is an option (445). Nevertheless, their potential application is limited when contrasted against the total number of transfusions.

Predepositing one's own blood requires knowledge in advance of the nature and extent of the elective surgery anticipated and, furthermore, the patient must be healthy enough to withstand the blood donation process (often entailing the donation of three units of blood in the month prior to surgery). The blood bank, for its part, must be prepared to meet the logistical requirements necessary to make the patient's own blood available at the time of the operation. And even when these steps are successfully undertaken, the process can be undermined should the patient require more blood products than he or she was able to predeposit.

Use of the patient's own blood has also been achieved through means other than deposits in advance. These efforts have primarily been undertaken for those, such as Jehovah's Witnesses, whose religious beliefs preclude them from accepting transfusions of blood products (121). Intraoperative salvage and postoperative collection of shed blood have been used in surgery following traumatic injury and in vascular, cardiac, and orthopedic surgery. Devices have been developed for collecting salvaged blood for reinfusion as whole blood or as "washed" red cells. The AIDS crisis has given new impetus to development of such techniques.

Fear of AIDS has also led to an increasing number of requests for "directed donations"; i.e., the transfusion of blood from specific individuals, usually family members or friends, rather than using a product from a general inventory. Directed donations were the standard mode of operation until technological advances in this century made storage and preservation of blood products possible through maintenance of a constant inventory, and typing and crossmatching of blood enabled safe exchange of blood between strangers with the same blood type. The director of one of the Nation's first blood banks described the importance of these advances in a 1938 article. "The advantage of the 'blood bank' over the previous method is obvious. [It] dispenses with the commotion occasioned by calling to the hospital a horde of excited relatives before a suitable donor can be found" (176).

Today, directed donations are viewed negatively by most blood bankers because of the potential for disruption of the blood collection and distribution system and because of lack of evidence that such donations are indeed safer. Opponents of directed donations have argued against setting up a two-tiered system of blood, one allegedly safer than the other. Furthermore, there has been concern about the effect on the donor pool; will prospective or regular donors refrain from giving in order to be eligible to give should an emergency arise for a friend or family member? Reflecting these concerns, the American Red Cross, AABB, and the Council of Community Blood Centers have issued a joint statement counseling against the establishment of directed donation programs (14) which was echoed by the College of American Pathologists (129) and the American Medical Association (38).

Individual hospitals and blood banks have had to grapple with the question of whether or not to allow requests for directed donations, either as a matter of institutional policy or on an ad hoc basis. Many hospitals have tried to discourage the practice either through scientific or moral suasion or bureaucratic intransigence. However, a few individual blood banks have instituted directed donation programs under pressure from patients, donors, and clinicians (445). In Philadelphia, Thomas Jefferson University's blood bank established a directed donation program at the urging of cardiac surgeons (whose patients commonly receive multiple units of whole blood or red cells).

Irwin Memorial Blood Bank, located in San Francisco, where AIDS has been a particular concern, adopted a program in June 1984 to allow directed donations as a matter of formal institutional policy to be made known to all prospective transfusion recipients. Irwin's somewhat grudging acceptance of the directed donation concept is reflected in its advice to patients and in procedural barriers it erects before allowing such donations to proceed. Patients are advised "that blood from directed (family and friend) donors is *at best no safer* than blood from other volunteer donors (and) there is actually a danger that directed donations may be less safe."

If patients insist on a directed donation, their physician must place the request at least a week prior to the anticipated transfusion and the patient's friend or relative must undergo an initial screening and testing procedure at the cost of an additional $15. If the potential donor passes the screening test, he or she must then return on a separate occasion to actually make the donation. The donor is told of the importance of forthright answers to screening questions and told that if use of the blood turns out not to be warranted for the particular individual, it will be turned over to the general inventory. Designated donors are encouraged to return and donate with no strings attached.

Special concerns about safety have also arisen in the pediatric context, especially with treatment of neonates in the intensive care setting. Blood replacement is a frequent occurrence in this population. In addition to such reasons for transfusions as hemorrhaging, arterial blood gas evaluations and other laboratory tests require the frequent withdrawal of blood for monitoring. Although this may be in small amounts of 5 or 10 ml at a time, in the aggregate it can amount to a significant proportion of the blood volume of tiny neonates. Particularly poignant cases of the deaths of very young children from transfusion-associated AIDS have received a great deal of media attention (325). As mentioned, the response to pediatric AIDS cases is complicated by problems in defining what actually constitutes AIDS in young children because of their naturally immature immune systems.

Some of the parents involved have emerged as articulate proponents of more vigorous donor screening methods, surrogate tests and limiting the number of donors for multiple transfusions when pediatric patients are involved. They have also criticized what they perceive as the dilatory response of the blood banking community (especially the voluntary sector) in adopting screening procedures, and an inadequate and delayed response in funding studies related to transfusion-associated AIDS, especially in pediatrics.

The impetus for directed donations from physicians or patients has also resulted from concerns that whatever the actual risks of contracting AIDS from a blood transfusion may be, the perceived risks may be no less important. A review of the directed donation program at Cedars-Sinai hospital in Los Angeles concluded that "[w]e function with a philosophy that incorporates a concern for the patient's psychological responses to illness, as well as his need for blood. . . . [B]y providing these very frightened patients with the knowledge that the blood to be received is from their chosen donors . . . [we] enhance their general well-being and eventual recovery" (452).

Directed donors have also been described as an additional source of donors; they may not have been active donors in the past. Family and friends can sometimes meet the majority of the patient's need for blood, thereby reducing the demands on the general inventory. And because the patient effectively supplies the donors, there is little or no cost associated with recruitment.

While directed donation programs may not be disruptive if limited to individual blood banks and for individual patients, a more serious case is one in which a donor gives blood but specifies that it may be used only for another member of one's organization. In this case, entire sets of blood might be tied up, which is somewhat reminiscent of the nonreplacement fee or blood credit system—but with the additional feature of restricting physical access to the blood and raising the specter of greatly increased outdating and wastage. According to the administrative director of the Greater New York Blood Center, "If people start to set up separate pools . . ., we'd see little packets of donors and eventually the blood banks would be destroyed" (341).

One example of blood banking's response to such suggestions was triggered when the president of a country club civic association in Long Island, NY, sent a letter soliciting members to join a special blood donor registry so that the risk of contracting AIDS might be reduced by "obtaining blood directly from people you know." When accounts of this effort appeared in the newspapers, local blood banking officials contacted the organizers, concerned about their basic idea of "establishing a registry of 'pedigreed donors' without knowing anything about the donors' actual medical background and history." When representatives of the civic association were given a tour of the local blood bank and apprised of the donor screening policies, they withdrew their suggestion and instead sponsored a conventional blood drive with no strings attached (432).

Directed donations built up around organizations instead of individual patients have great potential for disrupting the present, well-balanced system of blood supplies. In a recent AABB survey on public perceptions of AIDS and the blood supply, the largest percent of those who donated regularly did so to contribute to a company blood drive (33.6 percent)(25). Currently, companies allow employees to donate blood during working hours, and many firms give additional time off as a reward. Thus, the potential is present on the part of the company or even its employees to demand a directed donation program.

Legislators in several States (Florida, Georgia, Kentucky, Washington) have also introduced bills requiring blood banks to accept directed donations, but, in the face of concerted opposition by blood bankers, none of these legislative initiatives has progressed very far. (One related and similarly unsuccessful proposal from a New Jersey State senator would have made it a criminal offense to misrepresent one's health status or membership in a high-risk group.) The development and availability of a specific screening test for AIDS, however, should do much to alleviate the safety concerns that underlie much of the current interest in directed donation programs.

But while awaiting confirmation of the identification of the viral agent associated with the transmission of AIDS and the development of a definitive screening test, there remain a number of practical and ethical questions for blood bankers—and particularly for researchers tracking down the blood connection. Perhaps the most intractable questions involve how to deal with medical information which is riddled with uncertainty or information which fails to point up any possible therapeutic responses. Gerald Sandler of the Red Cross put it this way: "I have had 10 years of explaining tests to people. I want to know how you will deal with those 5 percent of the normal population who will be positive for anti-HBc. . . . How can you convince people that their blood is no good, but they're healthy?"

Questions of confidentiality and the need to balance privacy interests against public health concerns, while not unique to AIDS, are raised in sharper relief than in any other area of medical practice and research. Recent scientific breakthroughs may give these questions a new twist. In May 1984 the Red Cross announced plans to conduct pilot tests of donated blood for antibodies to the HTLV-III virus—the presumed agent of AIDS. Development of such a test carries with it immediate concerns about scale-up and availability, specificity and sensitivity, as well as ethical questions about the use of information revealed by the test. It remains to be seen whether the test will be simple and cheap enough to be readily available on a scale massive enough to obviate questions about who should have priority among potential users. In addition to blood banks generally, blood banks in high-risk areas and commercial plasmapheresis centers, additional millions of potential test users include members of groups at risk of contracting AIDS—male homosexuals, intravenous drug users, and Haitians.

Also unclear are the implications of a positive test. Red Cross officials have predicted that positive findings of an AIDS screening test will be dealt with much as hepatitis B findings have been in the past. Donors who tested positively would be informed by a letter, which would include an offer to make the information available to the donor's physician. The donor's name would then be added to a registry of permanently deferred donors, with the reasons for the deferral encoded in a format strictly limiting their availability. Additional questions arise because in a number of States, AIDS, like some other communicable diseases, must be reported by physicians to public health officials. Should these same reporting requirements apply in similar fashion to positive results of an AIDS test even if it is not a definitive diagnosis of the disease? These are among the issues confronting those who seek to develop, market, and implement an AIDS screening test. When announcing its plans for pilot testing, the Red Cross also stated that it was convening an ethics advisory panel to help sort through this thicket of questions.

Related dilemmas concern how to divulge information uncovered in the course of epidemiological investigations by public health officials. What should high-risk donors be told once they have been implicated in an AIDS case? Should other recipients of blood products from these same high-risk donors be told that they, too, are at risk of contracting AIDS (or as a way to prevent unwarranted fear, should the information be divulged only to their treating physicians)? Local public health officials have shared the names of AIDS victims in high-risk areas with local blood banks, so that it might be confirmed whether or not they donated and, if so, who received their blood products (e.g., the San Francisco Health Department and the Irwin Memorial Blood Bank). (Federal regulations require that records of blood donors who donate products for human use be kept for 5 years.)

Is this practice being conducted with the necessary degree of regard for the protection of patient confidentiality? Should it be expanded in scope? Do the proper authorities have access to names and other patient identifiers? Should social security numbers ever be used in this process? Are public health officials doing enough to assure that AIDS victims have not failed to mention if they were blood or plasma donors, either because they did not recall when and where they donated or because they fear further stigma?

These are representative of the kinds of ethical issues confronting blood bankers, public health officials, and especially researchers. (A task force of the bioethics research group, The Hastings Center, has recently completed a set of guidelines for confidentiality in AIDS research. These guidelines specifically eschew consideration of concerns specific to blood banking. These questions are being addressed by CDC and the National Heart, Lung, and Blood Institute in the course of designing protocols to test research hypotheses.)

Finally, while many areas experienced a decrease in blood donations in 1983, there does not seem to have been major or systematic shortages of blood supplies. The Red Cross, for example, had been experiencing yearly increases in collection of about 5 percent prior to 1983, but in 1983, no increase was noted. However, demand was about equal to supply, and Red Cross analysts noted that supply was dependent on demand, and that most of the decreased demand could be attributed to reduced hospitalization and surgery (302).

This decrease in demand was also noted elsewhere. The Gulf Coast Regional Blood Center reported a 5-percent decrease in red cell use and a 3.5-percent decrease in overall blood component use in 1983 compared to 1982. The single largest contributing factor was a severe economic recession in the gulf coast area, with decreased insurance coverage and elective surgery. But many patients were questioning physicians about transfusions, and AIDS played a large role in reduced use (527). Similar conclusions were made for the hospitals supplied by San Francisco's Irwin Memorial Blood Bank. Hospitals supplied by Irwin transfused 3 percent fewer whole blood and red cells in 1983 than in 1982, and there was no serious problem with supplies even though donations dropped 4.6 percent in the same period.

Some of the decline in demand probably reflected a tendency for patients to postpone elective surgery while the economy was poor. However, the steady decline in red cell use throughout all four quarters of 1983, when the economy was improving, suggests that fear of contracting AIDS may also have been a contributing factor in the decision to postpone surgery and in encouraging physicians to be slightly more conservative when ordering blood for transfusions (445).

PART 2: COORDINATION OF BLOOD RESOURCES

Coordination of blood resources is complicated by the pluralistic system of blood services that has developed in this country since World War II. To date, efforts at coordination have focused on two aspects of blood delivery. One is the coordination of all blood services within a given geographic area; this effort has been termed *regionalization*. The second area of coordination involves providing excess blood to other blood providers who are occasionally or chronically deficient; this phenomenon of cooperation is called *resource sharing*.

Regionalization is not acknowledged by all to be the best approach to managing blood supplies. One of the recurring questions is the benefit gained from participation in the American Blood Commission's regionalization recognition program. Another recurring debate centers on the issue of centralized blood services v. hospital-based services, or some combination of the two. In addition, there are external forces, such as health care cost containment efforts, which are just beginning to have an effect on regionalization efforts.

The need for resource sharing is probably the single aspect of blood delivery which is not seriously debated within the blood services community. Rather, the need for a single resource sharing system has been the issue, given the existence of two parallel, though largely successful, systems—run by the American Association of Blood Banks and the American Red Cross.

Regionalization

Essentially, regionalization is a term used to describe the local coordination of all facilities and organizations involved in blood collection, distribution, or use in a given geographic region. Generally, regionalization includes provisions for cooperation with other regions, thus linking regional blood programs into a national resource sharing program.

Many regions have been able to meet their own blood needs completely, relying exclusively on volunteer donors and satisfying the demand for blood from local practitioners. While some areas of the country are still concerned about meeting local blood needs, other regions are concentrating on the *centralization* of blood services within regions (i.e., the consolidation of small-scale blood banking operations into a central blood center).

On the whole, within any region of the country, a patient who needs blood will receive it, but there still remain the questions of efficiency and cost. There are many groups operating within each region. Should the plurality of the present system be left as is, because it produces acceptable products at a sufficient level, or is there a better organizational framework for the provision of blood products at lower cost?

Since the formation of the American Blood Commission in 1975, the ABC has supported regionalization as the most logical way to improve blood services in the United States. The ABC recognized that there were effective, high-quality, regional blood programs in a few areas of the country, but felt that a national program was needed to improve the fragmented and uncoordinated blood services in other areas. From the start, the ABC regionalization program was conceived and implemented so as to preserve the roles of the many participants in blood banking. It has improved relations in regions in which a strong central blood service needed more formal and effective communications with its clients, and in doing so, maintained the autonomy of all participants with respect to management of the regional blood resources (507). But in less centralized regions, changing the roles of the participants or closing small operations have often been opposed.

Since the ABC has no enforcement mechanism, participation in the regionalization program has always been voluntary. In order to support the regionalization program, the ABC charges application and recertification fees to regions desiring to receive recognition.

The regionalization program sets forth criteria for **regional associations** which distinguishes regional associations from **regional blood programs** and provides a mechanism for areas wishing to be recognized to form such coooperative arrangements. The recognition criteria contain specifications in the following areas:

- governance,
- management,
- donor recruitment,
- inventory control,
- service area,
- interregional relationships, and
- range and quality of services.

For instance, the criteria require that the governance of a **regional association** shall provide for active participation of five interest groups:

1. donors;
2. blood centers, or the facility(ies), in the re-

gion which perform the functions of collections, processing, storage, and distribution of blood;
3. hospital transfusion services;
4. physicians who provide direct patient care; and
5. the patients who receive blood.

Participation by these five groups is in contrast to a **regional blood program**, which usually involves only blood collection and distribution programs and perhaps hospital transfusion services. Participation of all these groups is often considered to be the essential difference between a recognized region and other regional blood programs.

Among other goals, the criteria state that the regional association should take an active role in inventory control and the redistribution of blood according to need within the region, and provide for cooperation with other regions in cases of unexpected need. Also, rather than require a particular approach, the criteria specify that donor recruitment should be philosophically coordinated within a region (i.e., either individual or community responsibility,) so as to prevent donor confusion. The regions are also required to provide a specific range of services within acceptable quality limits (e.g., the provision of a physician available for consultation on difficult blood problems on a 24-hour basis) and to do as much as possible to promote good transfusion medicine (34).

In order for a region to receive official ABC recognition, it must pass through a four-phase application procedure evaluating a variety of operational and organizational criteria. In addition to an application fee of $1,500, regions must supply application materials—including bylaws, financial statements, operating reports, etc.—and host a site visit by members of the ABC regionalization committee. Once recognized, a region must be recertified every 5 years (30).

As of October 1983, the ABC had fully recognized 43 regions, with 29 additional regions somewhere in the application process. These regions are located all across the country, and the ABC estimates that 50 percent of the Nation's blood supply is collected through regions participating in the regionalization program (31b). Despite these accomplishments, however, there are questions as to the need for and the effectiveness of the ABC regionalization program.

Many criticisms of the ABC regionalization program stem from ABC's lack of power. ABC was conceived as a "private sector" organization "charged with carrying out public policy but lacking enforcement powers." The ABC never received a Federal charter. As a result, ABC programs are voluntary, and ABC recognition carries with it no legal status. The fact that "recognition" rather than certification is used to achieve compliance testifies to the difficulties of the ABC as an unofficial body in exerting its influence (601). Nevertheless, the ABC contends that the program provides an incentive to regions who voluntarily choose to regionalize and provides the technical assistance and advice to complete the project successfully.

The New York Blood Center (NYBC), one of the largest blood centers in the country, has opted not to pursue ABC recognition. In 1958, the New York Academy of Medicine Committee on Public Health realized that there were serious deficiencies in the safety of the blood supply and transfusion practices. Foremost among their recommendations were the steps which resulted in the NYBC. Years later, when the ABC was beginning its regionalization program, the NYBC was thriving and chose not to participate.

Few would argue that the NYBC is in any way inferior as a result. However, in 1978, the same committee of the New York Academy of Medicine examined the progress made toward the goals enunciated 20 years earlier. The main problem which remained to be solved was attainment of a good cooperative working relationship between the Blood Center and the hospital transfusion services; hospital blood bank directors felt that they did not have any voice in the operation of the blood center. Despite the appointment of advisory committees to the Blood Center, the NYBC management tended to accept only advice with which it agreed. Thus, hospital blood bank directors felt obliged to form their independent incorporated Council of Blood Bank Directors.

In an attempt to resolve this problem, the same New York Academy of Medicine committee convened a subcommittee to explore the possibilities for developing a regional association more or less in accordance with ABC regionalization recommendations. Over the course of the next year, a compromise proposal, introduced by the representative of Blue Cross/Blue Shield of Greater New York, was finally approved by all participants, excepting the representative of the NYBC. The Blood Center objected to the portion of the proposal which called for a Council with its governance independent of the NYBC. To date, the impasse remains.

In the meantime, the New York Academy of Medicine Committee on Public Health has appointed a subcommittee to observe and report annually; this committee's charge is sufficiently broad to monitor all aspects of blood supply and transfusion services. This situation provides an example of a region which functions effectively in most respects but lacks a mechanism to resolve problems between the blood bank and its users (360).

Further, due to the cumbersome and expensive four-phase application procedure, some regions with strong regional blood programs had little incentive to gain ABC recognition, given the costs and effort required to acquire it. Some strong regional systems, such as the Puget Sound Blood Program, have not seen a need for such formal recognition, while other areas have not applied but have benefited from the information made available through the program and the knowledge gained from activities, successes, and failures of other regions. Because of this latter fact, perhaps the ABC regionalization program deserves more credit than the statistics indicate; and perhaps the program has provided assistance to those who needed it most (517).

Others have criticized the inconsistency with which the ABC confers recognition. For instance, in some places, autonomous functioning of small local blood banks which refused to be integrated into larger regional programs continued, but the regions were "recognized" nevertheless (601). In other areas, regions were allowed to apply for recognition without the participation of many of the users of blood.

In one notable instance, a region was allowed to apply for ABC recognition without the inclusion of the region's major blood supplier, the Red Cross, in the formal regionalization plan. The Washington, DC, Metropolitan Region has largely resolved its blood supply problems. Now, the Red Cross supplies the majority of blood in the area, supplemented by the Metropolitan Washington Blood Bank (MWBB), and some hospitals continue to be largely self-sufficient in the collection and processing of whole blood, red blood cells and platelets, as well as basic laboratory services. Only 2 percent of the area's blood supply is imported from outside the region. Several groups in the Washington area have applied for ABC recognition in an attempt to solve the problem of local coordination, but have reached an impasse as the major area supplier, the Red Cross, sees itself as a successful regional blood program (509).

In other instances, attempts at obtaining ABC recognition have stalled because of continuing territorial battles between blood programs. For instance, both the South Florida Blood Service and the Broward County Blood Center have expressed interest in the ABC regionalization program, but the two blood centers are still in the midst of a dispute over blood collection within Broward County. The competition for donors between the two blood centers has attracted the concern of the community, and efforts are under way to encourage a compromise. As a result, attempts at recognition have been tabled until the dispute is resolved (465;532).

A report completed in 1981 under contract to NHLBI, evaluating the first 2 years of ABC's regionalization program, arrived at a much more positive conclusion. The analysis concluded that the regionalization program did provide incentives to improve, and the associations recognized by the ABC did meet the regionalization criteria, which were consistently and fairly applied. It concluded that the regional associations demonstrated evidence of both interregional resource sharing and regional self-sufficiency, and that "most regional associations include a high proportion of the total number of blood service establishments in the region." Generally, the regions do not conform to political divisions, but rather are built around existing blood center operations. The report also noted that plasmapheresis centers do not participate, although they may conduct substantial operations within a region (32).

Finally, there have been some concerns about possible antitrust allegations of "price-fixing" or "restraint of trade" on the local level as a result of regionalization (364), although there has been no litigation on this issue to date. The problem of antitrust action on a national level as a possible consequence of the Resource Sharing Agreement is currently being addressed by the ABC and its legal counsel. (See subsequent discussion.)

In conclusion, now that supply has been largely stabilized and inventory is not the central concern, efficiency and participation in decisionmaking by more than representatives of blood banks have become primary goals in regionalization efforts. The role of ABC's regionalization program has been to provide the catalyst and information for such regional efforts. It appears that each region will solve its problems on an individual basis, gaining from the experience of other regions and not necessarily pursuing ABC "recognition" as an end in itself.

Resource Sharing

Over the past 30 years, there have been several attempts at interorganizational resource sharing. The first system has operated under the auspices of the AABB since its beginning in 1951 and is called the Clearinghouse Lifeline Program. In essence, the Clearinghouse serves as a facilitator in the exchange of blood or blood credits between blood banks, blood centers, and hospital blood banks or transfusion services. For the most part, the Clearinghouse serves regional blood centers, although it serves any AABB accredited facility which agrees to the conditions of participation, including facilities which are not members of the AABB.

In 1955, the Joint Blood Council, a short-lived group formed by the AABB, American Red Cross, American Medical Association, American Hospital Association, and the Society of Clinical Pathologists, attempted to develop a cooopperative interorganizational reciprocity blood program between the AABB and the ARC. The committee's proposal was never enacted, as the Red Cross representative indicated that the ARC Board of Governors would not approve the plan (18). The Red Cross then instituted its own national reciprocity plan for Red Cross blood centers, the Central Exchange Program, based in Washington, DC.

In 1958, negotiations reopened between the AABB and the ARC in another attempt to reach a sharing agreement. Finally, in 1960, an agreement for an interorganizational reciprocity program was reached between the AABB and the ARC. The agreement became effective May 27, 1961, and the two organizations operated under a series of sharing agreements which differed only in terms of fees, until 1976, when the Red Cross withdrew over concerns about nonreplacement fees. Upon the withdrawal, ARC formalized its sharing program, which acquired the name "Compass."

Most recently, the major collectors of blood in the voluntary sector, and the American Blood Commission, attempted to arrive at a comphrehensive resource sharing agreement. The Resource Sharing Agreement (RSA) was a proposal for a coordinated blood distribution arrangement between the American Blood Commission (ABC), the American Association of Blood Banks (AABB), the Council of Community Blood Centers (CCBC), and the Red Cross.

In late 1979, the Red Cross requested a Business Review from the Department of Justice for the proposed Resource Sharing Agreement (328). The antitrust considerations relevant to the RSA were price-fixing and illegal boycotting. The agreement contained provisions for shipping, processing, and other charges involved in the movement and sale/exchange of blood and blood products. Further, the system included an indemnification account and replacement deposit fee (responsibility fee, or nonreplacement fee). As a result, the Red Cross was concerned that a civil suit might be brought against it.

Representatives of the Justice Department's antitrust division expressed the view that the RSA would not be challenged because it contained no enforcement mechanism for violation of the agreement. Litigation would be difficult, and a plaintiff would be forced to prove a boycott (330).

The boycotting concern was raised by ABRA in a letter from its general counsel to the general counsel of the American Blood Commission. The letter of May 3, 1983, charged that the RSA would implement a group boycott against producers of nonvoluntary blood products (meaning source plasma collected and/or fractionated by ABRA members). ABRA's argument was that as long as the FDA licensed these products, any contract limiting their purchase would be in violation of the antitrust statutes. The February 19, 1982, draft of the RSA stated that "only blood obtained from voluntary donors and labeled in accordance with applicable law will be shipped." The December 15, 1982, draft replaced the volunteer clause with ". . . (blood) procured and processed in conformity with the National Blood Policy . . ." However, ABRA maintained that the National Blood Policy was and is synonymous with volunteer blood and that the result would be the same.

Because of the threat of civil litigation, the Red Cross refrained from joining in the RSA during the May 3, 1983, meeting at which the agreement was to have been signed. The December 1982 draft of the agreement was signed by the ABC, the AABB, and the CCBC but has not been implemented, although individual members of the AABB and the CCBC utilize the Clearinghouse. In addition, the Resource Sharing Council, under the auspices of the ABC, continues to meet in an effort to continue the dialog between the organizations on resource sharing. Despite the Red Cross' decision not to participate, the Resource Sharing Council invited them to attend as observers, if they so desired, but the invitation was declined. Most recently, representatives of the ABC and the CCBC attended a regular meeting of the AABB Clearinghouse committee as observers.

Even without implementation of the Resource Sharing Agreement, and without a single coherent national sharing system, regions with blood shortages are able to meet their needs. Individual blood centers contract with other blood centers outside of the formal mechanisms of the Clearinghouse or the Red Cross, as well as within them. For instance, the South Florida Blood Service (SFBS) has been undergoing a huge transition over the past 5 years in its switch from paid to volunteer donors. As part of the transition, the region began importing exclusively volunteer blood from other regions in order to supplement the growing local collections from volunteer donors.

Over the years, the SFBS has decreased its percentage of imported blood, completely eliminated the use of paid blood, and increased its local collections from volunteer donors. The management of the SFBS managed to meet the region's blood needs through a combination of contracts with both Red Cross centers and independent regional blood centers, use of the AABB Clearinghouse, and supplementation via ad hoc shipments.

In some regions, there are even local clearinghouses which serve functions similar to the AABB's. For instance, the Metropolitan Washington Blood Bank (MWBB) was formed by hospitals over 20 years ago to receive daily inventory reports and to coordinate blood movement between the hospitals. Today, the MWBB continues to serve that function; in addition, it imports needed blood from outside the region and participates in the AABB Clearinghouse. In August 1983, the MWBB, after deciding that the region's blood needs were still not being met locally, as evidenced by the net import of blood into the region, began its own blood collection program. The Metropolitan Washington region continues to be dominated by the American Red Cross, which controls approximately 90 percent of the local blood supply.

American Association of Blood Banks

In 1979, the AABB National Committee on the Clearinghouse developed its current program, whereby blood banks may participate on a blood credit-debit and/or fee-only basis. The Clearinghouse Lifeline Program consists of two alternative plans for members: the Blood Replacement Exchange and the Blood Cooperative Programs.

Participants in the Blood Replacement Exchange Program ship and receive blood under a debit/

credit accounting system, and accept and issue blood credits, if applicable. Routine inventory surpluses and shortages are reported daily to the District Clearinghouses, which match up compatible blood banks for inventory adjustment shipments. Also, members who charge nonreplacement fees may transfer credits through the Clearinghouse. In addition, the resources of the Clearinghouse are available to alleviate emergency shortages. Transactions are settled via monthly statements, which yield a net debit or credit balance owed by the participant. In 1982, 96 percent of the Clearinghouse transactions were through the Exchange Program, as opposed to the Cooperative Program. In the Blood Cooperative Program, blood banks operate on a fee-only basis.

The Clearinghouse also coordinates payment for any exchanged blood or credits. The Clearinghouse charges a $0.40 fee for each transaction to both the shipper and the recipient of the blood (or credits) in order to cover the costs of operating the service (16). Payments for blood are made directly between the shipping and receiving blood banks, although the Clearinghouse maintains records of all transactions and provides monthly statements which summarize the amount of blood credits or money owed by individual participants.

The Clearinghouse sets a standard fee for blood obtained through it, unless both parties to a transaction agree to another fee (usually the slightly higher regular unit charge of the shipping blood center). Transportation costs, as of fiscal year 1984, must be split between the parties of a transaction. This change was instituted by the AABB Board of Directors on the premise that both facilities benefit from the shipment. The shipping bank is able to outlet surplus blood that may otherwise outdate on their shelves, and the receiving bank is able to obtain type-specific blood needed to meet a blood shortage (259). The Clearinghouse will also arrange for long-term inventory shipments to provide assistance to regions who need time to build their donor recruitment programs toward the goal of self-sufficiency.

The Clearinghouse has a national office (relocated from Irwin Memorial Blood Bank, San Francisco, CA, to AABB National Headquarters, Arlington, VA, in June 1984) which oversees five districts/regions covering the whole United States. Requests are first referred to the regional offices, and only referred to the national office if the region is unable to comply with the request. The 1984 American Association of Blood Banks budget allocates $459,000 for operation of the Clearinghouse, including $39,000 for the move of the national office (21).

In addition to coordinating the movement of blood and blood components, the Clearinghouse transfers credits for blood donation between blood banks and between regions where such programs exist. Individuals giving blood in one region may receive credit for their donation in another area of the country, thereby canceling nonreplacement fees for themselves or in the name of another patient. Blood banks settle their accounts in one of two ways, depending on which program they participate in. (All payments for platelets, cryoprecipitate, and fresh-frozen plasma are handled on a cash basis; replacement fees only apply to whole blood or red cells.)

Members of the Blood Replacement Exchange may settle a debit balance by paying a $15 replacement fee per debit or by shipping the appropriate unit(s) of blood. Centers choosing to settle via actual blood shipments also receive $30 compensation per unit from the receiving center for processing expenses, raised from $25 in January 1984 by AABB Board of Directors, effective in May 1984. Conversely, centers with blood credit balances either receive cash compensation (at $15 per credit) or replacement blood shipments (and pay the $30 processing fee). Blood replacement shipments must be type-specific and in the same type proportion as the general population. An approximately equal number of credit balances are settled by replacement blood shipments and cash payments.

Participants in the Blood Cooperative Program may outlet and receive blood and blood components on a fee-only basis (as opposed to maintaining a debit/credit balance sheet) to or from any member of the Clearinghouse. Accounts are settled monthly based on the net total of fees owed. Cooperative banks do not exchange blood credits, but may make a replacement shipment or remit the $15 replacement fee in the name of a specific patient. (Members of the Replacement Exchange Program may accept blood or credit on behalf of a specific patient, but they may not ship blood in the name of a patient, as the mechanism already exists to transfer credit) (16).

In both the Blood Cooperative and Replacement Exchange Programs, blood banks are charged or credited for blood receipt or shipment according to a standard fee schedule set by the AABB Board of Directors. Cooperative members are charged a straight monetary fee according to the applicable fee schedule, while Exchange members are charged/credited according to the current breakdown between replacement and service fees. The Clearinghouse fee schedule covering inventory shipments effective January 1984 is provided in table 35.

In 1983, 47 percent of the transactions coordinated by the Clearinghouse were for actual shipments of blood or blood components. The remaining transactions consisted of issuing and/or transferring blood credits (25 percent) and payment of nonreplacement fees (28 percent). The relative proportions of the different types of transactions have changed very little in recent years [table 36]. Similarly, the volume of blood moved through the Clearinghouse has changed very little over the years, with the most noticeable change occurring in 1977, after the withdrawal of the Red Cross from the Clearinghouse [table 37].

Table 35.—Resource Sharing Inventory Shipment Fees

	Shipment to a cooperative bank	Shipment to an exchange bank	
	Unit fee	Replacement fee	Service fee
Whole blood and red blood cells............	$40.00	$15.00 +	$25.00
Washed and frozen red blood cells............	$65.00	$15.00 +	$50.00
Deglycerolized red blood cells	$90.00	$15.00 +	$75.00
Platelets, cryoprecipitate, or fresh-frozen plasma..	$20.00		$20.00

NOTE: The fee and replacement ratio for other components shipped under the Blood Replacement Exchange are based on mutual agreement between the shipping and receiving blood banks.
SOURCE: AABB, *Guide for the National Clearinghouse Lifeline Program of the American Association of Blood Banks*, July 1984.

Table 36.—AABB Clearinghouse Transactions by Type

Year	Blood shipments	Replacement fees	Credits
1983....	47%	28%	25%
1982....	41	28	31
1981....	38	28	33
1980....	42	24	33
1979....	36	25	33
1978....	33	30	37
1977....	34	29	38
1976[a]...	35	13	52
1975....	33	13	54
1974....	28	12	47
1973....	32	11	56

[a]In late 1976, the American Red Cross withdrew from the Clearinghouse.
SOURCE: AABB Clearinghouse Transaction Reports, 1973-83.

American Red Cross

In addition to the AABB Clearinghouse program, which is available to any user or provider of blood, the Red Cross has its own "Compass" system for resource sharing. Based on past surpluses or shortages, and predictions for future demand, the American Red Cross annually coordinates the exchange of blood between its regions on a contractual basis. The majority of the Red Cross sharing is internal; i.e., between Red Cross regional centers. In addition to contracted exchanges, the Red Cross arranges some sharing on an ad hoc basis, some with blood banks outside of the Red Cross.

Each Red Cross region contracts to buy from or sell to a given center a certain amount of blood on a weekly basis. That blood is committed to the contracted recipient (after the needs of the collecting region are met). Although all contracts are reported and monitored by the American Red Cross Blood Services headquarters, many agreements are initiated and completed directly between the regional centers, without the intervention or assistance of the national office.

For the 1983-84 fiscal year, the Red Cross had contracts with 33 regions for the provision of 6,729 units on a weekly basis (349,908 units annually) to 31 different recipients, both Red Cross regional centers and non-Red Cross blood banks, at a total estimated value of $14.2 million (based

Table 37.—Utilization of AABB Clearinghouse, 1973-83

Year	Shipments of blood and blood components	Percent change previous year	Total transactions	Percent change previous year
1983	278,032 units	+31.6%	587,679	+15.0%
1982	211,296	+22.5	510,853	+13.7
1981	172,426	−15.9	449,397	− 8.0
1980	205,263	+21.0	488,300	+ 4.8
1979	169,668	+ 2.3	466,074	− 5.8
1978	165,905	−11.7	494,982	−10.6
1977	187,930	−28.2	553,859	−25.6
1976	261,696	+11.6	744,583	+ 4.9
1975	234,448	+19.5	709,571	+15.2
1974	196,176	− 5.0	615,915	− 4.5
1973	206,536	—	617,779	—

NOTE: Total number of transactions includes both the Exchange and Cooperative Programs; transactions include shipment of blood (both inventory and replacement), issue of blood credits, payment of nonreplacement fees, and returns (under 1 percent annually).
SOURCE: AABB Clearinghouse Transaction Reports, 1973-83.

on the contracted weekly volume and the fee schedule for whole blood provided by each supplying region). Of the total contracted blood supply, approximately 65 percent, or 4,344 units per week (225,888 units annually at an estimated value of $9.25 million), are committed to 10 other Red Cross regions. Thirty-five percent (124,000 units annually) will be provided to 21 non-Red Cross blood banks.

In addition to the weekly contracts, 20 centers had an additional weekly surplus estimated at 1,500 to 1,700 units, and 5 regions had consistent surpluses (approximately 500 units/week) for which they desired exportation contracts. Both types of noncontracted weekly surpluses amount to approximately 100,000 units annually. These noncontracted surpluses are provided on an ad hoc basis.

Red Cross regional centers report any daily surpluses or shortages to the national headquarters of the American Red Cross Blood Services. If a region needs blood, the American Red Cross will match up a request with a surplus. However, regional centers often know from experience who might have a surplus and will contact another center directly. All blood exchanged through the resource sharing plan is shipped prepaid. All blood is provided at the cost of the processing and no credits for donation or blood replacement are given or exchanged. All fees are paid directly between blood centers; the American Red Cross does not handle any billing or paperwork for exchanges of blood or blood components.

The vast majority of blood or blood components moved through Compass is whole blood or red blood cells, although there is some movement of fresh-frozen plasma and cryoprecipitate, and an increasing demand for platelets. Through both the contracted and ad hoc arrangements, 71,682 units of whole blood, 469,640 units of red blood cells, 43,885 units of platelets, 21,728 units of fresh frozen plasma and 91,805 units of cryoprecipitate were actually moved in 1982-1983 (table 38). These amounts represented a decrease of 3 percent from the 1981-82 movement.

Volume of Sharing

In describing the movement of blood in this country, it is useful to know what proportion of the total blood supply is involved. In 1980, 17.1 million units of blood or blood components were produced in the United States (518). In that year, the AABB Clearinghouse coordinated the movement of 205,263 units of blood or blood components, while the American Red Cross moved 445,433 units, yielding a total of 650,696 units, or 3.8 percent of the total available supply. This percentage represents only those units that were moved through the formal mechanisms of one of the two systems. It is impossible to estimate how much blood is moved on a local level, or through informal networking, locally or long distance. Judging from the existence and expansion of local clearinghouses such as the Metropolitan Washington Blood Banks, and the success of temporary programs such as the informal network of sup-

116 • *Blood Policy and Technology*

Table 38.—Blood and Blood Components Moved by American Red Cross Regional Blood Centers in 1982 and 1983

	Moved in 1983	Moved in 1982	Increase
Whole blood:			
to other RC centers	21,653	45,763	−53%
to blood banks	50,029	73,021	−31%
Total	71,682	118,784	−40%
Red blood cells:			
to other RC centers	318,365	307,992	+ 3%
to blood banks	151,275	137,051	+10%
Total	469,640	445,043	+ 6%
Platelets:			
to other RC centers	24,493	21,742	+13%
to blood banks	19,392	19,018	+ 2%
Total	43,885	40,760	+18%
Fresh-frozen plasma:			
to other RC centers	6,029	8,537	−30%
to blood banks	15,699	18,334	−14%
Total	21,728	26,871	−19%
Cryoprecipitated AHF:			
to other RC centers	74,313	67,068	+11%
to blood banks	17,492	21,995	−20%
Total	91,805	89,063	+ 3%
All blood and blood components:			
to other RC centers	444,853 units	451,102 units	− 1%
to blood banks	253,887	269,419	− 6%
Total	698,740	720,521	− 3%

SOURCE: American Red Cross Blood Services Operating Reports, 1982 and 1983.

port for the South Florida Blood Service, it appears that there is a substantial amount of blood which moves "off the record."

In addition, the charging and payment of nonreplacement fees, and the issue and exchange of blood credits, continue at a strong rate. In 1983, over half of the Clearinghouse transactions were for the exchange or issue of credits (25 percent) or for the payment of nonreplacement fees (28 percent). While the individual responsibility philosophy is not universally accepted, it is still widely used in this country.

The figures of the American Red Cross for the past 5 years indicate an absolute increase in the amount of blood and blood components which were produced but fail to suggest a trend toward or away from increased blood movement (table 39). The lack of a pronounced increase in the percentage of blood moved denies a widening gap between surplus and shortage areas. Similarly, the net volume of blood and blood components moved through the AABB and the ARC has continued to rise (table 40), although the pattern

Table 39.—Movement of Blood and Components Through the American Red Cross, 1979-83

Year	Volume moved through ARC	Total production by ARC	Percent total production moved
1983	698,740 units	14,331,858 units	4.9%
1982	720,521	13,045,189	5.5
1981	562,431	12,052,017	4.7
1980	445,433	11,233,274	4.0
1979	332,971	10,465,129	3.2

SOURCE: American Red Cross Blood Services Operating Reports, 1980-83.

seems to reflect the influence of variables such as the change in number of members in the Clearinghouse, and the amount of sharing arranged outside of either formal network, rather than an increasing demand for imported blood within deficient regions.

Conclusion

The blood collection organizations are largely in agreement about the need for resource sharing. The current lack of cooperation between the AABB and the Red Cross appears to be due to concerns about antitrust violations. There is lit-

Table 40.—Total Movement of Blood and Blood Components in the United States, 1979-83 (including both the AABB and the American Red Cross)

Year	Clearinghouse	Red Cross	Total	Percent change from previous year
1983	278,032 units	698,740 units	976,772 units	+ 4.8%
1982	211,296	720,521	931,817	+26.8
1981	172,426	562,431	734,857	+12.9
1980	205,263	445,433	650,696	+29.5
1979	169,668	332,971	502,639	NA

SOURCE: AABB Clearinghouse Transaction Reports, 1979-83; and American Red Cross Blood Services Operating Reports, 1980-83.

tle evidence to support the notion that the Red Cross, or any of the other blood collecting organizations, sought to block the most recent resource sharing agreement in hopes of retaining organizational control over its blood supply. Concerns about nonreplacement fees remain to a lesser extent but are superseded by concerns for a well-managed blood supply. The nonreplacement fee continues to be supported for recruitment reasons in selected areas of the country; in other areas, the fee is adamantly opposed. The trend, however, is away from the nonreplacement fee, and it will likely become a nonissue in terms of logistics and sharing of blood resources. The philosophical objections to cooperating with organizations operating under different recruitment strategies have subsided.

Even without a single coherent national sharing system or the implementation of the Resource Sharing Agreement (the one attempt at formalized resource sharing between the major organizations in the voluntary sector: the AABB, ABC, CCBC and the ARC), regions with blood shortages are generally able to meet their needs, either through long-term contracts for blood provision or ad hoc arrangements to compensate for unexpected demand or shortages. Individual blood centers often contract with other blood centers outside of the formal mechanisms of the Clearinghouse or the Red Cross, as well as within them. For instance, in 1983, the South Florida Blood Service received 70 percent of its imported blood through long-term contracts, 21 percent through ad hoc arrangements, and only 9 percent through the formal mechanisms of the Clearinghouse.

Contrary to the situation in past years, the supply of blood in the United States is no longer a critical concern. Blood is managed and shared effectively, as witnessed by low outdate rates and consistent interregional movement of blood. Efforts at coordination by the private sector have been largely successful.

On the local level, many areas have coordinated their blood services, either through the ABC Regionalization Program or through individualized approaches. In the remaining areas, discussion has at least been initiated on the means for regional coordination. Nationally, the two voluntary sharing systems provide an effective means for moving blood from "place of plenty" to "place of need." In addition, blood bankers are predisposed toward assisting in times of blood supply emergencies and temporary shortages, so many ad hoc arrangements are made between individual blood service facilities. Thus, the combination of formal and informal sharing works, though it might be more efficient in individual instances.

PART 3: IMPACT OF HEALTH CARE COST CONTAINMENT

The rising cost of health care has been a persistent and growing problem for a number of years. In the past several years, a number of cost containment efforts have been adopted; for example, greater use of health maintenance organizations and home health care services and more extensive coinsurance requirements. Perhaps the most far-reaching effort at health care cost containment was Medicare's introduction in October 1983 of a new system for hospital reimbursement based on a prospective per-case payment using diagnosis-related groups (DRGs). Under this form of payment, hospitals will be paid a specific amount for each patient treated in a particular group, regardless of the number or types of services provided.

Until October 1983, Medicare employed a retrospective cost-based reimbursement approach whereby hospitals could recover from Medicare most of what they spent for Medicare beneficiaries. Any costs incurred in treating Medicare patients, including costs of blood products, were effectively "passed through" to Medicare (or to patients and any other insurance they may have had). Similar cost-based reimbursement systems covered many non-Medicare patients. There was little incentive for hospitals to control costs. Under the new system, however, hospitals will be rewarded for reducing the cost of treating a patient over the entire course of the hospital stay. The new system is likely to have an effect that reaches far beyond the Medicare system if it is adopted by other third-party payers. Per-case payment encourages the hospital and its physicians to consider explicitly the benefits of any services against their added costs. Thus, Medicare's prospective payment system is likely to affect all health care suppliers, including the blood services complex.

Per-case payment systems such as DRGs provide a number of incentives to hospitals which are not present under cost-based systems. Two general incentives to hospitals in any per-case payment system are: 1) to reduce the cost to hospitals of each inpatient stay, and 2) to increase the number of inpatient admissions. Cost per case can be reduced by decreasing the number of inpatient days, but it can also be reduced by using fewer technological services or attempting to provide them at lower cost. In addition, because outpatient care is excluded from the current DRG system, hospitals may be encouraged to arrange to provide more services, including ancillary services, on an outpatient basis. Finally, hospitals may seek to increase profitable admissions by manipulating case load.

The direction and strength of these incentives for any particular hospital will be altered by key features of the DRG payment system (e.g., the proportion of the hospital's case load covered by DRG payment, the treatment of costs as passthroughs), as well as by other system constraints (e.g., physicians' incentives to practice high-quality medicine, community pressure to provide certain services), so that specific outcomes of implementing the DRG system for any part of the health care system, including blood services, are difficult to predict.

One result of hospital efforts to contain costs that is already being felt by some blood suppliers is a tendency for transfusion services to "shop around" for blood products. Although there are some indications of product preference (e.g., 308), the safety and efficacy of blood products are for the most part standardized. Thus, the only factors differentiating blood products are cost and availability. As shown in chapter 3, fees for blood services vary widely among blood suppliers; thus, it is possible for blood users to compare costs. The use of preservative systems for blood components, and the computerized communications systems now in place, make availability less of a problem, except perhaps for components with short shelf lives, such as platelets.

Assuming that availability needs can be met, comparative shopping may lead to increased use of the AABB Clearinghouse, greater price competition among blood suppliers, and a breakdown of regionalization programs (383). At a minimum, competition should result in more contract negotiation between blood suppliers and transfusion services. In the long run, the result could be either lower prices across the Nation or more negotiation about prices among blood suppliers—resulting, perhaps, in a standard price for blood products. DRGs may have little effect on the plasma derivatives market, which is already highly competitive (see ch. 3).

One manifestation of hospitals' comparative shopping on the basis of price may be increasing questioning of the cost structure of blood suppliers' processing fees. As discussed in chapter 3, blood suppliers have not devised a uniform industrywide system to account for the costs of their blood products. Blood suppliers have recently experienced steady increases in the excess of revenues over expenses, often attributing such increases to needs for capital expansion or research. Where competition is not a viable option, hospitals may exert pressure on blood suppliers to bring down costs by limiting or seeking other avenues for funding research projects or capital expansion. Demands for price concessions may have particular adverse effects on independent (i.e., non-Red Cross) blood centers which have built part of their reputations on research.

DRGs are most likely to have the effect of revitalizing hospital transfusion and pharmacy committees' monitoring of physicians' use of blood products. This effect may not be limited to the whole blood sector. In general, hospital utilization reviews and quality audits are likely to increase under DRGs (550). As discussed in part 4 of this chapter, the appropriate use of blood products has been a topic of concern, primarily because of safety considerations, but sometimes (e.g., albumin), for reasons of cost. The implementation of DRGs will give hospitals both an added incentive to monitor individual physicians' use of blood products and a systematic means for monitoring hospitalwide use. The implementation of DRGs is expected to increase the reliability of patient discharge data, because payment will rely on the accuracy and timeliness of discharge abstracts (550). It will also provide a systematic way to match blood use to specific diagnoses, an area in which national blood data are particularly lacking.

Methods to correlate patient outcome with aspects of hospital care are also being devised (551), and these may be useful for studies of efficacy of blood components. Studies of the relationships between use and patient outcome will be important because utilization reviews have often focused on cost containment to the exclusion of concerns about quality of care (545), although such studies will add to administrative costs.

The cost of blood products may come to affect hospitals' case mix, and as a result, blood suppliers' production schedules. There is speculation that for certain patients (e.g., post-heart surgery, post-vascular surgery, oncology patients), DRG allocations may be depleted on blood demands alone (see, e.g., 12). For example, in a bleeding patient the cost of platelet concentrates alone may be as high as $360 for 1 day. Under the DRG system, hospitals may become more specialized in their care, treating only certain groups of patients. Presumably, the rise of specialized care centers will make for more rational adjustments in per-case reimbursement rates, rather than affecting patient access to care—although this may be a short-term effect. Patients may have to travel farther to specialized care centers.

The net long-term effect of these changes may benefit patients, assuming the appropriate adjustments in DRG reimbursement rates are made so that specialized care hospitals are not adversely affected by serving large-volume blood users. Recent research has shown that patients treated in hospitals serving large numbers of specific diagnoses have better outcomes (188). Blood suppliers, however, may have to adjust collection and production schedules as client hospitals change their case load mix. For example, regions with transplant centers may require increased donations.

It is difficult to determine whether DRGs will affect the present balance between hospital blood bank and community blood center collections. Community blood centers have come to dominate blood collections (see ch. 3). There is speculation, however, that hospitals may set up their own donor rooms in an attempt to contain and control costs of blood services. Although the question of economies of scale in community blood centers remains open, it is doubtful whether hospitals would enjoy any economies of scale from collecting and processing their own blood products. For example, Wallace and Wallace/ABC (576) found that collecting hospitals charged more for blood (although it is difficult to determine whether higher charges actually reflected higher costs of collection).

Small-volume hospitals would find it particularly difficult to maintain the necessary levels of expertise in donor recruitment, collection, and processing, in addition to being unable to make the necessary space available. What may happen is that a selected number of highly specialized hospitals may begin to provide for their own special needs (e.g., for platelets and granulocytes from pheresis; see 372). Because outpatient services do not currently come under DRG regulations, DRGs may temporarily favor transfusion services that are independent blood centers. For example, all Red Cross blood services have applied for Medicare provider certification.

The extent to which blood centers will be able to be reimbursed as Medicare providers is limited, however. The Health Care Financing Administration (HCFA) recently rescinded the Medicare provider certification of a blood bank, noting that, "as the law now stands, a blood bank cannot be paid directly for services it renders" (412). The intermediary had originally considered the blood bank in question as eligible for direct Medicare payment on the assumption that the blood bank would be considered a physician-directed clinic. According to HCFA, under current law the blood bank is only allowed to bill for physicians whom the blood bank employs or has a contractual arrangement with, and who administer blood, but not for services rendered by paramedical personnel.

Similarly, HCFA refused to make an exception to the Medicare provision limiting therapeutic apheresis procedures to inpatient or outpatient settings (172). The blood bank in question wanted to be granted an exception on the basis that it was a physician-directed clinic. Thus, a move by blood centers to be considered comparable with outpatient units and increase their service base, as well as help hospitals take advantage of anomalies in the current reimbursement system, may meet resistance from HCFA. It is expected that eventually outpatient care will also be covered by a prospective payment system.

Multi-hospital chains, both profit and nonprofit, are another response to government scrutiny of health care costs. Such chains are believed to provide more efficient management (98). There was some speculation that multi-hospital chains might find it in their interest to take over functions such as blood services, but apparently blood services were not considered profitable enough to get involved in (270), and blood collection and distribution will be left to the largely not-for-profit sector.

Apart from DRGs, private efforts at cost containment may result in changes in the blood services system, such as an increase in the use of nonreplacement fees, or similar credits applicable to processing fees. Self-insurers (and participants in corporate donor programs), such as Wells Fargo Bank in California, have expressed concern that the cost of blood may be inordinately high because donors effectively subsidize nondonors (259). It may be that such corporations will request some form of credit for their employees in exchange for holding mobile collection drives.

To summarize, the effects of DRGs and other cost containment efforts are difficult to predict. A special commission has been established to monitor the effects of the DRG system and devise necessary modifications. Health care providers, including those in the blood services complex, are watching and hoping to influence developments in the Medicare reimbursement system (e.g., 24). It is unlikely that there will be a significant change in the organizational structure of blood collections—i.e., blood center collections should continue to predominate and perhaps increase their influence. However, hospitals may exert pressure on blood collectors to reduce charges for blood products, and blood centers in some areas may have to change their product mix. The greatest impact of DRGs may be on the ability of independent blood centers to conduct research and expand their facilities. DRGs will certainly provide an opportunity for more stringent monitoring of blood product utilization.

PART 4: APPROPRIATE USE OF BLOOD PRODUCTS

Introduction

Both blood suppliers and users agree that blood is overused and used inappropriately, but they differ about the extent to which it is misused and about the means to promote more appropriate use. Estimates of the amount of blood products which are inappropriately used are high: 20 to 25 percent for red cells (204); up to 90 percent for albumin (8); and 95 percent for fresh-frozen plasma (457). However, data by which to evaluate the overall appropriate use of blood products do not exist, in many cases because of lack of scientific precision concerning when a component or derivative should be administered.

In addition, while some data exist on the number of patients transfused with particular blood products (e.g., 518), national data on the reasons why transfusions were given are harder to come by. Studies such as Friedman's (204) of the diagnostic categories for which red cells were transfused (as well as the relationship between such transfusions and geographic location, patient age and gender) have not been conducted for other blood products.

Perhaps as important as overall trends in the use of blood products are instances of bad transfusion practice which are believed to occur (19). As with appropriate use, national data on the extent of such bad practices do not exist.

What is known is that there are wide geographic variations in the rate of transfusions. For example, transfusion rates for red cells and whole blood varied from a high of 15.3 patients per thousand population in the Mid-Atlantic States to 12.9 per thousand population in the Mountain States. Hospitals in the New England region transfused 50 units of red cells per thousand population, compared to only 36 units per thousand population in the Mountain States (518). The reasons for these variations are not known. Although general guidelines exist (e.g., 17), in many cases transfusion decisions, like many other medical decisions, rely on clinical judgment. In addition, handbooks widely used by physicians (e.g., 425) may contain information which is inconsistent with guidelines written by experts in transfusion. There are wide variations across the United States in other areas of medical practice, such as lengths of hospital stays, that are not adequately explained by demographic differences or differences in health outcomes (553).

Concerns over misuse have focused on different blood products over time. Initially, questions centered on the widespread practice of infusing whole blood instead of packed red cells. Current questions involve albumin solutions, fresh-frozen and single-donor plasma. For example, a National Institutes of Health Consensus Development Workshop on fresh-frozen plasma indications and risks was held in September 1984.

Whole Blood

Whole blood transfusions decreased from 67.4 percent of total blood component transfusions in 1971 to 13.0 percent in 1980, and from 78 percent of transfusions involving red cells to 19 percent (see fig. 6 in ch. 3). More recent nationwide information on transfusions is not available, but Red Cross data indicate that production of units of whole blood continues to decrease: by 12.2 percent between 1980 and 1981; by 11.6 percent between 1981 and 1982, and by 20.7 percent between 1982 and 1983. For the year ended June 30, 1983, only 893,791 units of whole blood were produced in the Red Cross system, compared to 5,328,403 units of red cells.

In addition to the normal range of transfusion hazards, risks specific to the use of whole blood are circulatory overload as a result of rapid and excessive infusion, and immunization to platelets and granulocytes. Circulatory overload can result in pulmonary edema and congestive heart failure, especially in patients whose cardiovascular status is precarious or compromised (273,388). Transfusions of whole blood are also viewed as not cost effective. Two or more components can be made from every unit of whole blood. Recovered or salvaged plasma can be sold by the blood center for additional revenue.

For some physicians, the only valid indication for the use of whole blood is when a patient needs red blood cells and plasma simultaneously; i.e., for the active, massively bleeding patient (e.g., some surgical procedures and major trauma with continuing hemorrhage) (407,500). Others (e.g., 395) see no need for either fresh or stored whole blood in clinical practice, and believe that all uses of whole blood should be replaced by a "three-tiered" combination of: 1) volume expansion with a fluid; 2) red blood cell replacement; and 3) replacement of clotting factors, if necessary.

There are also different guidelines on the percentage of blood loss indicative of transfusion with either whole blood or a combination of other components (e.g., 17,500); the type of fluid replacement to use if whole blood is not used (see discussion of albumin below); and the amount of whole blood to transfuse, in particular the requirement for a single unit of whole blood (e.g., 202,369).

Aside from the misuse of whole blood to restore volume and oxygen-carrying capacity, whole blood is also believed to be transfused inappropriately when used to provide "general support," to treat hypoproteinemia with some degree of concomitant anemia, or to prepare a nutritionally deficient patient for some form of stressful treatment. According to one textbook of transfusion medicine, the latter represent "serious misconceptions about the efficacy of blood transfusion, the dynamics of blood cell protein turnover in disease and malnutrition, the optimal management of the undernourished patient, and even more serious misconceptions about the risks of transfusion." In addition, transfusion to promote wound healing is "usually a florid example of poor medical practice" (407). The idea that whole blood is preferable to other blood products because it contains all components is also believed to be mistaken. Whole blood stored over 24 hours contains few viable platelets and granulocytes, and levels of Factors V and VIII are reduced (17).

Red Cell Concentrates

Red cell concentrates are seen as preferable to whole blood in many instances, because red cells have the same oxygen-carrying capacity as whole blood, but are without some of its dangers. Risk of circulatory overload is reduced, as are risks of citrate and ammonia intoxication; metabolic acidosis; acid/base imbalance; and some forms of allergic and febrile reactions (369). Another important clinical advantage of red cell concentrates is their use in situations where donor blood identical with the recipient's ABO type is unavailable, and use of the universal type O is indicated (407). In such circumstances, the use of whole blood has the risk of infusion of large amounts of donor plasma containing antibodies directed against red blood cells, which may result in severe hemolytic transfusion reactions (171). In addition, a volume of red cells provides twice the increment in hematocrit as does infusion of an equal volume of whole blood (17). However, red cell concentrates carry all the infectious risks of whole blood, and the use of multiple components exposes the patient to multiple risks of hepatitis (17).

Use of red cell concentrates has been found to vary considerably by geographic location, age, gender, operative status (i.e., operated v. nonoperated), diagnostic category, and even by month of transfusion (see 202,203,204; and, for a more limited analysis, 518). In studies of 1974 and 1977 hospital data, Friedman and his associates found that women, particularly surgical patients, receive more red cell transfusions than men do, apparently because of their lower hematocrit levels (204). However, for all diagnostic groups except one, males received a higher mean amount of units.

Not surprisingly, surgical patients were transfused more often than nonoperated patients, and older patients more than younger patients. Patients over 65 years of age constituted 44.3 percent of transfused patients, and received 43.7 percent of all units transfused (204). The major disease categories accounting for most units transfused in Friedman's study of 1977 data were malignant neoplasms, cardiovascular disease, nonmalignant diseases of the gastrointestinal tract, fractures and traumatic injury, and anemia (see table 41). The largest single group of units transfused were those transfused to operated males for cardiovascular disease, which Friedman, et al., attributed to coronary bypass surgery.

Table 41.—Blood Utilization by Major Disease Categories Ranked by Total Units Transfused and Percent of Units Transfused: Operated Males, Nonoperated Males, Operated Females, Nonoperated Females, and All Patients in Each Category

Major disease category	Operated males Total units transfused	Operated males % of units transfused to all patients	Nonoperated males Total units transfused	Nonoperated males % of units transfused to all patients	Operated females Total units transfused	Operated females % of units transfused to all patients	Nonoperated females Total units transfused	Nonoperated females % of units transfused to all patients	All patients Total units transfused	All patients % of units transfused to all patients
1. Malignant neoplasm	10,166	5.7	6,687	3.8	9,516	5.4	6,728	3.8	33,097	18.7
2. Cardiovascular disease including cerebrovascular disease	14,957	8.4	2,792	1.6	7,217	4.1	3,678	2.1	28,644	16.1
3. Nonmalignant disease of the gastrointestinal tract	5,807	3.3	8,947	5.0	5,415	3.1	7,607	4.3	27,776	15.7
4. Fractures and traumatic injury including soft tissue injury	9,946	5.6	889	0.5	9,570	5.4	892	0.5	21,298	12.0
5. Anemia including acute hemorrhagic, hemophilia, and other diseases of the hematopoietic system	447	0.3	3,383	1.9	673	0.4	4,750	2.7	9,253	5.2
6. Obstetrical procedures and complications	0	0	0	0	6,392	3.6	1,289	0.7	7,681	4.3
7. Bone and joint disease excluding fractures	2,134	1.2	157	0.1	3,421	1.9	423	0.2	6,135	3.5
8. Disease of respiratory tract and lungs	1,386	0.8	1,605	0.9	776	0.4	1,275	0.7	5,042	2.8
9. Liver disease, portal hypertension, and esophageal varices	1,352	0.8	1,692	1.0	519	0.3	1,234	0.7	4,797	2.7
10. Disease of the kidney, urinary bladder, and urethra	1,501	0.8	882	0.5	1,389	0.8	953	0.5	4,725	2.7
11. Nonmalignant gynecologic disease including uterine leiomyomas and breast disease	8	0.005	0	0	4,230	2.4	416	0.2	4,654	2.6
12. Complications of surgery and medical care	1,171	0.7	200	0.1	1,276	0.7	201	0.1	2,848	1.6
13. Perinatal conditions	497	0.3	1,002	0.6	348	0.2	854	0.5	2,701	1.5
14. Benign tumors excluding uterine leiomyomas	390	0.2	16	0.01	2,164	1.2	116	0.1	2,686	1.5
15. Gall bladder and bile duct disease	778	0.4	72	0.04	1,207	0.7	109	0.1	2,166	1.2
16. Disease of prostate gland and other male genital organs	1,925	1.1	125	0.1	0	0	0	0	2,050	1.2
17. Nutritional, congenital, and metabolic disease	670	0.4	151	0.1	691	0.4	237	0.1	1,749	1.0
18. Disease of skin, soft tissue, connective tissue, and muscle, excluding traumatic injury	436	0.2	124	0.1	670	0.4	269	0.2	1,499	0.8
19. Infectious disease including viral hepatitis	257	0.1	455	0.3	307	0.2	377	0.2	1,396	0.8
20. Hernias	505	0.3	106	0.1	397	0.2	168	0.1	1,176	0.7
21. Diabetes mellitus including complications	300	0.2	122	0.1	414	0.2	299	0.2	1,135	0.6
22. Disease of the pancreas	352	0.2	138	0.1	173	0.1	112	0.1	775	0.4
23. Disorders of central and peripheral nervous system excluding vascular and psychiatric disease	161	0.1	112	0.1	185	0.1	199	0.1	657	0.4
24. Disorders of fluid, electrolyte, and acid-base balance	25	0.01	127	0.1	59	0.03	190	0.1	401	0.2
25. Disease of endocrine glands other than pancreas	135	0.1	27	0.02	69	0.04	82	0.05	313	0.2
26. Disease of the eye and ear	22	0.01	52	0.03	38	0.02	59	0.03	171	0.1
Totals (this table)	55,328	31.2	29,863	16.8	57,116	32.2	32,517	18.3	174,824	98.5
Miscellaneous (no category assigned)	368	0.2	724	0.4	529	0.3	953	0.5	2,574	1.5
Totals (all patients)	55,696	31.4	30,587	17.2	57,645	32.5	33,470	18.9	177,398	100.0

SOURCE: B. A. Friedman, T. L. Burns, and M. A. Schork, A Study of National Trends in Transfusion Practice, 1980.

Stored red cells, whether packed or in whole blood, do not contain functional platelets or granulocytes. However, the nonfunctional platelets and granulocytes contained in red cell concentrates (and whole blood) can result in alloimmunization. Thus, for patients who have already indicated reactions to transfusions—in particular, urticarial reactions—or for patients likely to be receiving frequent transfusions, washed or, less frequently, frozen-thawed-deglycerolized red cells are indicated (17). These prepared components are 1.5 to 3.5 times as expensive as unprocessed red cells. They account for very little of total red cell production. In the Red Cross only 46,802 units of frozen red cells and 50,952 units of washed red cells were produced in 1983.

A major textbook of transfusion medicine notes that: "Despite a large and longstanding experience, the indications for transfusion of red blood cell products are not always easy to delineate." There is a wide variety of available transfusion products, wide variation in the homeostatic capabilities of patients, and a multiplicity of clinical situations. Thus, while providing some general principles, the textbook suggests that "rules of thumb about when to transfuse, optimal hematocrit levels, and other such notions are unrealistic" (407). Others (e.g., 201) suggest that more objective clinical criteria for blood transfusion can and should be developed.

One of the most controversial areas concerning red cells is the matter of the "transfusion trigger," or the hemoglobin level which indicates to physicians that a patient will be injured by oxygen deprivation, requiring a transfusion of red cells. Patients vary considerably in their tolerance of anemia. For example, women naturally have lower hematocrits than men, but surgeons appear to use the same support and ceiling hematocrit levels to regulate blood transfusion for both genders (202). Similar practices exist for patients in diagnostic categories such as chronic renal failure and chronic obstructive pulmonary disease (232). A hemoglobin of less than 10 g/dl has been the traditional "transfusion trigger" most often used by physicians (204).

Recently, alternatives have been suggested. While clinical judgment of the patient's condition is suggested most often (e.g., 17,407), Gould (232) suggests combining clinical status with an evaluation of a patient's ratio of oxygen consumption to oxygen delivery ("oxygen extraction ratio" or ER) rather than a hemoglobin count.

Red cells are sometimes used instead of a more appropriate nonblood therapy. For example, Friedman and his associates found that iron deficiency anemia was the fifth leading blood-user diagnosis group in the United States among nonsurgical patients (204). This condition rarely warrants blood transfusion (201). Rather, it is treatable with dietary change or iron supplements.

Platelets

Patients most likely to require platelet transfusions are those suffering from malignancies involving the bone marrow (e.g., leukemia and lymphoma), those suffering from bone marrow depression as a result of chemotherapy, drugs, infection or other causes (e.g., 481), and those suffering from drug-induced thrombocytopenia (platelet loss). Deaths due to leukemia have significantly declined since the introduction of platelet therapy. Surgical patients suffering from thrombocytopenia may also require platelet transfusions (199,533).

The risk of hepatitis and other transmissible infectious diseases from platelets is the same as for whole blood. As with whole blood transfusions, circulatory overload can occur, especially in children. In addition, because platelets are stored at room temperature, the risk of bacterial growth is greater than that of whole blood. Risks specific to random-donor platelet transfusions include alloimmunization resulting in a refractory state, transfusion reactions as a result of incompatibility between antibodies in the platelet concentrate and red blood cell antigens of the recipient, and graft v. host disease as a result of the collection of lymphocytes along with the platelets. When sensitivities develop, single-donor transfusions are substituted for random-donor platelet concentrates, although these are not without their problems (533).

It is generally recognized that there are large gaps in knowledge of the proper use of platelets (481). There is general agreement that platelet transfusions are of limited benefit in patients suffering from idiopathic thrombocytopenic purpura and other forms of rapid platelet destruction (264,533). There are different opinions concerning the use of platelet transfusions when other forms of platelet dysfunction (thrombocytopathy) are present. For example, the AABB Physicians Handbook indicates that platelet transfusions are indicated for thrombocytopathy. Daly (145) indicates that such transfusions are rarely necessary.

As with other components, the proper dosage of platelets is a matter of unresolved clinical concern. Aster (55) notes that treating the "platelet count" rather than the patient may result in waste. Other questionable uses of platelets are for open heart surgery, irrespective of a patient's own platelet level and clinical status (on the assumption that a qualitative platelet defect exists), and in patients who develop a hemorrhagic diathesis after renal transplantation (55).

Most significantly, some question the prophylactic use of platelets in patients with malignancies. Clinical trials investigating this question have led to different conclusions (481); another clinical trial is currently under way (533). The resolution of this question will have a major effect on the blood supply and economics of blood services (520).

Granulocytes

Granulocyte transfusions may be indicated for patients who have an inadequate supply of white cells (granulocytopenia) and a life-threatening infection which is unresponsive to antibiotics. Candidates for granulocyte transfusions include patients with acute leukemia, aplastic anemia, solid tumors and auto-immune diseases, and transplant recipients. Granulocytopenia can result from chemotherapy or primary bone marrow depression.

Granulocyte transfusions carry the same risks of infectious disease as whole blood. In addition, immunosuppressed or immunodeficient recipients may be at risk of developing graft v. host reactions. Allergic, febrile or hemolytic reactions, HLA and red cell antigen immunization, and severe pulmonary insufficiency can occur (17, 369). Granulocyte transfusions are expensive because of the complexities of cell procurement, storage and administration and the requirement for close day-to-day cooperation between clinicians and the transfusion service. For example, granulocytes must be obtained, crossmatched, and administered within 24 hours of donation, putting enormous pressure on blood banks and transfusion services. Granulocyte donors may be particularly at risk because granulocytes must be obtained via pheresis and alloimmunized patients may rely on a small pool of donors.

Indications for use of granulocytes are perhaps the least clear of all the components, with the exception of fresh-frozen plasma (199,481). As a result of several clinical investigations, including clinical trials (e.g., 191,482,590), the prophylactic use of granulocyte transfusion has been judged to be of questionable therapeutic value, at a minimum (17). Some say the use of prophylactic granulocytes should be considered a strictly investigational procedure not to be utilized outside of research settings (e.g., 481). The therapeutic value of granulocytes has been difficult to judge because of the seriously compromised clinical status of candidates for granulocyte transfusions (e.g., 190). The use of granulocyte transfusions has been declining nationwide. In general their use to combat infections seems to be a therapy of last resort.

Cryoprecipitate

Cryoprecipitate contains large amounts of Factor VIII and von Willebrand's factor, in addition to concentrated amounts of fibrinogen, fibronectin, and Factor XIII. The major clinical disadvantage of cryoprecipitate is the individual variation in Factor VIII from bag to bag, resulting in unpredictability of the required therapeutic dose (397). Cryoprecipitate has all the infectious risk factors of whole blood. Other risks include febrile and allergic reactions, and hemolysis as a consequence of incompatibility between antibodies in cryoprecipitated AHF and antigens of recipient red blood cells.

Indications for cryoprecipitate vary. It is recommended for the treatment of Hemophilia A and von Willebrand's disease, congenital fibrinogen deficiency, and other conditions associated with consumption of fibrinogen (e.g., obstetrical complications, disseminated intravascular coagulation) and Factor XIII deficiency (e.g., 17,282). Others do not mention Factor XIII deficiency (369). The most recent use of cryoprecipitate has been for fibronectin replacement in infection or shock. This use has been questioned, because clinical indications have not been adequately tested, and administration of excess fibronectin may be harmful to the recipient (497).

The major controversy surrounding the use of cryoprecipitate is its use in preference to lyophilized Factor VIII concentrate. Preparation of cryoprecipitate is a labor-intensive process. Administration is more difficult because, unlike lyophilized Factor VIII, cryoprecipitate must remain frozen to retain its therapeutic value. As already noted, the Factor VIII content of cryoprecipitate varies from unit to unit and is largely unknown. While the conventional wisdom is that cryoprecipitate is less likely to transmit infectious disease because fewer donors are involved, in fact a severe hemophiliac treated with cryoprecipitate would be exposed to 500 to 1,000 donors a year. If one of the units is contaminated with a low-prevalence virus, the hemophiliac receives all of it. In a commercial pool, a low-prevalence virus would be diluted and might be inactivated by antibody in the pool.

Fresh-Frozen and Single-Donor Plasma

Single-donor plasma, fresh-frozen (usually called fresh-frozen plasma, or FFP) contains all the coagulation factors found in native plasma. Single-donor plasma (not frozen) contains all of the stable coagulation factors but reduced levels of the labile coagulation Factors V and VIII. Both fresh-frozen and single-donor plasma have all the risks of infectious disease that whole blood has, as well as the risk of allergic or febrile reactions and incompatibility between plasma antibodies and recipient red cell antigens. Transfusion of plasma to correct for coagulation deficiencies carries with it the risk of fluid overload (17).

The dramatic increase in the use of fresh-frozen plasma over the last decade has prompted concerns that the uses of it "are often vague and without scientific basis," and that it is "likely that other products are available that are equally effective as and safer than fresh-frozen plasma" (567). Most FFP is administered as replacement for deficient coagulation factors in postoperative patients and in a variety of medical bleeding disorders. Some also is used as a replacement for fluid and colloid loss in patients with burns and shock. As with other components, systematic data on the purposes for which fresh-frozen plasma is used are not available.

Recommended indications for FFP and single-donor plasma vary. The most frequently cited indication for fresh-frozen plasma is the situation in which a specific factor deficiency has not been established (17,282,369,397,497). *Harrison's Principles of Internal Medicine* (425) indicates that fresh-frozen plasma ("and cryoprecipitate") is necessary for treatment of coagulation disorders, especially hemophilia, a suggestion that most experts in transfusion do not agree with. There is disagreement over the use of FFP and single donor plasma in other situations, in particular for the treatment of low plasma volume (17,282,369,397, 497). The use of other solutions for fluid replacement would obviate the risk of infectious disease.

Other indications on which there is disagreement include the use of FFP: as a protein-containing medium (282); as a source of Factor IX (282); for disseminated intravascular coagulation and when deficiencies of multiple clotting factors exist, as in liver disease (397;497); the preparation of hemostatically deficient patients and intra- and postoperative correction of bleeding problems (497).

Albumin and Plasma Protein Fraction

The primary indication for administration of albumin (and a similar product, plasma protein fraction [PPF]) is for plasma volume expansion in shock and trauma. Because albumin and PPF are heat-treated, they are safer than whole blood with respect to transmission of infectious disease. Most adverse reactions are due to technical accidents during manufacture (520) or to inappropriate or incorrect administration (494,538). Recipients of albumin run the risk of fluid overload.

Like fresh-frozen plasma today, the overuse of albumin was once a topic of great concern. Although its use remains controversial (see below), public concern about the use of albumin appears to have subsided. Cost was a major element in the controversy. Albumin is considerably more expensive than crystalloid solutions such as saline and Ringer's lactate. A liter of Ringer's lactate solution costs approximately $1; an amount of albumin required to produce a comparable result costs $130 (394). One estimate is that as much as 10 percent of the total drug budget for an acute hospitalization may be related to use of albumin and other blood products (112).

In 1975, indications for the use of albumin were the subject of an NIH Workshop (494). Following the workshop, guidelines for the use of albumin were published (538), and a number of attempts were made to modify physicians' use of albumin (e.g., 8). As late as 1977, however, Alexander, et al. (8), found that albumin was being used inappropriately in 71 percent of surgical cases and 41 percent of nonsurgical cases. Worldwide U.S. production and consumption continues to rise (see ch. 3). A recent international study (including the United States) found that clinical uses of albumin covered many uses not recommended by health and regulatory agencies—e.g., for nephrosis, in detoxification, and as part of the treatment of malignancies (260). An indication of the confusion about the amount of albumin that is needed in clinical practice is the significant variation among countries, even countries similar in levels of medical sophistication (388).

Despite the guidelines published as a consequence of the NIH workshop, textbooks continue to disagree on some of the uses of albumin; e.g., in adult respiratory distress syndrome (17, 112, 349, 520) and coronary bypass pump priming (388, 520). The latest edition of *Harrison's Principles of Internal Medicine* (425) cites the use of albumin in severe malnutrition, nephrosis, and certain gastroenteropathies. Use of albumin for malnutrition is not advised in manuals written by blood bankers (e.g., 17). The international study referred to above suggested that the needs of patients were reflected better by clinical use than by agency recommendations. Thus, use of albumin remains controversial.

Factor VIII

Until the AIDS crisis, there was little controversy in this country concerning the appropriate use of Factor VIII, particularly since it is readily available. There is now some movement from use of lyophilized Factor VIII to use of cryoprecipitate, at least for less severe hemophiliacs. Use of lyophilized Factor VIII has reportedly decreased substantially in the past year. In countries where Factor VIII is less available, prophylactic use of Factor VIII is an issue. Mollison (388) reports the results of a randomized clinical trial conducted in Great Britain (54) which showed that reducing the incidence of bleeding in severe hemophiliacs by 15 percent would require the use of 73 percent more Factor VIII than would be used by simply treating episodes of bleeding. Reduction of bleeding by 66 percent would involve an increased usage of approximately 160 percent.

Methods to Change Usage Patterns

To some extent, then, controversy surrounds the appropriate use of all blood products. A key element in the controversy is that criteria for clinical use are often unclear. Thus, practice at the bedside relies on anecdotal reports and evidence from inadequate trials (567). However, even when medical guidelines are generally accepted, local practice varies and may sometimes be inappropriate. Past attempts to change medical practice have relied largely on educational efforts. Although systematic data do not exist to adequately test their effectiveness, these attempts appear to have been largely unsuccessful. Currently, a number of new efforts to curb the misuse of blood products, described below, are under way. Perhaps the most effective push in the direction of more appropriate use will be the impact of Federal cost containment efforts.

Education

As noted above, past attempts to change medical practice have relied largely on educational efforts such as seminars and textbooks. For example, the American Association of Blood Banks has published a series of books based on seminars and workshops at their annual conventions. Three textbooks are available (Huestis, Bove, and Busch [three editions]; Petz and Swisher, 1981; and, Mollison [seven editions 1951-83]). It is unclear, however, to what extent these efforts have reached practicing physicians. Medical schools devote little attention to transfusion practice. The result is that medical students and residents learn most of what they know about blood transfusion by the practice of "chaining" (520): "The chief resident passes along what he has learned, gathered in an entirely unsystematic way, to the assistant residents, who then in turn teach the interns and medical students as they rotate through the various clinical services." Results of formal teaching exercises such as having blood center personnel speak at grand rounds, staff meetings, or in-service training programs, have been varied (262). As discussed with respect to fresh-frozen plasma and albumin, textbooks in general use by physicians do not always follow the guidelines promulgated by blood bankers.

The rise of component therapy has exacerbated the need for clinicians to become more sophisticated about the use of blood. As a consequence, several books of guidelines directed at practicing physicians have been published. A pocket-sized book published by AABB seems the most accessible (i.e., in addition to being pocket-sized, it has brief chapters, is indexed, and costs only $3). An AMA guide, *General Principles of Blood Transfusion* (39), has gone through several editions (1970, 1973, 1977) and is being revised. Currently, the AABB is engaged in a more active attempt at physician education. Its *Physician's Handbook* is to serve as the basis for a new physician self-assessment program, the *Transfusion Medicine Self-Assessment Program* (26). Other attempts at continuing medical education include the American College of Surgeons' recent postgraduate course, *Pre- and Postoperative Care: Blood and How to Use It* (36).

Perhaps the most encouraging trend in physician education is the institution by the National Institutes of Health of "Transfusion Medicine Academic Awards" (403; see app. A), and other efforts concerning appropriate use. Recipients of Transfusion Medicine Academic Awards will work with local medical schools to incorporate transfusion medicine into the curriculum. Currently, five such awards, at $50,000 per annum for 5-year periods, have been granted. The program will be announced each year until needs in transfusion medicine are fulfilled. Perhaps as important as the awards themselves is the fact that current transfusion medicine award recipients are communicating with each other about their experiences in inculcating local changes (534). In addition, applicants for National Research and Demonstration Center in Transfusion Medicine (NRDC) awards are encouraged to design projects directed at testing and evaluation of strategies to affect health management practices and physician and health-professional knowledge.

As encouraging as these attempts at more physician education are, a limiting problem is that many indications for transfusion are based on "soft" scientific data. Thus, guidelines conflict and experts conclude by saying that it is impossible to provide rules of thumb. There is a need for more objective evidence, but few randomized clinical trials have been conducted. For example, even though NIH has stressed the need for clinical trials and applicants for NRDC and Specialized Centers of Research in Transfusion Medicine (SCOR) awards are encouraged to conduct controlled, carefully monitored trials, support for such trials **alone** is explicitly prohibited by the awards. Currently, however, clinical trials are under way on the appropriate uses of platelets (at Puget Sound), Factors VIII and IX (at the San Francisco Veterans Administration Medical Center), and fibronectin (Albany, NY) (532).

Blood Center and Hospital Controls

Attempts to educate physicians and blood bank personnel as to the appropriate uses of blood products, while useful, typically have had limited impact. Accordingly, some blood centers and hospitals have made more direct attempts to modify the use of blood products. At Puget Sound Blood Center, for example, requests for more than eight units of a blood component must be cleared through a blood center consultant before the blood is released. This consultation process is an example of the extent to which blood center physicians have gone from laboratory to clinical aspects of transfusion (532).

Such a practice, however, is only made possible because Puget Sound maintains a central crossmatching laboratory, and all orders for blood and its products are received in that lab; thus, they are aware of requests for small amounts of blood products. Other blood centers respond to large requests from hospital transfusion services and so are not aware of individual clinical practices. In addition, some clinicians bristle at blood centers' intervening in clinical practice. Attempts have been made to organize clinicians to reduce the power of blood centers (360,591). In most situations, however, blood centers are not aware of the use to which the components they supply are put (295). Thus, except for decisions about production (e.g., the supply of whole blood relative to other components), they have little control over the appropriate use of blood products.

It also may not be economically sound for blood centers to discourage use of blood products (457), so transfusion committees may be another answer. Current JCAH (Joint Commission on the Accreditation of Hospitals) guidelines on this requirement are very general, however, and hospital transfusion committees have been regarded as largely ineffective. JCAH is developing new guidelines for hospital transfusion committees (245). In response to requests from local hospitals, the New York State Council on Human Blood and Transfusion Services is also preparing a set of guidelines for transfusion committees, but this too will be fairly general (316).

A new AABB Committee is developing guidelines for hospital transfusion committees (245). These guidelines will not focus on specific indications for appropriate use of particular products, or, as is currently the case, statistical reviews of overall blood use. Rather, they are intended to provide suggestions for ways for hospitals to monitor systematically physician practice, in the hope that bad practices will be detected and controlled. A system for such monitoring has already been implemented in at least one hospital (242). Even without promulgation of guidelines by outside parties, however, it is expected that hospitals will begin to more closely monitor blood use as a consequence of cost containment measures such as DRGs (275). These monitoring systems will not necessarily provide indications of national trends in appropriate use, but implementation of the DRG system may provide a base for such national monitoring if it is deemed necessary.

Finally, the American Blood Commission is considering applying for an NIH grant to study the appropriate use issue, but one previous such request was not granted.

Conclusion

Clearly, the issue of appropriate use of blood products is receiving a great deal of attention as a result of the AIDS crisis and Federal cost containment efforts. Attempts to educate practicing physicians and to curb misuse of blood products through review of transfusion practices are increasing. In the absence of objective scientific criteria on many aspects of blood use and data on the current extent of inappropriate use, the effects of these efforts will be difficult to evaluate.

6.
Alternative Technologies

Contents

	Page
Part 1: Alternative Sources of Blood Products	133
Introduction	133
Stem Cell Culturing	134
Red Blood Cell Substitutes	136
Platelet Substitutes	150
Part 2: Alternate Source for Plasma Products—Use of Recombinant DNA Technology	152
Introduction	152
Application of Recombinant DNA Technology to Large-Scale Production of Plasma Proteins	159
Other Applications of Recombinant DNA Technology	172

LIST OF TABLES

Table No.	Page
42. Composition of Fluosol-DA (20)%	139
43. rDNA Companies That Are Working on Cloning the Gene for Serum Albumin	160
44. Companies Working on Cloning the Gene Coding for Factor VIII	164

LIST OF FIGURES

Figure No.	Page
12. Schematic Diagram of Cell Replication and Differentiation	134
13. Oxygen Dissociation Curve	136
14. Perfluorochemicals	138
15. Crosslinked Hemoglobin	143
16. Liposomes	146
17. Structural Map of the pBR322 Plasmid DNA Molecule	153
18. Common Methods for Inserting Foreign DNA Into the pBR322 Plasmid	155
19. The Filter Hybridization Technique of Grunstein and Hogness, 1975	156

6. Alternative Technologies

PART 1: ALTERNATIVE SOURCES OF BLOOD PRODUCTS

Introduction

Substitutes and alternative sources of therapeutic blood components are likely to eventually make the entire spectrum of human blood products obsolete, but it will be at least 3 to 5 years before any one of these new products becomes commercially available. Within the next decade, virtually all plasma derivatives will be synthesized using recombinant DNA technology. Substitutes for blood's cellular elements such as red blood cells (RBCs) and platelets will be much more difficult to develop, but present research activities, although in their infancy, suggest that all of the problems are likely to be resolved. The most probable order of availability is that alternative sources of plasma derivatives will be developed first, followed by red cell substitutes, and eventually by platelet substitutes.

As in the current blood industry, there is a division within the development process of alternative blood sources and substitutes. Most work in cellular substitutes has concentrated on an RBC substitute, with the recognition that such a product may really be an additional transfusion product or adjunct solution, rather than a replacement for RBCs. Most of the research is being performed by academic investigators or at military research institutes, although commercial organizations are also involved, ranging from plasma fractionation companies (e.g., Alpha Therapeutics) and large industrial concerns (e.g., Monsanto Corp.), to small biotechnology firms which have focused on specific preparations (e.g., hemoglobin synthesis).

In contrast, nearly all of the research on new sources of plasma derivatives is being conducted by biotechnology companies. There is substantial R&D in progress, in which the goal is to clone clinically useful plasma proteins utilizing recombinant DNA technology.

Impetus to develop blood substitutes and alternate sources comes from several factors. First, there has been increasing use of component v. whole blood therapy, which means that blood substitutes need only duplicate the specific property of the desired blood product. Second, recent advances in biotechnology, particularly in the field of recombinant DNA technology, have suddenly raised the prospect that alternative sources for blood products, particularly plasma proteins, can be attained. There is therefore a new technology which can be exploited for its potential for profitable commercialization.

Another major impetus to develop these products lies in their anticipated safety. Frequent blood recipients, such as hemophiliacs, invariably develop viral hepatitis, and nearly 10 percent of all blood recipients develop some posttransfusion viral hepatitis. Blood-transmitted AIDS is the most recent safety problem, and substitutes and alternative sources would avoid the problem of blood-transmitted infectious diseases.

The costs of transfusion may also be lower, because such requirements as special storage conditions and compatibility testing may be avoided. Although the price of a unit of blood currently ranges from about $35 to $60, this charge does not include a hospital crossmatch and/or transfusion fee, which can often double the total charge for a blood transfusion. "Artificial blood" offers the hope that the direct cost of transfusions will be less. And with the plasma derivatives, current R&D activities are in many cases based on the hypothesis that these products can be produced at far less cost then the blood-extracted products they would replace.

Current availability of blood products also varies considerably as a function of the supply of donors. Shortages still occur in the summer months and around the Christmas holidays. Onsite, resuscitative solutions in large quantities are needed for civil disasters and battlefield casualties. Although U.S. hemophiliacs now have access to adequate supplies of Factor VIII, very few hemophiliacs in developing countries receive or have access to this treatment.

Blood substitutes may also be preferred over blood-derived products, such as for patients who for various reasons will not or cannot receive blood from other individuals; or in organ or tissue perfusion, where the greater oxygen delivery capacity of a blood substitute may better maintain tissue viability.

In sum, most of the impetus to develop alternate blood sources and substitutes is based on economic, safety, and availability considerations. None of these products has yet reached the marketplace, and developmental efforts are still at the stage of laboratory investigations or animal testing; clinical trials with humans have not begun except for oxygen-transport substitutes. Thus, it should probably be at least 3 to 5 years before the first of these products will be approved for human use.

Stem Cell Culturing

Red blood cells, platelets, and granulocytes are mature blood cells that have a limited lifespan and are incapable of self-replication. Replacement of these cells takes place in the bone marrow, where less differentiated cells exist with capabilities to differentiate into different cell types. These "'stem cells" in the marrow possess both the ability to replicate (multiply) as well as to differentiate into specific hematopoietic cell lines (commitment). Figure 12 is a schematic diagram of stem cell replication and differentiation.

It is conceivable that stem cells could be grown in culture so that a continuous supply of cells for transfusion would become available. But at this time, stem cell culturing for the production of mature, transfusable blood cells is not possible.

Although it has been known for over a century that mature blood cells were derived from the bone marrow, it was not until 1961 that an assay was developed which proved that bone marrow cells are capable of forming colonies of hematopoietic progenitors (530). Other studies have conclusively shown that the colonies are derived from a single cell and that the responsible cell was a true multipotential stem cell (596). Having an extensive capacity for self-replication, stem cells comprise only 0.1 percent of the total cell population in the bone marrow. Stem cells also circulate in the blood stream, albeit in much lower concentration than in marrow. Thus, it is possible to obtain stem cells from two sites (marrow and

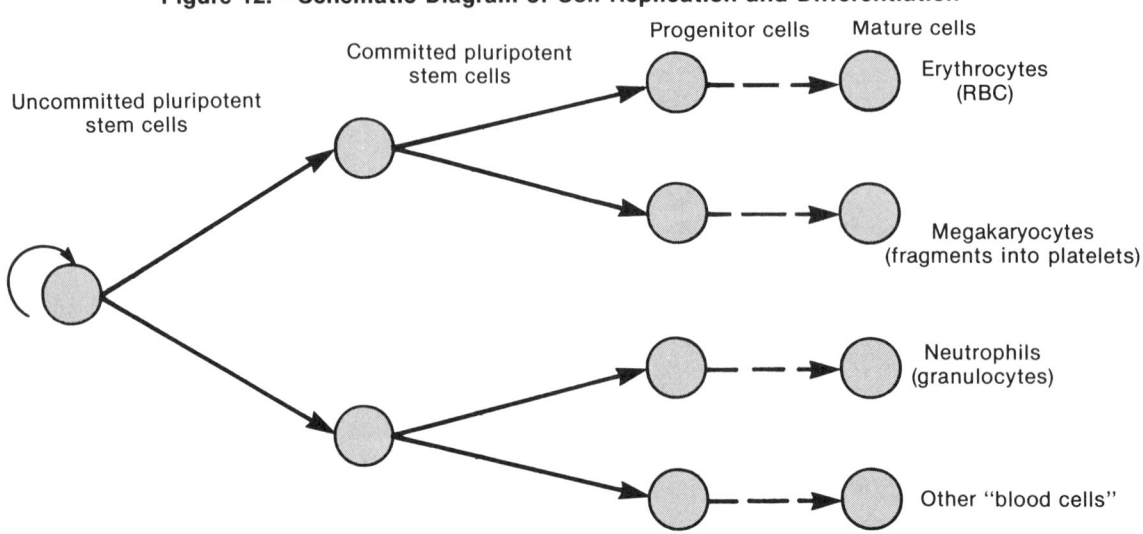

Figure 12.—Schematic Diagram of Cell Replication and Differentiation

SOURCE: R. Kahn, et al., *Alternate Sources*, 1984.

blood), and their self-replicative capacity obviates the need for large numbers of cells to initiate a culture.

Stem cells have also been shown to differentiate and form colonies in tissue culture (92). Mouse stem cells that produced granulocyte progenitor cells and pluripotent stem cells have been cultured (159), and mouse bone marrow cultures have been induced to generate stem cells for more than a year (358), with documented red cell, granulocyte, and megakaryocyte (precursors to platelets) production.

The specific conditions needed in maintaining a long-term bone marrow culture vary with the species from which the cells are derived, but in general they include an optimum cell density, the proper nutrient medium, regular maintenance (i.e., changing the medium), and a specific incubation temperature. A number of investigators have successfully established long-term cultures of human bone marrow cells (135,213,266), but the culture methods developed are clearly suboptimal. The cultures survived for only 2 and 6 months; while hematopoietic differentiation was observed, it is uncertain whether there was significant stem cell replication. Differentiation also did not proceed along all cell lines. For example, mature, even functional, granulocytes have been produced (239), but mature megakaryocytes have not been seen.

The list of culture supplements is long and varies significantly between investigators (e.g., some use vitamins and others do not). Such culture supplements as fetal bovine serum, horse serum, and steroids have been used with very little knowledge of the active ingredient(s) or mechanism of action. The optimal temperature for growth is also unresolved. Some cultures require 33° C, while others are maintained best at 37° C.

Last, cultures of human stem cells have properties that cultures of mouse stem cells (which live far longer) do not, and it is uncertain whether the differences represent suboptimal conditions or are unique to the species used. For example, bone marrow cultures usually consist of a layer of cells adherent to the culture dish as well as a nonadherent layer. In the mouse system, stem cells are released from the adherent layer into the nonadherent layer, where they differentiate (158). This progression of stem cells from the adherent to the nonadherent phase is absent or significantly impaired in human cell cultures (135).

Future Directions

A considerable number of unresolved issues and problems must be addressed before stem cell culturing becomes an attractive method to produce transfusable blood cells. At the very least, much more needs to be learned regarding hematopoiesis in general. For example, there is little knowledge of the factors that tell the uncommitted stem cell to differentiate into progenitor cells, and then into the mature blood cell (124). At the very least, a complex series of cellular and environmental interactions govern the differentiation process (399,411). Some are known, such as the hormones erythropoietin for RBC production and thrombopoietin for platelet production, once progenitor cells have developed. Control mechanisms must be known in order to provide confidence that the cells produced are indeed normal, rather than products of an uncontrolled bone marrow malignancy. It will also be essential to determine those factors that govern stem cell replication as opposed to commitment, if mature blood cell production is to be sustained.

Even with greater understanding of the events governing hematopoiesis, several major problems remain. First, how will production be amplified from culture flasks producing millions of cells to production of sufficient numbers (10^{10} to 10^{12}) for transfusion? For example, the cumulative production of granulocytes in primary mouse marrow cultures reaches a maximum of 6×10^7 cells over a period of a year (10^6 cells/culture/week) (358), and therefore about 10,000 cultures would be necessary to generate 10^{10} granulocytes, or the number of cells found in one granulocyte transfusion product. It is conceivable, however, that maintenance of a culture for longer periods, accompanied by secondary culturing of the primary culture as well as by the addition of growth enhancement factors, could shorten production time considerably.

Second, how will the mature cells be harvested so that unwanted contaminants are eliminated?

Blood cells derived from a cell culture must be free of nutrient media, which contains proteins that can elicit an immune response in the recipient. Other supplemental factors (e.g., steroids) may also cause adverse reactions.

Third, will end-products of the culture be functional cells? It is likely that compatibility testing between "donor" and recipient will have to continue, thus negating the advantage of a universally compatible product, which other blood substitutes are likely to be. Last, there is evidence that long-term cultures will sometimes contain malignant cells (354). This would, at the least, require stringent precautions to purify the transfused product; it might prohibit use of those products altogether.

Stem cell culturing offers the potential of producing transfusable blood cells in a laboratory environment rather than from routine blood donations. This approach to blood cell production, however, is in its infancy; much more research is needed before an accurate assessment of its usefulness can be made.

Red Blood Cell Substitutes

Most of the research on substitutes for the cellular components of blood have focused on RBCs, with some research on platelet substitutes. Of the many different white cell populations, only the granulocyte is currently used for transfusion. As granulocyte transfusions are now used primarily for combating bacterial infections in an immunocompromised patient, the most practical substitute has been to administer antibiotics. The increasing availability of new, potent, and specific antibiotic preparations has contributed to the decline of granulocyte transfusions over the past few years, and development of other antibiotic preparations should obviate the need for granulocyte transfusions.

Function of Red Blood Cells

Red blood cells are biconcave discs that are, for all practical purposes, bags filled with hemoglobin. Each molecule of hemoglobin contains four polypeptide chains: two alpha chains and two beta chains. Each alpha chain has 141 amino acids and each beta chain 146 amino acids, and all four molecules comprise the globin portion of hemoglobin. Each of the four chains contains an iron atom to which oxygen binds in a reversible fashion. Thus, a hemoglobin tetramer binds four molecules of oxygen.

The four chains, which form a loose tetrameric structure, can readily dissociate to form two dimers. The formation of tetramers is favored when hemoglobin is contained within the red cell. When hemoglobin is free in solution, dimer formation is favored, which has poor oxygen binding characteristics.

The interaction between oxygen and hemoglobin in erythrocytes can be described by what is called an oxygen dissociation curve (fig. 13), which depicts the degree to which hemoglobin is saturated with oxygen. At 50 percent saturation (i.e., P_{50}), and under normal physiological conditions, the y-axis of the curve is near 26 mm of mercury, or 26 torr. When the affinity of hemoglobin for oxygen is increased and oxygen is therefore less able to dissociate from the hemoglobin molecule, the oxygen dissociation curve is shifted to the left and the P_{50} decreases. In other words,

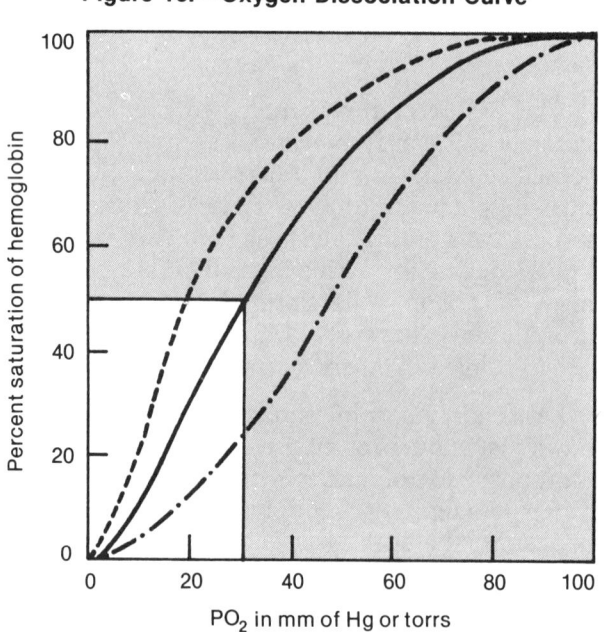

Figure 13.—Oxygen Dissociation Curve

SOURCE: Kahn, R., et al, *Alternate Sources*, 1984.

less oxygen is needed for 50 percent of the hemoglobin to be saturated, but oxygen is less able to be released from hemoglobin. Alternatively, if hemoglobin's affinity for oxygen is decreased and oxygen can more readily dissociate from hemoglobin, more oxygen will be needed for 50 percent of the hemoglobin to be saturated. This is represented by a shift in the oxygen dissociation curve to the right and an increase in the pressure of oxygen needed to saturate 50 percent of the hemoglobin with oxygen. A shift of the oxygen dissociation curve in either direction is unwanted, because the ability of hemoglobin to pick up oxygen in the lungs and to unload it in the tissues will be adversely affected.

The affinity of hemoglobin for oxygen is influenced by many factors. For example, pH, carbon dioxide levels and the intracellular molecule 2,3-DPG affect the position of the oxygen dissociation curve and hence the P_{50} value. A decrease in pH reduces the affinity of hemoglobin for oxygen and shifts the oxygen dissociation curve to the right. This change is referred to as the "Bohr effect" and is seen following substantial muscular action, which is associated with production of lactic acid. The decrease in pH helps in delivering oxygen to the exercising tissues. Carbon dioxide also binds to hemoglobin and, by displacing oxygen in the hemoglobin molecule, results in reduced affinity of hemoglobin for oxygen and a shift of the oxygen dissociation curve to the right.

Physiologically, however, the molecule 2,3-DPG has the most important influence on P_{50} levels. It decreases the affinity of hemoglobin for oxygen (right shift) by shifting the equilibrium between the deoxygenated and the oxygenated forms of hemoglobin. It stabilizes the deoxygenated form, causing oxygen to be released. However, when the oxygen concentration is high—as it is in arterial circulation—the equilibrium is shifted toward the oxygenated form of hemoglobin, thereby negating the influence of 2,3-DPG. At low oxygen pressure (e.g., in tissues), 2,3-DPG displaces the oxygen on hemoglobin, causing oxygen to be released.

The function of hemoglobin can be altered in many ways that ultimately reduce its ability to transfer oxygen. For example, the iron of the heme group can be oxidized from the ferrous to the ferric form, producing methemoglobin, which is incapable of combining with oxygen. Such oxidization readily occurs to hemoglobin in solution, but protective effects within RBCs prevent this alteration from happening. Hemoglobin function also decreases when RBCs are stored, mainly because of a reduction of 2,3-DPG, thereby causing the P_{50} to decrease (left shift). Fortunately, 2,3-DPG levels are largely regenerated through metabolic processes within the first few hours following transfusion.

Although a left-shifted oxygen dissociation curve indicates a decreased capability of hemoglobin to unload oxygen, its occurrence does not necessarily mean that tissue oxygenation will be adversely affected. The body can effectively compensate for decreased oxygen availability by increasing cardiac output, heart rate, or the efficiency with which tissues can extract oxygen.

While oxygen is chemically bound to hemoglobin, it also is physically dissolved in plasma, but the concentration of oxygen in plasma is far less than in oxygenated hemoglobin, and plasma is normally an inefficient medium for oxygen delivery to tissues.

The ideal RBC substitute should have six properties: 1) an oxygen dissociation curve and oxygen-carrying capacity similar to that of intact RBCs; 2) be nontoxic and nonantigenic; 3) have good flow characteristics; 4) remain in the circulation for a long period of time; 5) have a long shelf life; and 6) be cost effective in comparison to present RBC transfusions.

While no substitute as yet fulfills all of these criteria, four approaches to achieving the ideal substitute have been explored. One approach is to utilize a class of synthetic compounds called perfluorochemicals. Purified hemoglobin has also been chemically modified to prolong its circulation and enhance its oxygen binding/dissociation properties. A third approach has been to synthesize analogs of hemoglobin that, as in the native molecule, chemically bind oxygen. Last, investigators have attempted to assemble a red cell by encapsulating hemoglobin in lipid vesicles called liposomes.

Each of these substitutes has problems and drawbacks, some in common with one another and some unique to a particular substitute. Nevertheless, at least one clinically useful RBC-like preparation should become available by the close of this century.

Perfluorochemicals

Perfluorochemicals (PFC) are compounds in which all the hydrogen atoms have been replaced by fluorine atoms (fig. 14). They are chemically inert and not metabolized by the body. Unlike other RBC substitutes, PFC transports oxygen only in solution. Because the molecules of PFC do not strongly interact with one another, they have more room for gas to occupy the spaces between each atom and molecule. Thus, PFC can dissolve 40 to 70 percent oxygen per unit volume, almost three times the oxygen-carrying capacity of blood. It is this relatively high solubility of gases that make these compounds attractive as red cell substitutes.

Figure 14.—Perfluorochemicals

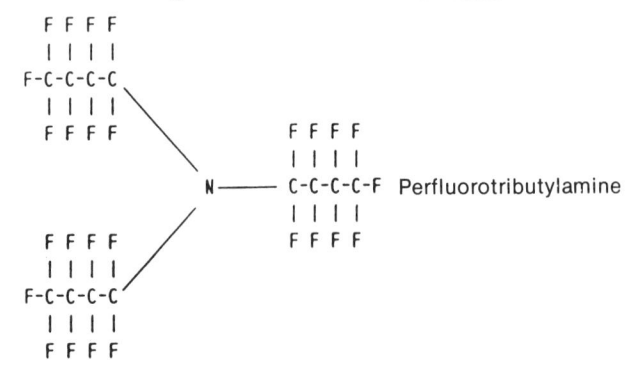

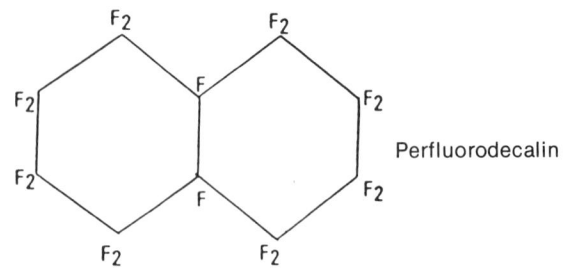

SOURCE: R. Kahn, et al., *Alternate Sources*, 1984.

The concentration of physically dissolved oxygen in a PFC solution is linearly related to the concentration of the PFC in the solution. As the PFC concentration increases, its contribution to oxygen delivery and consumption also increases (235). However, the oxygen-carrying capacity of a PFC is also directly proportional to the concentration of oxygen in the environment. At room air oxygen levels, PFC will hold little oxygen; it therefore must be given in a high oxygen environment in order to be effective.

Pure PFCs, however, are immiscible with blood, and, without any alteration, would act as an embolus when injected into the bloodstream. Since PFCs are not easily converted to finely dispersed stable emulsions, they must be emulsified to produce a very low viscosity and surface tension. PFCs can be emulsified with surfactants known as Pluronics, and in this form they can be mixed with blood. Because PFC must be used in an emulsified form, formulation and preparation of emulsions are at the center of studies on these blood substitutes. The emulsifying agent most widely used in dispersing PFC is Pluronic F-68. The preparation has the appearance of either a clear solution or a suspension resembling diluted milk, and the size of the particles can be as small as 0.1 to 0.2 microns, or 1/70 the size of an RBC.

The emulsification process and the size of the particles produced are important for stability and potential toxicity. PFCs that are rapidly eliminated from the circulation do not form stable emulsions, and conversely, those PFCs that can be easily emulsified have been found to have long body retention times. Since the body does not metabolize PFC, those particles not excreted have been shown to aggregate in the liver and spleen.

In an effort to find a PFC that is both stable in emulsion and rapidly cleared from the body, there has been a systematic effort to screen a great number of PFCs for their utility as blood substitutes. In 1973, a combination of two PFCs were formulated, one with a short half-life in the body, and the other with a much longer half-life. It was this new PFC combination that was distributed by the Green Cross of Japan to its American subsidiary, Alpha Therapeutics, and used in the United States in recent patient studies. Called Fluosol-DA, it consists of 20 percent (weight to volume) PFCs; perfluorodecalin (14gm/dl), with a half-life in the body of 7.5 days but with only a moderate emulsification capacity, and perfluorotripropylamine (6gm/dl), with a half-life of 65 days but with excellent emulsification.

Among perfluorocarbon preparations, Fluosol-DA is the most thoroughly studied and received the widest publicity. Besides containing the two PFCs and the emulsifying agent Pluronic F-68 in a balanced salt solution, hydroxyethyl starch is added to maintain blood volume and to enhance the flow characteristics of the solution (table 42) (219). The preparation has a circulation half-life of about 13 hours and a tissue half-life of 9 days as measured in animals (218).

Because they are biologically inert, PFCs contain no antigens, and therefore typing or crossmatching is unnecessary. The emulsions may be frozen and refrozen, and they can be autoclaved for sterility. They are also easily synthesized from readily available materials.

Other than as a substitute for red blood cells, PFCs have advantages in other areas of medicine. For example, carbon monoxide interferes with oxygen transport because hemoglobin's affinity for carbon monoxide is 250 times greater than its affinity for oxygen. In contrast, PFCs do not carry carbon monoxide at all, and PFC administration could provide oxygen to a carbon monoxide victim until the patient replaced his abnormal red cells. Another potential use for PFC relates to their small particles, which can easily penetrate vessels that have been constricted, such as in cerebral ischemia, myocardial infarction, or by abnormal blood cells (e.g., sickle cell crisis).

Uptake of oxygen by PFC in the lung depends entirely on the concentration of oxygen in the alveoli. PFC does not preferentially extract oxygen from the air as hemoglobin does, and the oxygen level in a PFC solution equilibrates with the oxygen level in the atmosphere. Since PFC preparations at ambient oxygen levels (air contains 21 percent oxygen) will carry very little oxygen, PFC therapy requires that the patient be given concurrent administration of 60 to 100 percent oxygen in order to deliver enough oxygen to the tissues.

PFC administration in a high oxygen environment is required because the highest achievable concentration of PFC in blood is about 20 percent; higher concentrations are unstable. Consequently, in order to efficiently utilize the oxygen carrying/delivery capacity of PFC, the patient must be exposed to the risks of a high oxygen environment, which can result in highly reactive oxygen metabolites that can in themselves inactivate cellular enzymes, damage DNA, and destroy cell membrane architecture (195). The concentration of oxygen in inspired gas (i.e., the FiO_2) at which significant damage after short-term exposure (24 hours) is first seen is about 70 percent, which is only slightly greater than the minimal concentration of 60 percent oxygen that has been successfully used for PFC administration (233). Thus, the advantages of PFC must be weighed against the potential toxicity of the high oxygen environment in which they must be given. This cumbersome and costly requirement for PFC administration may prove to be the limiting factor in its use as a substitute for blood transfusion.

Animals have also been known to survive a total exchange transfusion if they inspired 100 percent oxygen without PFC infusion (233). This demonstrates that plasma can be a very effective oxygen carrier at high oxygen concentrations, and questions whether the benefits seen with PFC infusion resulted from the use of this material or were merely due to the animals' breathing a high concentration of oxygen.

Table 42.—Composition of Fluosol-DA (20%)

Perfluorodecalin	14.0[a] %
Perfluorotripropylamine	6.0
Pluronic F-68	2.7
Yolk Phospholipids	0.4
Glycerol	0.8
NaC1	0.6
KCL	0.034
MgCL₂	0.02
CaCL₂	0.028
NaHCO₃	0.210
Glucose	0.180
Hydroxyethyl starch	3.0

[a]Composition expressed as percentage of weight to volume.
SOURCE: T. Mitsuno, H. Okyanagi, and R. Naito, "Clinical Studies of a Perfluorochemical Whole Blood Substitute (Fluosol-DA)," Ann. Surg. 195:60-69, 1982.

Another disadvantage of PFC emulsions relates to the need to freeze them for storage because of the emulsion's instability. A surfactant that will make stable emulsions at room temperature with a variety of PFCs has recently been studied (123). The new emulsifier also enabled the PFC concentration to be increased to over 50 percent, compared to current PFC concentrations of 20 percent.

Clinical studies.—The first human volunteers were given the PFC emulsion, Fluosol-DA, in 1979. Initial clinical studies were performed in Japan and reported a high degree of safety and efficacy (272,384,413).

In April 1980, Alpha Therapeutics Corp., the American subsidiary of Green Cross of Japan, began clinical trials of Fluosol-DA in California. Seven severely anemic patients were given Fluosol-DA before surgery to determine its effectiveness in supplementing oxygen transport. When the patients breathed low levels of supplemental oxygen (slightly more oxygen than ambient air levels) the PFC carried only a small amount of oxygen, as expected, and had virtually no benefit. When patients received pure oxygen, their arterial oxygen content rose significantly and the PFC provided 24 percent of the oxygen consumed (537).

Japanese experience with Flurosol-DA and reports from some American investigators have generally given the substitute high marks for safety and efficacy. But the frequency of such reactions from Fluosol-DA administered to Japanese patients has been significantly less than reported in Americans. This could be due to a number of factors such as racial differences (e.g., lipoprotein levels differ between Japanese and Americans), different patient populations, medical practices, or monitoring procedures. Nevertheless, there is a definite reluctance to extrapolate the Japanese experience with Fluosol-DA to American usage. Moreover, in the last 2 years an increasing number of reports have begun to document a variety of toxic affects attributed to its administration.

Adverse effects.—PFCs are chemically inert and do not appear to be degraded biologically. Their principal avenue of escape from the body is via the lungs and to a small extent through the skin. Because of the particulate nature of the emulsion, however, it was suspected, and later confirmed, that clearance also involved the reticuloendothelial system (RES). Both animal and human studies have shown that some of the material is retained by the liver and spleen for at least 2 years after a single administration (312). Small PFC particles coalesce intracellularly, but with time these larger particles undergo further change to become smaller again. Most droplets of PFC eventually disappear. The exact mechanism(s) by which PFCs move from the RES to the lung, or from the lung to the airway, is unknown at present. Macrophages (a type of scavenger white blood cell) may play a role, since they readily take up PFCs and could carry the material to the lungs.

Because the RES is involved in PFC clearance, it was anticipated that saturation of the RES would reduce the body's ability to clear other foreign substances, notably bacteria or viruses. This hypothesis was confirmed in mice challenged with a bacterial toxin simultaneous with PFC administration, in which the lethality of the toxin rose nearly eightfold (350). These results suggested that PFC administration would be contraindicated in patients who are likely to have infections (e.g., trauma patients) or a weakened resistance to infection.

Of greater concern, however, and as yet unaddressed, is the possibility of chemical carcinogenesis as a result of the long retention time. Although there is no data that would support such a hypothesis, the fact that these chemicals remain in the body for some time is disturbing, and the issue will have to be addressed before general use is permitted (197).

Early studies on the effect of PFC infusion occasionally noted pulmonary reactions, which were attributed to a variety of physical properties of the chemicals (122,218,502) that affected either platelets or plasma proteins (334). Recent evidence, however, suggests that alterations in the immune system may be the triggering event. The transient hypoxemia and pulmonary congestion seen upon Fluosol-DA infusion (537) is similar to the effect of infusing activators of the body's complement system. Stimulation of white blood cells is also often associated with pulmonary reactions. Thus, it seems likely that PFC emulsions cause pulmonary dysfunction by activating complement and/or white cells. Release of a substance(s) from damaged leukocytes may then result in both leukocyte and platelet aggregation.

The first patient treated in the United States with Fluosol-DA developed a pulmonary reaction after receiving 30 milliliters of material over 15 minutes; no reaction occurred with a subsequent infusion after premedication with steroids (572). Laboratory studies indicated that Fluosol-DA activated the complement system, thereby resulting in macrophage aggregation, which was a reasonable explanation for the pulmonary reaction (chest tightness, shortness of breath) that was seen upon infusion. Further studies suggested that the component of Fluosol-DA responsible for the effect was the emulsifying agent, Pluronic F-68. This finding is not unexpected, since PFCs are very unreactive and, in emulsified form, are probably coated with the surfactant. It is therefore likely that any interaction with blood components involves the surfactant rather than the PFC itself.

The recent effect of another commercially available PFC emulsion on macrophages was studied and the material found to be cytotoxic to these cells (101b). Although the study was performed on cells kept in culture, where exposure to PFC is likely to be higher than in actual use, it reinforces concern over the effect of these compounds on the body's immune system. More evidence of toxicity is the finding that PFC emulsions can disrupt the phagocytic function of peripheral blood neutrophils and monocytes (574). These reports clearly suggest that further studies are needed to clarify the mechanism and consequences of the leukocyte dysfunction that are seen upon exposure to PFC preparations, and that more detailed evaluations of the effects of PFC on host immune defenses are also needed.

Concerns surrounding use of PFCs as blood substitutes prompted the Blood Products Advisory Committee of the FDA to disapprove Fluosol-DA for human use at one of its recent meetings (561). The committee heard presentations from the manufacturer of the product, including a summary of the results obtained from approximately 100 patients in the United States and Canada who were given Fluosol-DA under an Investigational New Drug (IND) permit issued by FDA. Although few reactions were noted in these patients, all of the subjects were premedicated with relatively high doses of corticosteroids.

The committee's concerns over the possible masking of immune reactions by steroid administration, the potential toxicity of the high oxygen environment in which the PFC was administered, the relative paucity of data regarding the effect of Fluosol's emulsant (Pluronic F-68) on the recipient's own blood cells and tissues, and the lack of convincing data that PFC administration to anemic patients was efficacious, were the key factors that led to the committee's decision (197,383).

Other emulsions having more favorable characteristics than Fluosol-DA (599) are being developed. Current PFC emulsions appear unsatisfactory for use as a blood substitute; their safety is far from established and their utility is hampered by the high oxygen environment in which they must be given, and a PFC that is stable as an emulsion at room temperature and that is quickly excreted needs to be developed.

Even if these issues can be resolved, it seems unlikely that clinicians will choose daily infusions of a PFC emulsion until the patient's red cell mass returns to normal over a red cell transfusion. The high oxygen environment requirement precludes use of PFC transfusions in the battlefield or at the site of an accident and would even discourage its use in a hospital setting. Resolution of the safety and efficacy issues may lead to use of PFCs for specific indications such as in patients with religious objections to blood transfusion, in carbon monoxide poisoning, sickle cell crisis, or cerebral ischemia. If its use is limited to these clinical situations, PFC emulsions will never have a significant effect on the blood transfusion industry.

Hemoglobin Solutions

Early studies on the use of unpurified hemoglobin solutions were disappointing in that their administration to animals and man were often associated with renal abnormalities and coagulation defects (10,56,93,251,453,454,498), although the effects appeared to be dose-related (175,224, 381,418,492).

Removal of RBC membrane fragments (i.e., stroma) from hemolyzed RBCs to produce "stroma-free" hemoglobin eliminated many of the renal and coagulation problems (74,75,125,455).

Stroma-free hemoglobin is produced by slowly lysing washed RBCs with a buffered solution of water (rather than unbuffered water), followed by high speed centrifugation and micropore filtration (424,454,455).

To further purify a hemoglobin solution, other investigators have altered the conditions of hemolysis, or the centrifugation and filtration steps (95,155,240,257,396,490).

Although it is possible to prepare at least limited quantities of a hemoglobin solution that has no known contaminants, questions regarding the safety of the preparation still remain. Coagulation abnormalities, renal dysfunction and alterations in cardiovascular function appear to be the most common effects (83,197), but do not always appear together. Liver necrosis is sometimes observed.

Severe hematologic alterations have occurred in the first few hours after infusion of purified hemoglobin in dogs, but not in monkeys and pigs (82). These results have raised many disturbing questions. Is it possible that contaminants below detectable levels can still cause adverse reactions? If so, how will the safety of a clinically useful preparation be determined prior to its infusion? Second, what animal species should be used for extrapolation to humans? Differences in response between species make interpretation of safety data confusing and the choice of animal model for experimentation extremely important. Variations in response **within** animal species have also been seen. For example, infusion of a presumably pure hemoglobin solution into a group of rabbits has caused severe, acute toxicity (even sudden death) in some of the animals, but no adverse effect in others.

Variations in the response to infusion of a hemoglobin solution into eight normal volunteers have been reported (477), and other investigators have noted unexplainable variations in the toxicity seen **between** preparations that were made using the same recipe (83). Such findings have recently prompted the Army Research and Development Command, the sponsor of the vast majority of research on hemoglobin solutions, to issue a request for proposals to obtain a supply of hemoglobin solution in sufficient quantity to study the nature of the interspecies variability, and to determine those factors which result in batch-to-batch variability.

If presumably "pure" hemoglobin can cause adverse reactions, is it possible that hemoglobin itself can be toxic under certain conditions? Hemoglobin has been shown to activate the body's immune system (i.e. complement system), although it was possible that the preparation used was impure (589). It is also possible that the configuration of hemoglobin in solution is conducive to binding bacterial endotoxins, either in vitro (during preparation of the solution) or in vivo as the molecule passes through the gastrointestinal circulation (357). Unpublished observations (83) suggest that endotoxin may indeed be the primary factor contributing to the toxicity seen.

The fact that inter- and intraspecies variability exists emphasizes the need for standardization and complete documentation of the methods used to prepare the hemoglobin solution. Careful selection of the species used for testing and attention to the conditions of the experiment are also key issues. Unfortunately, the literature on this subject is, in general, much less thorough and exact. A wide variety of species under an equal variety of experimental settings have been utilized, with hemoglobin solutions whose preparation and properties are incompletely described.

Fate of infusion.—In addition to obtaining a nontoxic solution, other significant problems have been that: 1) free hemoglobin normally persists in the circulation only a short time with a half-life of only 2 to 4 hours (75,87,455,477); 2) free hemoglobin has a significant oncotic effect; and 3) its affinity for oxygen is unacceptably high.

The short circulation time of free hemoglobin is due to the tetrameric form of the molecule easily dissociating into dimers and monomers, with rapid clearance of these subunits by the kidney. Hemoglobin also readily binds to the plasma protein, haptoglobin, which is then rapidly cleared by the reticuloendothelial system, primarily the liver (101a,212). If the amount of hemoglobin transfused exceeds the haptoglobin binding capacity, unbound hemoglobin is filtered through the kidney, where it is reabsorbed. If the filtered amount exceeds the reabsorptive capacity of the kidney, hemoglobin then appears in the urine.

Free hemoglobin's significant oncotic effect severely limits the maximum amount that can be given. While the concentration of red cell enclosed hemoglobin in blood is 14g/dl, only 7g/dl of free hemoglobin can be administered without exceeding the normal oncotic pressure of plasma. Increasing the amount infused to achieve the oxygen-carrying capacity of the blood lost will raise the risk of volume overload in the recipient. Therefore, significantly less oxygen transport capacity is attainable with hemoglobin in solution compared to an equal volume of blood, and it cannot be used as a 1:1 replacement fluid.

Several approaches have been taken to stabilize the hemoglobin molecule and thus slow its disappearance from the circulation, as well as to decrease its oncotic effect so that more can be given. One way is to crosslink (or "modify") hemoglobin molecules (386) either intermolecularly or intramolecularly (fig. 15). The former type of crosslinking produces hemoglobin of high molecular weight, while the latter stabilizes the tetrameric form of the molecule. Although the intravascular half-life using either method is prolonged (to 15 to 30 hours) and the oncotic effect of the polymer becomes similar to that of hemoglobin in RBCs, the oxygen affinity of modified hemoglobin remains extremely high, and therefore its ability to deliver oxygen is still greatly impaired.

Another potential problem with many modifying agents is that hemoglobin molecules become crosslinked both intra- and intermolecularly, resulting in a wide assortment of hemoglobin polymers of different sizes. Thus, batch-to-batch reproducibility of a preparation is extremely difficult, and the ability to determine which polymers, if any, are undesirable is a difficult task. Recently, however, crosslinking agents have been found that result in well-characterized, reproducible polymers of hemoglobin. One such agent is the adenine nucleotide, adenosine triphosphate (479).

Figure 15.—Crosslinked Hemoglobin

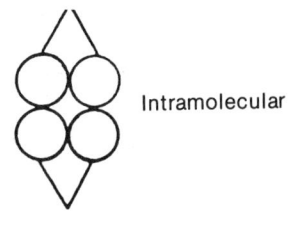

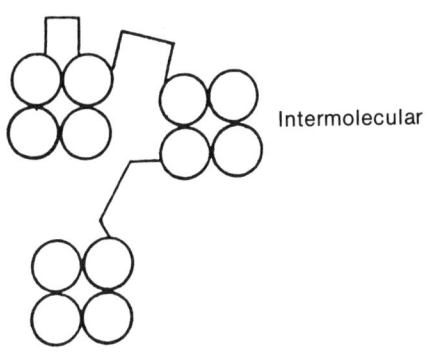

SOURCE: R. Kahn, et al., *Alternate Sources*, 1984.

Another new crosslinking agent is the chemical 3,5 dibromosalicyl-bis-fumarate (540), which is nontoxic, inexpensive, and capable of crosslinking hemoglobin at specific sites in a reproducible manner, and thus is attractive for high-volume production of a modified hemoglobin solution.

Another approach to stabilize hemoglobin is to attach it to a larger molecule which persists in the circulation for longer periods (113,525,526). Hemoglobin has been attached to the sugar, dextran, with longer circulation times, but the relatively high viscosity of the complex severely limits the amount that can be given (113,525,526).

Another major drawback of native hemoglobin is its high affinity for oxygen. Hemoglobin itself has a P_{50} of 13 to 18 torr, whereas the red cell P_{50} is 26 to 28 torr (234,396). This difference is mainly due to the intracellular molecule 2,3-DPG, which modulates oxygen affinity by binding to hemoglobin. This binding stabilizes hemoglobin's conformational state and enhances oxygen delivery (67,423).

Much research has centered on the search for molecules that could substitute for 2,3-DPG. Unfortunately, 2,3-DPG itself cannot be used because of its reduced binding efficiency to hemoglobin in solution (238). The most widely used, and most successful, attempts to normalize the P_{50} of hemoglobin solution have made use of the chemical, pyridoxal 5'-phosphate (P-5-P). This compound is an organic phosphate analog of 2,3-DPG (67,241,377) and has been shown to decrease the oxygen affinity of hemoglobin to essentially the P_{50} of RBCs (i.e., 26 to 28 torr). P-5-P functions by irreversibly binding to the beta chains of hemoglobin near the binding site of 2,3-DPG (68,69).

To achieve a P_{50} approximating that of RBCs **and** a longer circulation time, many investigators have both pyridoxalated and crosslinked hemoglobin. Pyridoxalated-polymerized hemoglobin does not have the oncotic pressure restrictions of unmodified hemoglobin, and it can be administered in a concentration of 14 to 15 gm/dl, the same hemoglobin concentration as in whole blood. The solution could be administered as a one-for-one replacement of blood, and the oxygen content per unit volume of circulating fluid would be unchanged. Because of these features, pyridoxalated crosslinked hemoglobin has been widely adopted as the preparation of choice, and it is the formulation currently being tested in animals and being proposed for future scale-up studies.

However, the P_{50} of such a preparation is really a composite P_{50}, since not all the hemoglobin will be pyridoxylated and crosslinked in a given preparation. Polymerized hemoglobin and unmodified hemoglobin are also eliminated by different mechanisms (89), and the contribution of each to any toxicity that is seen is difficult to resolve. Future studies are likely to focus on methods to prepare homogeneous preparations of modified hemoglobin, which could then be used to more easily determine the etiology of any toxic effects. The true benefits of transfusing a hemoglobin solution are difficult to assess, because, as mentioned previously, cardiovascular and tissue compensatory mechanisms occur when the concentration of hemoglobin in blood is moderately decreased. This does not imply that hemoglobin solutions are of little value, but rather that the clinical efficacy of one preparation over another will be very difficult to prove, and testing in animals will have to closely simulate the clinical condition in humans, for which its use is intended.

Other problems.—Three other potential problems with hemoglobin solutions as a blood substitute are related to the source of the hemoglobin, how it will be stored, and whether the infused material will invoke an immune response with the formation of antibodies in the recipient.

Hemoglobin solutions are currently being made from outdated human blood. If all the outdated blood in the country could be channeled into hemoglobin solution production, only approximately 600,000 units would be available (or 5 percent of the 12 million units collected).

An alternate source for hemoglobin is through recombinant DNA technology. **The hemoglobin molecule has been cloned** (see later discussion) and therefore it is possible that sufficient amounts could be prepared to satisfy all hemoglobin solution production requirements. Alternatively, it is conceivable that an animal hemoglobin could be substituted for the human molecule. Crosslinked and pyridoxalated bovine hemoglobin has the equivalent circulation time and oncotic pressure as its human counterpart and has a more favorable P_{50} than does human hemoglobin (156).

Injections of bovine hemoglobin into rabbits have resulted in antibody formation (185), and it seems likely that antibody formation would occur in humans. Even if only one "unit" were given, the ability to track such recipients and insure that they would not receive another unit at a later date would be very difficult. Whether human hemoglobin given to humans will be proven non-immunogenic is also unknown, and it is possible that modifying the configuration of the molecule upon crosslinking may enhance its immunogenicity.

A final concern regarding hemoglobin solutions is their stability during storage. Refrigerated or frozen storage may be suitable in a hospital environment, but is not satisfactory for use as an emergency resuscitative fluid, particularly in the battlefield. The most suitable form of the product for this purpose is as a freeze-dried powder that could be kept at room temperature. It is not certain that long-term storage of clinically suitable freeze-dried hemoglobin can be achieved. But other equally complex, large proteins have been successfully freeze-dried and reconstituted without loss of function, and there is no reason to assume that the ability to freeze-dry and reconstitute a functional hemoglobin preparation will be any more difficult to resolve.

Clinical studies.—Although nearly all the work done on hemoglobin solutions has utilized animal models, there have been published reports in which no more than a few milliliters of a hemoglobin solution was transfused into humans (10, 93,109,175,212,224,333,381,415,418,430,477, 492). All but the most recent report (477) used a crude preparation of hemoglobin that was uncharacterized. All of the studies were performed on volunteers who had normal cardiovascular parameters, and in all of the reports adverse effects were noted.

In the most recent study (477), a microporefiltered hemoglobin solution was administered to eight volunteers, all of whom experienced cardiovascular, renal and coagulation abnormalities lasting several hours. Another unpublished study using presumably pure hemoglobin was sponsored by the Biotest Corp. (88). The study began in the late 1970s but was terminated prematurely after the first two volunteers who received the unmodified preparation developed severe side effects and had to be hospitalized. Although the etiology of the reactions was thoroughly investigated, no explanation was uncovered.

Since 1978, no clinical trial has been initiated in the United States. The Army Research and Development Command hopes to initiate a clinical study in 3 to 5 years, but the starting time is dependent on whether the present safety issues can be resolved (83). Ability to reproducibly prepare large batches of a homogeneous hemoglobin solution is a fundamental requirement for such a study to begin.

As a substitute for blood, the major shortcoming of hemoglobin solutions is their failure to circulate for an appreciable period. Current research so far appears unlikely to generate a molecule whose circulation time anywhere near approaches that of an RBC. Thus, hemoglobin solutions may be limited to use as an emergency resuscitative fluid.

The anticipated cost of the product will also be an important consideration. It is impossible to reasonably predict at this time what the dollar cost will be, since scale-up beyond laboratory use has not been accomplished. However, it has been estimated that preparing a unit of hemoglobin (equivalent in function to a unit of blood), may cost as much as $100 (83). If this estimate proves correct, the price would be significantly greater than the present price of a unit of whole blood. Thus, cost might be a drawback to its acceptance for civilian use. (The military is inclined to be less concerned with cost because of the emotional/emergency circumstances in which such hemoglobin products would be transfused.)

If the hemoglobin used in the preparation were derived from recombinant methods, the final cost of the product might be far less than if the starting material were human blood. This is because the purification of human hemoglobin from whole blood is a multi-step process with a 30 to 40 percent loss of starting material. However, cost issues at this point remain secondary, since the major hurdles of safety and efficacy have not been passed. Whereas the newer hemoglobin preparations have adequate retention times and oxygen transport properties for their intended use, the etiology of the sporadic adverse reactions seen in animals remains an enigma. The antigenicity of the solutions will have to be evaluated and, at worst, restrictions on the frequency of infusion may have to be put in effect.

Successful large-scale reproducible preparation and storage of these solutions have yet to be accomplished. The fact that polymerized preparations are composed of many molecular species poses major obstacles to characterizing just what will be transfused, how reproducible each batch will be, and what properties of a hemoglobin preparation are undesirable. Nevertheless, it seems likely that a hemoglobin solution will become available for transfusion eventually, and the Army's Medical Research and Development Command hopes to begin clinical trials of a hemoglobin solution in 3 to 5 years.

Synthetic oxygen binding chemicals.—Rather than use hemoglobin as an oxygen-carrying blood substitute, attempts have been made to synthesize organic chemicals that reversibly bind oxygen. Some compounds have been synthesized that do, indeed, bind oxygen reversibly (9,58,59). However, none of the compounds demonstrate a P_{50} that is appropriate for clinical application, nor have they been used in a biological system. If, however, one such compound should show promise, its small size would necessitate binding it to a larger molecule in order to achieve adequate circulation time.

It is likely, however, that availability of recombinant-made human hemoglobin will obviate the use of an organic analog. Moreover, it seems certain that the former development will succeed before a synthetic compound can be made and successfully complete all testing. Hence, research in this area is unlikely to yield a blood substitute of practical significance within the confines of a practical span of time.

Liposomes

Another approach to preparing an RBC substitute involves encapsulation of hemoglobin into liposomes. Liposomes are closed spheroidal vesicles which contain an aqueous phase. The internal volume is separated from the outside by a thin matrix composed of lipid molecules arranged in a bilayer structure as in a normal cell membrane (fig. 16). The composition of the aqueous internal compartment reflects the solution in which the liposomes are formed and can provide for entrapment of a wide variety of substances if so desired. Liposomes can be prepared from a single type of phospholipid, a mixture of phospholipids, or mixtures of phospholipids and neutral lipids; e.g., phosphatidylcholine plus cholesterol. Since these molecules are found in all mammalian cell membranes, liposomes are usually non-immunogenic to the host.

The properties of liposomes can be somewhat controlled by utilizing different lipids and/or different methods of preparation. For example,

Figure 16.—Liposomes

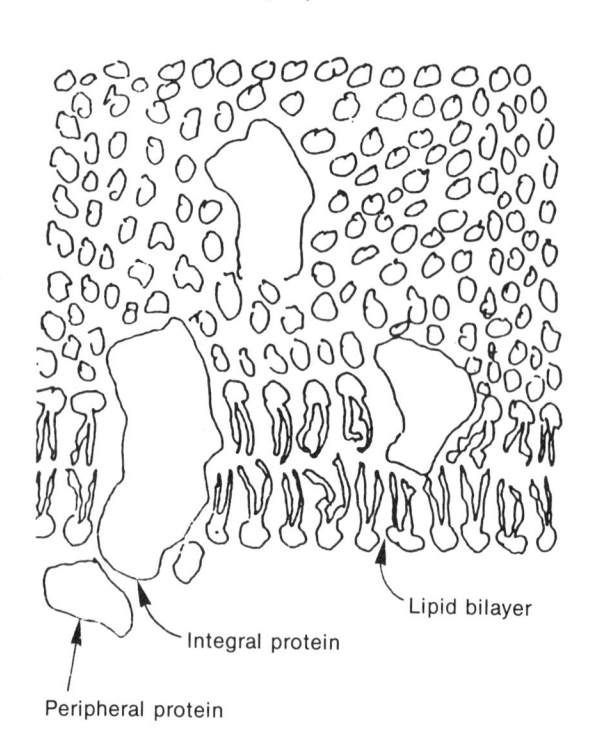

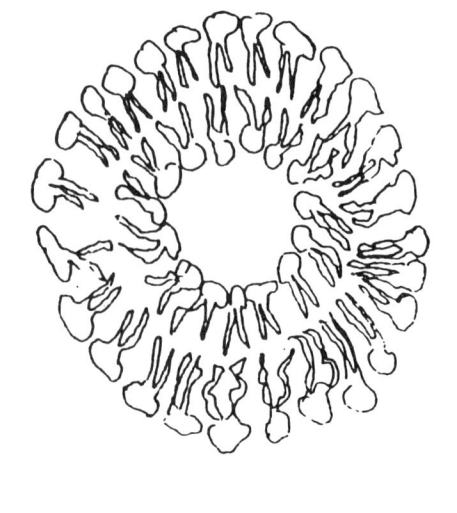

SOURCE: R. Kahn, et al., *Alternate Sources*, 1984.

whether the liposome will be multilamellar (i.e., vesicles composed of a series of alternating lipid layers separated from each other by an aqueous compartment) or unilamellar, or whether they are large or small, can be determined by the method of preparation. The net surface charge of the liposome can also be manipulated by the types of phospholipids used.

As an alternative to liposomes, vesicles can also be formed from synthetically made organic molecules (183). Since these vesicles contain only man-made molecules, their functional groups can be easily altered. They can be made to remain stable for months and have an extremely long shelf life. The size and permeability of small molecules can also be designed in the manufacture of the vesicles. The ability to control these properties make synthetic vesicles an attractive alternative to lipid containing vesicles but, at present, little work has been done with synthetic vesicles as biologically relevant macromolecules.

Preparation techniques.—Liposomes have been used in a variety of ways, such as model membrane systems for studying the mode of action of certain membrane-bound proteins, as carriers for enhancing the pharmacological activity of drugs, or to study the functional incorporation of macromolecules into cells. In all liposome preparations, special attention is given to the following characteristics: 1) captured volume (volume enclosed by given amount of lipid); 2) efficiency of the liposomes to encapsulate material; 3) ability to reconstitute cell membrane derived proteins; and 4) control of vesicle size.

Liposomes as synthetic red blood cells.—Although the overwhelming majority of research and development on liposomes has focused on their utility as a research tool to study cell membrane function, or as carriers of drugs, there has been a limited amount of work using liposomes as a blood substitute preparation. Hemoglobin has been successfully encapsulated into lipid vesicles at concentrations equal to that found in RBCs (160,177,276,285). The general approach has been to encapsulate concentrated hemoglobin solutions into liposomes made by mixing phospholipids and cholesterol. The liposomes contained no proteins (either inside or within the lipid bilayer) other than the encapsulated hemoglobin and, therefore, did not cause immune reactions (285).

The functional characteristics of the liposomal RBC substitutes were very similar to those of native red cells. In studies in which 2,3-DPG was also encapsulated, incorporation of 2,3-DPG resulted in an oxygen dissociation curve similar to that of whole blood (160,276). Liposomes with 2,3-DPG typically showed P_{50} values equal to 28 torr in one study (160,285) and 26 torr in another (276). Thus, with respect to their ability to carry oxygen from the lungs to the tissues, liposomes appear to be at least equal to other artificial blood substitutes. Unfortunately, they disappear rapidly from the circulation, with a half-life of only 5 hours (177).

Although data on storage of these liposomes are not extensive, they suggest the potential value of this technique. Suspensions of encapsulated hemoglobin were stable when frozen and stored at $-20°$ C. (160). The liposomes showed very little lysis and had P_{50} values similar to those before freezing.

Many investigators have performed exchange transfusions with rats using liposomal suspensions (160,276,285). However, it should be noted that a less than 95 percent exchange transfusion in animals can be tolerated simply by administering a colloid or crystalloid solution.

A different approach to preparation of vesicles has been taken by Davis and Asher (149). They recently patented a process whereby stroma-free hemoglobin was encapsulated in a polymerized hemoglobin membrane. The crosslinked hemoglobin membrane was permeable to oxygen and impermeable to hemoglobin. The vesicles were capable of reversibly binding oxygen and had diameters of less than 4 microns. Moreover, they were reported to be stable under conditions of normal blood flow. However, data supporting these claims have not been published, and the physiology of this liposomal preparation is unknown.

Although the above studies are certainly encouraging, many problems remain. First, the problem of rapid liposome removal from the circulation must be resolved before this substitute will find widespread acceptance. Several factors which govern removal of lipid vesicles from the circulation are: 1) irreversible binding of vesicles to tissues; 2) lysis of vesicles by plasma lipoproteins; and 3) clearance by the RES. Of these, removal by the RES (i.e., liver and spleen), is by far the dominant process (310,541). All studies reporting on the distribution of liposomes after intravenous injection have found that the liver is the site of liposome retention (111,309,449,514). Approximately 50 percent of the injected dose is found in the liver within a few hours after administration. The mechanism of uptake is not completely understood but may be related to the fact that the liver contains capillaries which allow small molecules to penetrate.

The rapid uptake of liposomes not only results in shortened liposome lifetime but also can saturate the RES and result in reticuloendothelial blockage. Thus, before liposomes can function as RBC substitutes, methods for limiting their uptake by the RES must be developed.

Recently, natural and synthetic glycolipids have been inserted into the liposomal membrane and tested for their ability to alter the final disposition of the liposomes. Incorporation of these glycolipids decreased uptake by the RES (104, 292,359,597). However, many glycolipids are antigenic and thus would not be suitable for insertion into a liposome that will be transfused. Alternatively, there are non-antigenic glycolipids that may also retard rapid liposome clearance. Hunt and Burnette (1983) have attached inert carbohydrates to lipids and incorporated the glycolipids into liposomes. They claimed to have reduced RES clearance and binding of liposomes to tissues, although complete studies were not published. Thus, it would seem that addition of inert carbohydrates may be one way to retard rapid liposome clearance.

The potential toxicity of a liposomal preparation is also of great concern. Initial studies (160, 177,276,285) indicated that hemoglobin-filled liposomes were non-toxic when infused into rats or rabbits. However, these studies did not address the long-term effects of the liposomal preparation, and toxicity of liposomes could potentially arise either from impurities present in the hemoglobin preparation, the lipids themselves, or impurities introduced in the encapsulation procedure.

Acute toxicity following administration of liposomes may not be seen, but adverse reactions may arise if the contents of the liposomes escape. Encapsulation of a toxin will essentially hide the entrapped material until the liposomes degrade, either by storage for long periods of time prior to use, or when they are exposed to destructive elements in the circulation (e.g., lipoproteins). There are, however, several approaches to prevent this potential problem. The most direct is to identify the impurities in the liposome preparation and eliminate them, which could be difficult and costly. A second approach is to design liposomes which retain their encapsulated material when stored or injected into the circulation. These approaches are not mutually exclusive but will likely have to be engineered into the liposomal preparation.

Lipids used in construction of the liposome are another source of potential toxicity. Although in vivo toxicity of liposomes is thought not to be a concern if proper care is taken in isolation and storage of the lipids, one study has shown that liposomes caused damage to the central nervous system in mice (4).

Another potential source of concern is contaminants in the lipids that can affect liposomal integrity. Changes in the structure of lipid molecules inevitably occur with time and can result in accumulation of lipid breakdown products in the preparation. These contaminants can facilitate liposomal degradation and loss of their encapsulated contents. To avoid this problem, the lipids will have to be purified prior to use. There does exist, however, a naturally occurring class of lipids (branched-chained dialkyl ethers) that are not subject to such breakdown (324). Another alternative would be to use synthetically made molecules that are not subject to these effects (183).

It will also be important to examine the effects of blood and blood constituents on liposomal disruption. It is known that serum lipoproteins can interact with phospholipid vesicles (393) resulting in their disruption (427,458,524). Since the loss of liposome integrity appears to be due both to the binding of plasma components to the liposomes and to exchange of vesicle components with plasma lipid constituents, any modification of liposomes that will prevent these events should increase their ability to retain entrapped material.

One such modification is the addition of cholesterol, which has been shown to dramatically decrease the permeability of liposomes in the presence of serum, plasma, or whole blood (311). Inclusion of specific, naturally occurring phospholipids has also been shown to increase the stability of liposomes in the presence of plasma proteins (261). These results are encouraging, but no detailed study has yet been carried out to determine the effect of plasma or whole blood on the long-term stability of modified liposomes.

As is desired for all RBC substitutes, red cell-like liposomes should have a long shelf life. Many investigators have examined the stability of several liposome preparations for their ability to entrap and hold drugs (361,522). All preparations, however, show some disruption after liquid storage, and storage of liposomes for extended periods is likely to result in some loss of membrane integrity.

A possible solution to many of the problems discussed above (e.g., toxicity, stability, and storage) may lie in the use of synthetically made vesicles, or so-called "membrane mimetic systems" (183,184) formed from synthetic surfactants. They can be stabilized by polymerization, which effectively seals the membrane surface. The polymerized vesicles are appreciably more stable than liposomes and have a shelf life of several months. Moreover, the size of the vesicles and their permeability properties can be engineered as desired. Although utilization of these vesicles has become a significant area of research in chemistry, biological applications have not been explored.

Last, scale-up to prepare large amounts of a liposomal preparation for transfusion using existing technology could be a formidable task. First, it will require isolation of large quantities of lipids and hemoglobin. The latter will undoubtedly be obtained by recombinant DNA technology (see following section). The majority of lipids could be isolated from crude preparations of egg lipids at a reasonable cost. However, it is known that liposomes which contain only these lipids would be cleared rapidly, and thus special masking lipids would have to be included in the final product.

Because the relationship between liposome composition/structure and clearance is not fully understood, it is very uncertain what the final product will contain and cost. But from the studies reviewed above, it is likely that some type of synthetically constructed lipid will be necessary. For example, a single synthetic surfactant may eliminate the need for purification and storage of lipids. Production of surfactants is also easier and less costly. Although no data have been collected concerning the potential toxicity of these preparations, it is entirely conceivable that the desired properties of stability and safety could be engineered into the surfactant's structure. This approach, however, is speculative; many years of basic research will be required before testing in humans can begin.

The second major problem in scale-up relates to preparation of the vesicles. Many of the methods for encapsulating materials were developed for drug delivery. Applications involved in drug therapy require relatively small amounts of vesicles compared with the large volume requirements for a blood substitute. In fact, difficulty in obtaining significant amounts of liposomes is likely to be the reason that extensive animal studies have not yet been reported with existing preparations.

At the outset, therefore, only those preparative techniques which can be easily scaled-up are likely to be considered. However, at the present time no suitable large-scale encapsulation procedure has been devised or tested to provide confidence that mass production of liposomes (or synthetic vesicles) can be achieved.

In sum, the use of encapsulated hemoglobin as an RBC substitute has received relatively little attention, particularly in comparison to the work on PFCs and hemoglobin solutions. While the technology is still in its infancy, encapsulation appears to be the approach most likely to lead to a blood substitute that has all the properties of an RBC. Certainly, major obstacles remain—particularly the toxicity, stability, and storage of such a preparation. But studies on liposomes or synthetic vesicles, while relatively new, are accelerating at a rapid rate, and technological advancements in this area will undoubtedly find solutions to the problems that remain. Even so, it is clear that many years of laboratory research will be required before clinical studies will be appropriate.

Platelet Substitutes

Under normal conditions platelets circulate in the blood for approximately 10 days as disk-shaped, formed elements, and do not adhere to other cellular elements, the vascular endothelium, or to themselves. But within a few seconds after injury to a vessel, platelets adhere to the exposed collagen surface. Such platelets become "activated" and release their internal constituents, resulting in a growing aggregate of platelets, and the simultaneous occurrence of clot formation. This growing mass literally plugs the hole in the damaged vessel wall. Thus, platelet function can be described in terms of the following reactions: 1) attachment at the site of the injury (adhesion); 2) aggregation of platelets to each other; and 3) release of substance(s) that facilitate blood coagulation.

Adhesion to a cut vessel wall is a complicated process that has been shown to require plasma factors as well as key platelet membrane molecules. Aggregation of platelets to each other is mediated by numerous exogenous platelet agonists such as thrombin and adenosine diphosphate (ADP). Each of these agonists has one or more receptors on the platelet surface. Binding of the agonist unmasks specific sites for plasma fibrinogen on the platelet membrane (70,355), which is thought to somehow serve as the "bridge" between platelets. Platelet secretion is also initiated by binding of agonists to the platelet membrane. Last, platelets have been implicated in the activation of several coagulation factors such as factor IX, factor X, and prothrombin (298,380,602).

Because of the complex role of platelets in the arrest of bleeding, it follows that the biochemistry involved in platelet function is also quite complex, and the mechanism(s) by which collagen, ADP, thrombin and other agonists result in platelet adhesion, aggregation and secretion are not completely understood. Thus, it is impossible at this time to fashion an artificial platelet which will mimic the entire physiology of the platelet. Nevertheless, two approaches have been explored as means to develop a suitable platelet substitute.

Platelet Fragments

The fact that platelets will clump to each other to form a plug and thereby seal broken vessels has been known for some time. Although the mechanism for this effect is still being unraveled, it might be hypothesized that intact platelets are unnecessary to achieve plug formation. Thus, it is not surprising that some early investigators examined the efficacy of transfusing platelet fragments. In one study (314) freeze-dried platelets were given to children who required platelet transfusion. Although substantial improvement was noted in certain coagulation tests, the clinical efficacy of the preparation in controlling bleeding was equivocal.

Another study by the same group utilized platelets disrupted by freezing and thawing, and again a transitory control of bleeding was seen (313). These somewhat encouraging results, however, were challenged by animal studies in which irradiation was used to create a clinical condition that warranted platelet transfusion. Three independent, well-designed studies employing this model showed that neither freeze-dried nor fragmented platelets were of value in control of bleeding (187,263,288).

These studies seem to have put to rest the notion that platelet fragments could adequately substitute for the intact cell. But in 1983 McGill and colleagues (365) examined the ability of platelet fragments to prevent bleeding in platelet-deficient rabbits. Their studies found that fragments appeared to have the same adhesive qualities as did intact platelets. In studies directed toward understanding platelet function in general, others observed that platelet membranes would interact with "activated" platelets in vitro but not with unstimulated platelets (446). Many investigators, however, remain skeptical that these recent observations warrant reopening this approach to obtaining a suitable platelet substitute. No clinical studies in humans using platelet fragments have begun or are even contemplated, and further studies by McGill in this area have been discontinued (366).

Even if such platelet fragments were effective, there would remain the question of the utility of such a preparation. The fact that platelet outdating is substantial in this country (i.e., greater than 10 percent of the units collected) implies that there is no chronic shortage, and the recently improved shelf-life of the component (from 3 days to 5) has greatly alleviated inventory problems that arise over weekends and holidays. Moreover, platelet fragments would still carry the risk of infectious disease and other adverse effects associated with traditional platelet transfusions. Thus, it is very unlikely that this substitute will ever see clinical use.

Liposomes as Platelets

Because of our understanding of the role many surface membrane constituents play in platelet function, it may be relatively easy to reconstitute one or two of these functions into liposomes. In fact, some progress in this area has very recently been achieved.

One of the platelet membrane glycoproteins which is thought to play a critical role in platelet adhesion has been reconstituted into lipid vesicles (499). When liposomes containing this protein were incubated with a plasma factor that is also important in platelet adhesion, liposome agglutination occurred, although the reaction did not entirely mimic that seen with normal platelets. In other studies the platelet membrane glycoproteins required for fibrinogen binding to intact platelets have been reconstituted into phospholipid vesicles (57,421). Both of these studies incorporated isolated platelet membrane glycoproteins into phospholipid vesicles and showed that the vesicles bound specifically to intact platelets in vitro. These data show that it is possible to reconstitute at least part of the platelet membrane constituents necessary for platelet function in vitro, although in no sense are the liposomal preparations used in these studies suitable for clinical use.

The fact that individual activities can be reconstituted, at least in this primitive fashion, offers promise that many activities can be reconstituted in a single liposome. All the necessary proteins would have to be reconstituted correctly. Since many platelet functions are interdependent, and since a completely reconstituted artificial platelet must also function in a similar fashion, the interactions between molecules must also be reconstituted. Although this might appear to be an impossible task, several cooperative membrane activities have been reconstituted in a stepwise fashion (294,456). Therefore, at least in theory, it should be possible to reconstruct many platelet functions.

However, virtually all of the problems discussed in relation to liposomes as artificial red cells are also relevant for development of liposomes as platelet substitutes. In addition, these liposomal preparations could be highly antigenic, since the reconstituted membrane proteins will be exposed on the liposome surface. Of concern is the observation that some cell membrane proteins have been found to be more antigenic when reconstituted into liposomes than they are in their native state in the cell membrane (300,495). However, the antigenicity of certain proteins can be modified by the lipid composition of the liposome (81), and it may also be possible to modify the reconstituted glycoproteins (e.g., remove the glyco- or carbohydrate portion) in such a way that they are no longer antigenic but still carry out their normal function. Neither of these approaches, however, has been studied so far.

It is impossible to estimate all of the difficulties that may arise for mass production of such a preparation. Very few of the membrane proteins critical to platelet function have been identified, much less isolated. However, when this information becomes known, production of significant amounts of the required proteins will no doubt make use of recombinant DNA technology. The rate-limiting step, however, as in the case of liposomal red blood cells, may be in the ability to generate significant quantities of liposomes.

Since membrane proteins will have to be incorporated into the lipid bilayer, the only suitable method known is the detergent removal procedure (57,421,499), which is very time-consuming and likely to be too expensive for mass production. New preparation procedures will likely need to be developed. Thus, it will be several years, at least, before a serious attempt will be made to construct a liposomal platelet substitute.

PART 2: ALTERNATE SOURCE FOR PLASMA PRODUCTS—USE OF RECOMBINANT DNA TECHNOLOGY

Introduction

Except for the oxygen-carrying function of RBCs, the physiological functions performed by the cellular and humoral components of blood are mediated largely through proteins. These proteins may act in a relatively specific and independent fashion, as in the case of antithrombin III and C1 esterase. Alternatively, a single species such as albumin may play a number of roles, alone or in conjunction with other factors, in maintaining homeostasis. Finally, a variety of proteins can interact in complex patterns to collectively carry out a function (e.g., coagulation).

All plasma proteins of therapeutic value have the potential of being produced by microorganisms carrying the genetic coding for the primary structure of the specific protein. The ability to construct a microorganism that can produce a useful product is possible because of recombinant DNA techniques that allow specific segments of DNA to be isolated and inserted into a bacterium, or other host, in a form that will allow the DNA segment to be replicated and expressed as the cellular host multiplies. The DNA segment is said to be "cloned" because it exists free of the rest of the DNA that, with it, constituted the genome of the organism from which it was derived.

A DNA clone can be prepared in a number of ways, but generally the process involves linking the desired DNA segment to a second piece of DNA known as the vector. The one feature all vectors have in common is that they are replicated independently inside a cell. The vectors commonly used for gene cloning in bacteria are of three basic types: 1) plasmids; 2) derivatives of the bacterial virus known as lambda; and 3) genetic hybrids constructed from plasmids and lambda, called cosmids. The vector chosen to prepare a gene clone will depend upon two primary considerations: 1) the size of the DNA segment to be cloned; and 2) whether or not the protein coded by the DNA is to be expressed (produced).

Plasmids used in cloning technology represent modified forms of DNA molecules that occur naturally in bacteria or yeast and generally confer a selective advantage to a cell harboring them (146). In the common bacterium *E. coli*, naturally occurring plasmids conveying resistance to antibiotics such as penicillin and tetracycline have been described (343,379,523). Another naturally occurring *E. coli* plasmid, known as Col E1, carries a gene coding for a protein that is secreted into the environment and inhibits the growth of other bacteria.

All plasmids have certain features in common. For example, their presence in a cell confers a selective growth advantage. In addition, they carry a specific sequence of DNA nucleotides that serves as a recognition signal for the host enzymes responsible for DNA replication. These enzymes will therefore not only replicate the chromosome as the cell multiplies, but will also replicate the plasmid molecule (and any foreign DNA linked to it).

The most commonly used plasmid for cloning foreign genes in *E. coli* is a derivative of the Col E1 plasmid known as pBR322 (84,85,86,91,519). The characteristics of pBR322 have been selected to optimize the plasmid for cloning DNA fragments up to approximately 5 kilobase pairs (kb) in length. The plasmid is efficiently replicated in the commonly used laboratory strains of *E. coli*, with multiple copies of the plasmid being present in a single bacterial cell (91). The pBR322 plasmid is diagrammed in figure 17 and can be seen to contain separate genes that confer resistance to the antibiotics penicillin (e.g., ampicillin) and tetracycline for the host cell.

The penicillin resistance gene codes for an enzyme known as beta-lactamase, which alters the structure of the penicillin molecule so as to inactivate it (11). The gene conferring resistance to tetracycline codes for a membrane protein that blocks transport of the drug to the interior of the

Figure 17.—Structural Map of the pBR322 Plasmid DNA Molecule

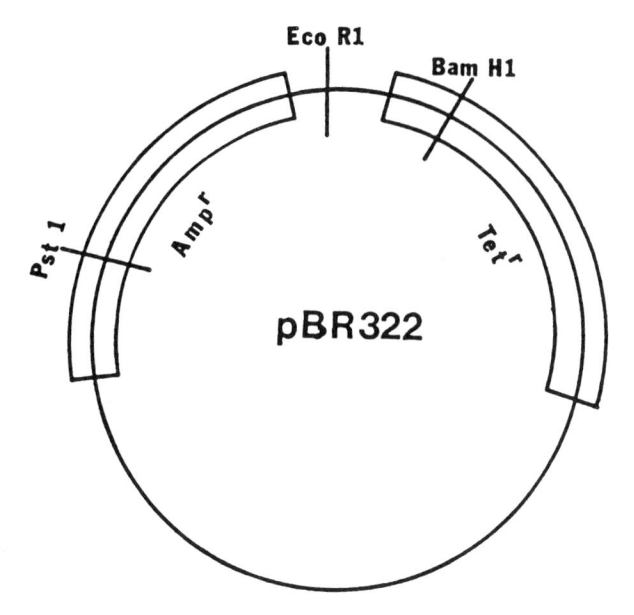

The entire plasmid is 4362 base pairs in length and exists in a circular form as shown. The relative location of the genes coding for tetracycline (tet^R) and ampicillin (amp^R) resistance are shown, as are the sites for the restriction endonucleases, Pst-1, Eco R1, and Bam H1.

SOURCE: R. Kahn, et al., *Alternate Sources*, 1984.

cell, where it exerts its inhibitory effect (523). Thus, *E. coli* cells harboring pBR322 will multiply on nutrient media containing penicillin and tetracycline, whereas cells not carrying the plasmid will die under these conditions. This difference is exploited in the cloning process.

One of the hallmark discoveries that has enabled molecular geneticists to splice DNA in a precise and premeditated fashion was the discovery of enzymes called restriction endonucleases (352,385). These enzymes recognize specific sequences of nucleotide bases in DNA and cleave the molecule within that sequence. To date, numerous restriction endonucleases have been identified from a large variety of sources, each with its own nucleotide base recognition sequence (352,385). Thus, a desired segment of DNA can be specifically excised from a larger piece of DNA if sites for particular restriction enzymes are known to flank the desired segment.

As shown in figure 17, pBR322 has several restriction enzyme sites that cleave the molecule once and have been used routinely for inserting pieces of foreign DNA. In addition to the single cleavage sites for restriction enzymes such as Pst-1, Bam H1 and Eco R1, pBR322 has numerous sites for a wide range of other enzymes that "cut" the plasmid molecule more than once (519).

Although pBR322 has been used extensively for cloning, a number of plasmids that are custom-tailored for a specific purpose have been constructed from pBR322 and other segments of DNA derived from a bacterial and/or bacteriophage genome. A modified plasmid may be desirable for a number of reasons, but most often they are used so that the information encoded in a cloned gene will be expressed by the bacteria carrying the gene. Several "expression vectors" have been constructed which are custom-tailored to express the protein product encoded in any piece of DNA inserted into the vector in a specific way (94,258,441, 573,581).

Other commonly used vectors for cloning foreign DNA are genetically modified derivatives of the lambda virus. As was stated previously for plasmids, lambda is a naturally occurring bacterial virus that infects *E. coli* cells (513). Once the cells are infected, their capabilities are commandeered by the virus such that viral particles are synthesized to the exclusion of other host macromolecules. Mature viral particles accumulate inside the cell until it finally lyses, at which time a large number of phage particles are released into the environment to repeat the process upon contact with other bacteria.

The modifications of lambda phage necessary to make it a useful cloning vector primarily require excising from the phage that part of DNA which is not involved in its growth cycle (586). The DNA excised from the natural genome is then replaced with fragments of foreign DNA. Replication of the cloned DNA is achieved by infecting a culture of *E. coli* cells with the modified lambda.

The one significant advantage to the use of a lambda vector for gene cloning is that very large DNA fragments can be cloned. Whereas most plasmids can accommodate only 3 to 5 kb of foreign DNA, lambda vectors can accommodate up to 20 kb of it (77,338,586). The main disadvantage to cloning with lambda is that the expression of the protein encoded in a eukaryotic (higher-order organism) gene is generally not efficiently expressed.

A third cloning vector, known as a cosmid (131,268,269) is actually a genetic hybrid between lambda virus and a plasmid. As with lambda, the primary advantage of cloning with cosmids is that very large pieces of foreign DNA (up to approximately 30 kb) can be cloned (269). Cloning in cosmids also suffers from the same disadvantages as cloning with lambda.

Choice of a particular vector to be used to clone a desired DNA fragment will depend ultimately upon what the investigator wants the cloning system to do. If the goal is to study the structural organization of a gene on a chromosome, the vector of choice would probably be one of the derivatives of lambda phage or a cosmid. Cloning with these systems would enable a large segment of a chromosome containing the entire gene and possibly flanking DNA to be studied in a single isolate. If, however, the aim of a cloning procedure is to engineer a cell to produce a protein product, cloning with a plasmid designed for expression of foreign DNA is the system of choice. Since the goal of cloning genes coding for therapeutically useful plasma proteins is to produce those proteins, the discussion that follows will focus upon cloning with plasmids rather than with the other vectors mentioned.

Eukaryotic genes, as they exist in the chromosome, are generally fragmented into regions of coding and non-coding DNA called exons and introns, respectively. In bacteria, genes do not consist of exons and introns but rather of a single coding sequence of DNA. If mammalian chromosomal DNA is cloned into a bacterial cell, the information will not be properly expressed, because the bacterium cannot decipher the complex exon/intron code of the mammalian DNA. In order to resolve this problem, messenger RNA is used to enzymatically synthesize a complementary DNA copy.

During the expression of a chromosomal gene in a mammalian cell, the information encoded in the separate exons is ultimately spliced together into a messenger RNA (mRNA) molecule. The mRNA is then transported from the nucleus to the cytoplasm, where it is translated into the amino acid sequence of the protein molecule (579).

Messenger RNA occupies a unique position in the flow of information from the nucleus of a cell, since it contains the entire coding sequence of the gene. Messenger RNA isolated from a mammalian cell can be used to program the synthesis of a double-stranded complementary DNA copy of itself in vitro. In many cases, cloning a complementary DNA (cDNA) copy of mRNA is the method of choice when cloning a gene that is to be expressed by a bacterial host. Since the cDNA form of a mammalian gene lacks the complex exon/intron organization of the nuclear DNA, it can be deciphered by a bacterium as if it were a bacterial gene.

The synthesis of cDNA from mRNA relies on use of an enzyme, isolated from avian tumor viruses, known as reverse transcriptase (60,528). This enzyme, under proper conditions, will synthesize a single-stranded DNA molecule that is the complement of an mRNA template. The single-stranded cDNA product can then be used in conjunction with another enzyme, DNA polymerase, to make a double-stranded cDNA molecule (353, 471), which can then be inserted into the vector. One method of insertion can be accomplished by chemically modifying the vector DNA and the cDNA so that the ends of both molecules are "sticky" (375,480). If the vector and modified cDNA are mixed, the sticky ends of both species can bind together, and the result will be the formation of a single, circular recombinant molecule (fig. 18) (126).

Another way to link cDNA to the vector is to attach a series of guanosine residues to the free ends of the vector DNA. Cytosine residues are also attached to the ends of the cDNA; when the vector and cDNA are mixed, the base pairing property of guanosine with cytosine allows the molecule to anneal into a single recombinant plasmid (573) (fig. 18).

The procedures for inserting foreign DNA into a plasmid do not yield a uniform product. When sticky ends of plasmids are generated, a certain percentage of the plasmids recircularize and thus do not recombine with the DNA to be cloned. It therefore becomes important to be able to dis-

Figure 18.—Common Methods for Inserting Foreign DNA Into the pBR322 Plasmid

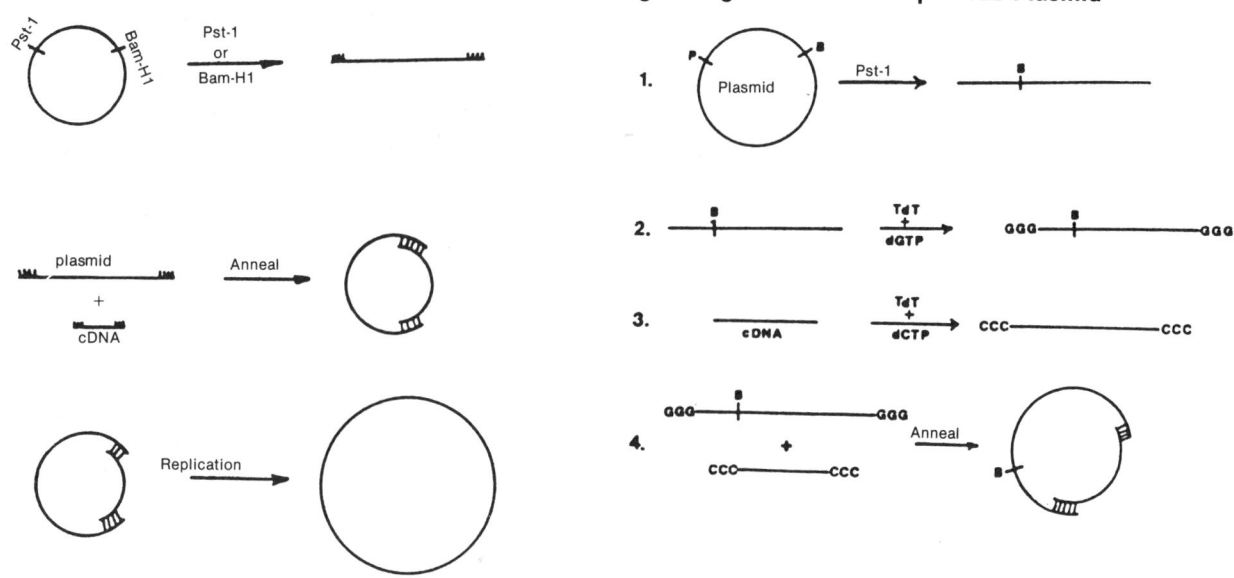

A. Insertion by annealing of sticky ends on plasmid and foreign DNA. In the example shown, the plasmid and foreign DNA have been modified with restriction enzymes to produce sticky ends. The two DNAs are then mixed together in the proper ratio and allowed to anneal. With a single replication of the recombinant molecule, the foreign DNA is recombined permanently into the plasmid.

B. Insertion by dG:dC tailing. Residues of guanosine and cytosine are added to linear plasmid and foreign DNA, respectively, using the enzyme terminal transferase (TdT). The dG and dC tails are complementary resulting in the recombination of the foreign DNA into the plasmid.

SOURCE: R. Kahn, et al., *Alternate Sources*, 1984.

criminate between plasmid molecules that have cloned inserts and those that do not. A sensitive method to screen for plasmids with inserts involves exploiting the presence of restriction enzyme sites located in the middle of the plasmid genes that code for resistance to the antibiotics penicillin and tetracycline (fig. 17). In general, when a piece of foreign DNA is inserted into a gene coding for resistance to an antibiotic, the gene is inactivated. Thus, foreign DNA inserted into the gene coding for penicillin resistance will inactivate that gene, and a penicillin-resistant bacterium will become sensitive to the drug. However, under these conditions the gene coding for tetracycline resistance will continue to function unaffected.

Inactivation of a gene following the insertion of foreign DNA provides a quick way to screen a large number of bacteria for those that harbor plasmids with foreign DNA inserts. If the DNA has been inserted into the gene coding for penicillin resistance, recombinant plasmids will no longer be resistant to penicillin but will continue to be resistant to tetracycline. Plasmids which do not contain DNA inserts should have resistance to both antibiotics. In practice, the plasmid mixture is added to bacterial cells that have been made permeable to DNA molecules and, following a brief incubation, the cells are plated on medium containing tetracycline. Under these conditions, bacteria that did not take up any DNA will not grow because they have no resistance to tetracycline, whereas bacteria that took up plasmid, with or without a DNA insert, will give rise to colonies.

An inoculum from each colony that grows on the tetracycline-containing plates is then tested for its ability to give rise to a colony on medium containing penicillin. Only those colonies that orginated from bacteria that took up plasmid without inserts will grow on penicillin, and thus are discarded. In this example, colonies that grow only on tetracycline and not penicillin represent bacteria that received recombinant plasmids harboring a foreign DNA insert.

Uptake of recombinant DNA molecules by competent *E. coli* bacteria (or other organisms) results in the appearance of colonies on agar plates within 24 to 48 hours of incubation. The collection of colonies (known as a library) will contain a representation of the cloned genes to which the bacteria were originally exposed, and therefore one or more screening protocols must be devised to identify the colony(ies) harboring the DNA sequence of interest.

In some cases, identification of the desired clone can be easily accomplished, as in the cloning of cDNAs coding for hemoglobin (353), or albumin (336). In these cases, the cDNAs were synthesized from mRNA extracted from the cell type primarily responsible for synthesizing the protein (i.e., reticulocytes and liver cells, respectively). In reticulocytes, most of the message present in the mRNA code is for hemoglobin; thus most of the bacterial colonies of the library will harbor cDNA that codes for hemoglobin. The result is that relatively few colonies will have to be screened before a cloned hemoglobin gene is identified. In most cases, however, the cDNA library will contain cDNA clones synthesized from a heterogeneous mixture of mRNAs, and thus the colony harboring the desired gene clone will be identified only after a large number of colonies have been screened.

Many methods are available to screen a library of colonies. Colony hybridization (247) is one method capable of examining hundreds of bacterial colonies quickly and easily. This method essentially involves growing colonies on nitrocellulose filter paper soaked in medium, lysing the cells and fixing the released DNA to the filter paper (fig. 19). Thus, a collection of DNA spots the exact size and shape of the colonies from which they were derived is left on a baked filter. The filter is then incubated with a buffered solution containing a nucleic acid probe that has been radioactively labeled.

Since the recombinant clones on the nitrocellulose are denatured, (i.e., the two strands of the DNA molecule have been separated) the single strands are immobilized on the filter and are capable of pairing to labeled complementary nucleic acid molecules present in the hybridization buffer. Colonies that hybridize to the probe can be easily detected by exposing the filter paper to X-ray film; positive colonies will appear as black dots on the developed film (fig. 19).

Maniatis et al (353) purified the mRNA coding for hemoglobin from reticulocytes and then hybridized labeled mRNA to a cDNA library. The success of this particular approach was due to the large amount of hemoglobin mRNA that was easily purified from reticulocytes. Success in identifying cDNA clones coding for albumin have also been reported using this technique (542). Once again, purification of the mRNAs was possible because of their large abundance in a particular tissue.

Identification of cDNA clones synthesized from less abundant mRNAs has also been possible using hybridization techniques. One approach that has repeatedly proven effective in identifying clones involves hybridization of a gene library to a chem-

Figure 19.—The Filter Hybridization Technique of Grunstein and Hogness, 1975

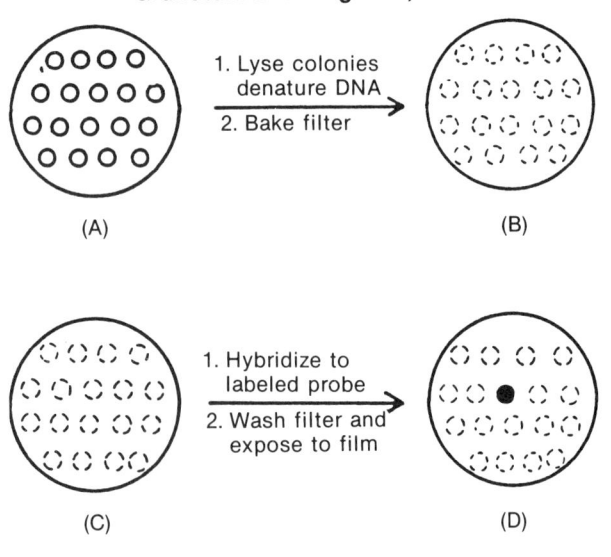

In this protocol bacterial colonies are grown on nitrocellulose filters that have been placed atop nutrient agar plates (A). The colonies are lysed and the DNA sticks to the filter (B). Baking the filter *in vacuo* results in the irreversible binding of the DNA to the filter in a form that is capable of hybridizing to a radioactive probe (C). DNA on the filter that hybridizes to the probe will become radioactive and expose the overlying area of the X-ray film (D).

SOURCE: R. Kahn, et al., *Alternate Sources*, 1984.

ically synthesized oligonucleotide probe (516b). Synthetic oligonucleotides of virtually any length and of a predetermined sequence can be easily and reliably synthesized by a variety of chemical means (516b). The longer the probe, the more specific it will be in hybridizing only to the clone of interest.

If the amino acid sequence of a limited part of a protein is known, a nucleotide sequence that will translate into that amino acid sequence can be deduced. Synthetic oligonucleotides have been used to identify gene clones for several plasma proteins. Edlund et al. (170) and Prochownik et al. (448) identified the genes coding for plasminogen activator and antithrombin III, respectively, using this methodology. The successful cloning of these and other genes emphasizes the effectiveness of synthetic oligonucleotides as hybridization probes for clone identification.

If the amino acid sequence of the desired protein is not available and its messenger RNA is in short supply, an antibody that reacts with the protein may be used for clone identification. In this technique, the antibody reacts with the antigenic site(s) on the protein synthesized by the bacterial colony harboring the clone gene. Immunological screening involves growing colonies on nitrocellulose filter paper and lysing the cells in a manner that will allow the cellular proteins to stick to the paper (258). The filter is then incubated with radiolabeled antibody and exposed to X-ray film. Any colony synthesizing immunoreactive protein will show up on the film as an exposed spot and thus presumably harbors the gene of interest. Immunological screening has been used to identify recombinant clones coding for the proteins proinsulin (94,573) and tropomyosin (258).

The advantage of the immunological screening approach to clone identification is that antibodies are more easily generated than oligonucleotides. Furthermore, colonies identified with this protocol are synthesizing the protein from the cloned gene in a correct fashion. The disadvantage to this approach relates to the requirement that the bacteria must express the cloned genetic information correctly and must synthesize enough of the protein to be easily detected by an antibody. These requirements may not be met by some colonies harboring the correct gene sequence, but not expressing the protein correctly or in sufficient amounts.

Once the desired gene clone has been isolated, it can be used in a number of ways. Since the gene is cloned, it can be produced in virtually any amount and in a pure form for study or further modification. For example, if the colony harboring the gene does not express the protein coded by it, the gene may be excised from the vector and reinserted into another vector that will allow the protein to be expressed.

Of all the applications of gene cloning technology, perhaps the most widespread use is destined to be in mass production of useful proteins. The hope is that existing protein products can be made more efficiently, more cheaply, and more cleanly by gene cloning than by current methods. Before these ambitions can be realized, however, several hurdles must be passed. The first involves applying the techniques discussed previously to identify the desired gene clone and to get the product of the gene expressed by the cellular host. As will become apparent, this step is probably the easiest task to surmount. Second, depending upon the product, some modification may be required to convert a precursor form of the protein, which may be inactive, into the activated form. The third requirement involves putting the recombined gene into a host that will be suitable for growth on an industrial scale. Finally, the protein product must be purified to meet safety and efficacy standards set by Federal regulatory agencies.

Insulin is a protein that has undergone all of these steps and is now marketed by Eli Lilly (Indianapolis, IN). It was one of the first pharmaceutically useful proteins for which the gene has been cloned and the protein expressed. Since the A and B polypeptide chains which comprise insulin are relatively short and the complete amino acid sequence of each was known, it was a straightforward task to chemically synthesize oligonucleotides that would separately code for each chain (227). The oligonucleotides were linked to the *E. coli* gene for an enzyme, beta-galactosidase, using a modified form of the pBR322 plasmid. The beta-galactosidase gene facilitated the expression of the insulin gene linked to it. Thus, insulin chains were synthesized in the form of a fusion product to beta-galactosidase. In other words, one long protein chain was composed of a portion of the beta-galactosidase protein and the entire insulin chain linked together end to end.

Ingeniously, the genetic code for the amino acid, methionine, was attached ahead of the code for the first amino acid of both the A and B insulin chains. Methionine can be destroyed by the chemical, cyanogen bromide, and thus this construction enabled the insulin polypeptides to be readily cleaved from beta-galactosidase. Since neither the A nor B insulin chain contains a methionine residue, the protein was not affected by cyanogen bromide cleavage.

The scheme to produce biologically active insulin was to isolate the A and B chains from the recombinant strains harboring the respective genes and then mix the polypeptides together. In the presence of mild chemical treatment, the chains were found to associate together correctly and the net result was pure, biologically active insulin (227). Subsequent clinical trials of recombinant insulin have shown the recombinant hormone to be as safe and effective as natural insulin in its physiological effects (303). However, the cost of the recombinant product is about twice the price of the hormone extracted from bovine/porcine pancreas, from which it has conventionally been derived.

Another recombinant product currently undergoing clinical trials is the antiviral agent, interferon. Interferon actually refers to a collection of three small proteins (known as alpha, beta and gamma) that apparently affords protection to cells from viral infection and some forms of cancer. Before it was produced by recombinant methods, interferon was isolated from lymphocytes, but the yield and purity was poor. Using recombinant methods, however, strains of E. coli harboring the alpha interferon gene have been developed that synthesize large amounts of interferon (153,228, 237,398). Preliminary results suggest comparable efficacy and side effects for the synthetic molecules as compared with the natural material isolated from lymphocytes (579). In addition to alpha interferon, the successful cloning of beta and gamma interferons has also been reported (153,154,237).

Although it should be clear from the foregoing discussion that pharmaceutically useful proteins can be produced in recombinant organisms, it should be noted that in each case a certain amount of serendipity was involved. For example, the techniques used to produce recombinant-made insulin can be used in only a limited number of cases. Since neither the A nor B chains of insulin contain the amino acid methionine, the cyanogen bromide treatment had no effect. However, if the protein did contain methionine, it would be cleaved by the treatment at each methionine site, resulting in a fragmented product that would probably be inactive.

Another potential problem that fortuitously was irrelevant for insulin or alpha interferon production is that neither protein needs modification after its synthesis before it can function. One common modification of proteins after their initial synthesis is the attachment of carbohydrate, termed glycosylation. Should glycosylation be a requirement for normal function, the product of recombinant bacteria will have to be glycosylated in some way in order to produce an active product.

One of the obstacles facing the biotechnology industry is the production scale-up of a recombinant product and its subsequent large-scale purification. To this end, strains of bacteria are continually being sought that synthesize a desired protein efficiently and in large amounts. The current maximum yield of product appears to be about one gram of protein per liter of ferment. With regard to the isolation of the desired protein from the bacteria, current methods generally involve treatment of the bacteria to release the protein. Treatment can include complete lysis of the bacterial cell or a milder procedure that makes the cell wall leaky. In either approach, a crude preparation of the protein is initially recovered.

Impurities of the preparation may not be very important, as in the case of industrial enzymes. Alternatively, one common contaminant of the lysed bacteria is cell wall fragments, which are pyrogenic (fever-causing) in humans. Other contaminants may be antigenic in humans and thus elicit an antibody response upon repeated therapy with the product. Any product to be infused into a human will have to meet FDA standards for purity and safety. Thus, novel procedures capable of substantial scale-up may have to be devised.

Because it is easier to purify a protein from culture medium than it is from a bacterial lysate, it would be advantageous if a recombinant-made protein were secreted into the medium. One of the shortcomings of *E. coli* as a host for cloning is that this bacterium does not normally secrete anything into its environment. This precludes harvesting the product from spent culture medium. Currently, a great deal of research is being done to modify *E. coli* so that it will secrete recombinant products.

Alternatively, other bacterial species such as *Bacillus subtilis* may be suited for scale-up, since this bacterial species already secretes a large amount of its own proteins into the external environment. Thus, the secretory machinery already operational in *B. subtilis* may be more easily exploited for more efficient production of plasma proteins. The fact that this feature of *Bacillus* strains has been exploited in the manufacture of industrially used proteins provides encouragement that the organism can be made to secrete recombinant plasma proteins.

Purification of protein products from recombinant organisms may be accomplished in a variety of ways. In many cases the purification scheme will depend in large part upon the biochemical properties of the protein to be isolated. One of the more specialized and successful methods available makes use of monoclonal antibodies (see subsequent discussion of "immunoglobulins" for an explanation of this new technology). If a monoclonal antibody produced against the recombinant protein is coupled to a solid matrix, it is possible to pass a crude mixture of proteins containing the protein of interest over the matrix, and only the protein recognized by the antibody will be retained. The desired protein can then be recovered by a variety of methods (72,587). This approach has proven successful for the large-scale, one-step purification of interferon from recombinant bacteria (428).

Application of Recombinant DNA Technology to Large-Scale Production of Plasma Proteins

The proteins currently recovered from the fractionation process are albumin, factor VIII, prothrombin complex and immunoglobulins. Other proteins with potential clinical application cannot be recovered in high yield from plasma or can be recovered only at the expense of another product. In addition, transfusion of many plasma fractionation products carries the risk of infectious disease, such as viral hepatitis and AIDS. It is for these reasons that recombinant DNA technology is believed to hold much promise. The gene sequences coding for a number of plasma proteins have been cloned, but numerous problems must be resolved before this new industry can effectively compete with conventional plasma fractionation.

The recombinant DNA industry will also likely attempt to clone genes coding for newly identified, clinically useful plasma proteins. This will probably be the easiest task facing genetic engineering technology, however, since the techniques discussed in the previous sections have proven so successful in the isolation of virtually any desired gene.

A major challenge facing gene cloning technology is scaling up production sufficiently to meet demand. It is likely, therefore, that large-scale production/purification capabilities must be available before genetic engineering can meet even the U.S. demand for plasma products. For some plasma products such as albumin, thousands of kilograms will have to be synthesized and purified. For products such as Factor VIII, such large amounts will not be required, but purification methods that will not inactivate this highly unstable molecule will have to be developed. Thus, scale-up will involve challenges in both the production of a recombinant plasma protein and its subsequent purification.

An additional problem to resolve will be to design biological systems for modifications after genetic expression for those plasma proteins that need such modifications to be functional. If the gene coding for a plasma protein that needs to have a carbohydrate molecule attached (i.e., glycosylation) is cloned in a bacterial cell which is incapable of doing so, a means of properly glycosylating the protein once it is purified from the recombinant bacteria must be devised. Alternatively, the gene may be cloned into yeast or mammalian cells which, under proper circumstances, may correctly glycosylate the protein. While glycosylation is perhaps the major form of post-translational modification, other modifications are sometimes necessary for protein activity.

Each plasma protein will, therefore, have its own specific problems. In the discussion that follows, the general status of cloning the genes that code for the plasma proteins of demonstrated or potential clinical value is reviewed.

Albumin.—Albumin is the major single protein species in plasma, with a normal concentration of approximately 70 mg/ml (371). It performs many functions, including maintaining the oncotic pressure of blood and serving as the carrier molecule for fatty acids and other small molecules in plasma (467). Albumin is synthesized in the liver and is the major protein product of that organ. The large amount of albumin synthesized by the liver is reflected in that tissue's abundance of albumin-specific mRNA, averaging 5 to 10 percent of the total mRNA in liver (474). With such a high concentration, it has been a fairly straightforward task to clone the cDNA that codes for albumin.

The gene for human albumin is probably the first plasma protein gene to be cloned, and numerous recombinant DNA companies have publicly claimed to have both recombinant yeast and bacterial strains carrying the human albumin gene (table 43). In addition to the companies listed, there are likely to be others that have all or part of the albumin gene cloned.

One company, Genentech, Inc., has also published the detailed construction of a recombinant *E. coli* that produces albumin (336). In these experiments, the albumin gene was linked to the DNA that regulates the utilization of the amino acid, tryptophan, in *E. coli*. In other words, the human gene was under the control of a segment of bacterial DNA that responded to the concentration of tryptophan in the medium. Under con-

Table 43.—rDNA Companies That Are Working on Cloning the Gene for Serum Albumin

1. Genentech, Inc., San Francisco, CA (in conjunction with Mitsubishi Chemical Industries, Japan)
2. Biogen, Inc., Cambridge, MA
3. Genex, Boston, MA (in conjunction with Green Cross of Japan and Kabi of Sweden)
4. Speywood Laboratories, England
5. Genetics Institute, Boston, MA (in conjunction with Baxter-Travenol)
6. Chiron Corp., Emeryville, CA

SOURCES: D. Clark, personal communication, 1984; and Marketing Research Bureau, Inc. (1982).

ditions of tryptophan starvation, the tryptophan genes as well as the albumin gene would be activated.

The majority of the albumin synthesized by the recombinant bacteria was found to be biochemically and immunochemically identical to native human albumin (336). However, the complex molecular configuration proposed for natural albumin (96,168) was not evaluated in the recombinant protein. Thus, the degree to which the natural and recombinant albumin molecules are identical in any way other than amino acid sequence and immunologic similarity remains unclear at this time. Interestingly, the recombinant *E. coli* of Lawn et al. (336) appeared to synthesize a small amount of albumin that was smaller in size than the native product, and may have represented incompletely synthesized albumin. Thus, not all the protein synthesized by this particular strain is comparable to native albumin.

The authors of the Genentech report do not give specific numbers for the rate with which albumin is synthesized by their bacterial strain(s). Rather, they state that the strain(s) make albumin at a "modest" rate (336). Other biotechnology companies claiming to have the cloned albumin gene have not published the biochemical properties of their product, its rate of synthesis by the host cell, or other technical information—all of which is regarded as proprietary.

In brief, it appears that the biotechnology industry has conducted the necessary initial research and development for production of recombinant albumin, and recombinant albumin production appears to be at the scale-up phase of production. But most companies appear to have this project on a back burner for the present, given the considerations discussed below.

The first obstacle to be faced in producing albumin by rDNA technology is whether the technology can produce enough protein to meet present needs, and in a cost-effective manner. Currently, most developed countries use between 100 and 400 kg of serum albumin per million population per year (62). In the United States in 1982, approximately 87,500 kg of serum albumin was used (356), or a rate of use of approximately 387 kg/million population/year. To address the feasibility of producing sufficient albumin to meet U.S. demand (as well as the additional 57,500 kg of albumin that was exported in 1982), an estimate of how much albumin could be synthesized by "state of the art" recombinant strains of bacteria or yeast is needed.

Although no rDNA company will divulge synthetic rates for individual proteins due to the proprietary nature of such information, it is general knowledge that in current expression systems the synthesis of a cloned gene product can constitute 10 to 50 percent of the total protein synthesized by the cell. The maximum achievable rate may vary significantly, however, for individual proteins (186,305,569). In general, the larger the protein the less efficiently it is synthesized by *E. coli*.

To determine how much fermentation will be necessary to meet the U.S. comsumption of albumin, two important assumptions must be made: 1) that 50 percent of the cellular protein synthesized by an optimized strain of bacteria will be albumin (in the optimized strains of *E. coli* producing human insulin, 50 percent of the cellular protein was insulin); and 2) that it will be possible to obtain 10 wet weight grams of bacterial paste from a liter of fermented culture (which, in fact, can readily be done). Of the 10 grams harvested, about 15 percent (1.5 grams) will be protein (340). Thus, 0.75 grams of albumin could be obtained per liter of fermented bacteria (i.e., 1.5 g protein/liter of fermented culture x 50 percent of total protein being albumin).

Extending the calculation further: 87,500 kg of albumin equals 87.5×10^6 grams of protein. Dividing 87.5×10^6 grams by 0.75 per liter of culture obtains 116.7×10^6 liters (or about 31 x 10^6 gallons) of fermented culture per year that will be necessary to produce sufficient albumin to meet U.S. demand. In order to supply the worldwide market, 193×10^6 liters (or about 51×10^6 gallons) of fermented culture will have to be produced.

Production capabilities already in place in this country could ferment this volume easily. For example, a typical bakers' yeast production facility may have 6 to 12 30,000 to 40,000 gallon fermenters in operation (286). These fermenters are capable (using yeast) of producing about $1-2 \times 10^6$ liters of ferment every day. Thus, if a recombinant strain of *E. coli* producing albumin at 0.75 g/liter of ferment and growing at a rate comparable to a yeast cell were given to such a production facility for albumin production, U.S. needs for albumin could be met within about 80 to 100 days of routine production. Worldwide albumin supply could be produced within a year.

The ease with which the albumin supply may be produced will, of course, depend upon the validity of the assumptions made. Once again, the assumptions were that a strain of *E. coli* is available that produces albumin at a rate comparable to the current rate of recombinant insulin production, and that this strain will multiply efficiently in a fermenter to yield 10 grams of cells per liter. In addition, it is assumed that the time necessary to re-seed a fermenter (i.e., the turnaround time) is comparable for yeast and bacteria. The first assumption regarding the albumin production rate is dependent upon the efficiency of the expression vector. But even if the maximum biosynthetic rate for recombinant albumin production were one-tenth that observed for insulin, the world market for albumin could be satisfied within a year by several companies with fermentation facilities comparable to those of Anheuser Busch in St. Louis.

Others, using more conservative numbers for the rate of recombinant albumin synthesis, arrived at a quite different conclusion; namely, that the current rDNA industry is not equipped to produce and process sufficient albumin to keep pace with worldwide, or even nationwide, demand (167). They estimated that 12.5 grams of albumin fractionated from plasma that currently sells for $25 will cost anywhere from $40 to $80 if produced by recombinant DNA technology. In their calculations, the rate of albumin production is assumed to be 10 percent of the bacterial protein, or a yield of about 100 mg/liter of ferment, compared to the previous calculation of 50 percent and 750 mg/liter.

Their conclusion, however, is based primarily upon processing considerations. For example, they assume that 50 gallons of water will be needed to process each liter of plasma by standard fractionation techniques. Based on the yield of recombinant albumin per gallon of water used, and extending water usage to an annual rate, they conclude that 10 billion gallons of water would be needed to produce the albumin that is currently fractionated from plasma with only 50 million gallons of water. They estimate that the cost of the additional water and disposing the effluent from the processing would greatly increase the cost of the product.

However, the entire contents of the fermenter will not have to be processed. Processing recombinant E. coli is not the same as plasma fractionation. First, the bacteria need to be separated from the media in which they are growing. Separation is achieved by continuous-flow centrifugation. This technique is commonly used in the fermentation industry and has the capacity to centrifuge cells from 30,000 gallons of ferment in about 2 to 4 hours (286). Thus, only the cell paste which is obtained from the fermenter is processed. The amount of water used, therefore, will be much less than in conventional plasma fractionation.

Since it costs only about $400 to produce a ton of bacteria or yeast in a fermenter (169) and 2,100 tons of cells will be needed to produce the world market of albumin, the costs incurred in the scale-up of albumin (or any other plasma protein) are likely to come from purifying the protein rather than from producing it.

Initial scale-up for recombinant products, however, is likely to be quite expensive. Although Eli Lilly will not divulge the scale-up costs for recombinant insulin, it has been reported that their costs were $70 million over expectations (584). This has resulted in an average of 50 to 55 cents per dose for recombinant insulin, whereas the price for mixed bovine and porcine insulin averages 28 to 35 cents and for highly purified porcine insulin 44 to 52 cents.

Perhaps the greatest difficulty in producing clinically acceptable recombinant albumin is the purification of the protein of bacterial contaminant. Several biochemical techniques to fractionate protein on the basis of size may be useful. Ultrafiltration is one such technique, in which a filter of controlled pore size retains molecules above a certain size while allowing smaller molecules to flow through. Thus, if albumin is significantly larger or smaller than the contaminants, it can be easily separated from them on a large scale by filtration. However, for a membrane filter to effectively separate two molecules, their respective molecular weights must differ by tenfold. Thus, in practice, ultrafiltration may prove incapable of purifying recombinant albumin. Alternatively, purification of albumin on a column containing a resin that separates molecules by size is a further refinement of the size-separation technique, although not so easily scaled-up.

Recombinant albumin may also be purified using techniques that exploit its affinity for specific molecules. For example, albumin is known to bind fatty acids, so chromatographic resins that are "fat-like" in their chemistry may prove useful. Likewise, electrostatic attractions between albumin and oppositely charged molecules (i.e., ion exchange chromatography) may prove effective for purification. In fact, this technique is currently being used by some plasma fractionaters in the purification of albumin (119). All of these methods can be scaled-up for industrial production, and should any one prove ineffective, a combination of two or more may purify recombinant albumin to an extent sufficient to meet safety requirements.

Scale-up in other countries may be more cost-effective. Japan, for example, has considerable experience in bioprocessing technology (549). In addition, there are extensive fermentation facilities in Japan, and many such corporations have ties with U.S. rDNA companies. Furthermore, the Japanese government has targeted biotechnology as a key industry and has provided tax incentives and other subsidies to bioprocessing. Thus, it may be cost-effective to produce high-volume products like albumin in Japan, and import the product to the United States.

Finally, the cost considerations discussed above were based on the rate with which the protein product is synthesized and how the product is recovered from the recombinant organism. It is very likely that further R&D will result in more efficient protein production, thus reducing the cost of the final product.

One possible method to increase the efficiency of production involves use of other strains of bacteria, such as *Bacillus subtilis*, or yeast. *B. subtilis* is a common, non-pathogenic, soil bacterium that has been used industrially for large-scale production of proteins used in detergents and in the processing of corn starch. The annual production of these proteins by *B. subtilis* ranges in the thousands of tons. *B. subtilis* has attracted the interest of the rDNA industry because of its great biosynthetic capability. When grown under suitable conditions, it can produce up to 10 to 15g/liter v. 1.5 gram/liter for *E. coli* (186,265). In addition, products made by *B. subtilis* are excreted into the medium rather than accumulated intracellularly, as is the case with *E. coli*.

Thus, if the gene coding for albumin were expressed in *B. subtilis*, the yield would be far greater than with *E. coli*, and the product would accumulate in the medium rather than in the cells. This would facilitate subsequent purification and processing and possibly continuous fermentation without re-seeding. To date, however, the use of *B. subtilis* for production of recombinant proteins is still several years behind the *E. coli* system.

Expression of recombinant albumin in yeast also lags behind the *E. coli* system, yet offers certain advantages for scale-up. Yeast, like *B. subtilis*, have been grown industrially for years, and considerable experience exists in large-scale bioprocessing techniques. In addition, the wet weight yield of yeast in a fermenter is about 2.5 times the wet weight yield of *E. coli*. Since current strains of recombinant yeast can accumulate protein to a level comparable to *E. coli* (569), the yield of recombinant protein should be increased 2.5 times per liter of ferment.

Also, yeasts have the capacity to secrete certain recombinant proteins into the medium. For example, a group from Chiron Corp. (543) synthesized the gene coding for the hormone urogastrone, and were able to get the gene expressed in a yeast system. In their report, the protein accumulated intracellularly to a level of approximately 30 mg per liter of non-fermented yeast culture. The Chiron group has now extended its early work and has linked the urogastrone gene to a gene coding for a yeast protein that is secreted into the medium (214). Thus, there is successful exploitation of a natural process in yeast, resulting in secretion of the recombinant protein.

Success of the secretion process also depends upon the individual properties of the recombinant protein, with small proteins being more efficiently secreted than larger ones. The secretion rate for the small hormone urogastrone, for example, is in the range of 20 mg per liter of ferment. But according to industry spokemen, a protein as large as albumin would not be secreted by this mechanism. Thus, different methods will have to be developed for successful secretion of albumin and other larger proteins by yeast cells. But even if the protein is not secreted, yeast offers an attractive approach to producing albumin in a very cost-effective manner.

One potential disadvantage to use of the yeast system in which the recombinant product accumulates intracellularly is the difficulty encountered in breaking yeast cells open to recover the recombinant protein. The yeast cell wall is very resistant to treatments such as detergent, osmotic shock and even sonic disruption, thus complicating initial processing procedures. Furthermore, the harsh procedures employed to break open the cells can have a denaturing effect on the biologic activity of the protein to be isolated.

In summary, current technology employing *E. coli* is capable of producing recombinant albumin to meet worldwide demand. Attention is now focused on the purification of recombinant albumin and whether this can be accomplished in a cost-effective manner. It is possible that sophisticated purification techniques will be efficacious but not cost-effective. Alternatively, albumin may be produced in a more cost-effective manner in other cloning systems (e.g., *B. subtilis*) where removal of hazardous contaminants may be less of a problem. However, these systems are not as well developed as is *E. coli*, and more research and development will be required. However, the ability to produce albumin by recombinant technology in a cost-effective manner will probably be achieved; exactly when this will happen is uncertain.

Coagulation Proteins.—Blood coagulation involves a large number of plasma proteins, at least one tissue protein, phospholipid membrane surfaces, calcium, and platelets (148,287). Coagulation of blood can occur via one of two mechanisms, known as the intrinsic and extrinsic pathways. The end result of both pathways is the conversion (activation) of the plasma protein prothrombin to thrombin, which then converts the soluble plasma protein fibrinogen to an insoluble fibrin clot.

Factor VIII.—Currently, most Factor VIII is obtained by fractionating fresh-frozen plasma. Factor VIII is generally quantitated in "units of activity" and in the United States in 1982, approximately 500 million units of Factor VIII were prepared by plasma fractionation (356). The 500 million units of Factor VIII have been estimated to constitute only about 280 grams of purified protein.

The Factor VIII molecule itself appears to consist of at least two proteins (63,178,339,378). One of these is known as Factor VIII:von Willebrand's factor (VIII:vWF). Deficiency of this protein is the underlying cause of the bleeding disorder known as von Willebrand's disease. The other component of the Factor VIII complex (VIII:C) appears to be a glycoprotein with an apparent molecular weight of around 200,000 (178,287). It is VIII:C that is lacking in hemophilia A patients and the molecule that the rDNA industry hopes to produce using gene splicing techniques. The world market for recombinant Factor VIII:C has been estimated to be as high as $2 billion (255).

The site of synthesis of factor VIII:C is not conclusively known, but recent evidence points to the cells lining the hepatic sinusoids (516a). The normal circulating concentration of factor VIII:C is approximately 100 nanograms per milliliter of plasma, and the protein is very unstable. Information regarding the molecular nature of factor VIII:C has been slow to accumulate. Consequently, the approach that has been taken to obtain recombinant-made Factor VIII:C has been to synthesize an oligonucleotide probe based on the amino acid sequence of the molecule, which was then used to screen bacteria containing human DNA (535). Using this technique, segments of human chromosomal DNA that code for portions of factor VIII:C have been identified, and the approach has been to splice these segments together to construct the complete factor VIII:C gene. A list of the companies claiming to have cloned at least a portion of the factor VIII:C gene is shown in table 44.

The clones identified in this manner were constructed with chromosomal DNA, and, therefore, the factor VIII:C gene exhibits the exon/intron gene structure characteristics of mammalian chromosomal DNA, which are not present in bacterial DNA. Recall that bacteria are incapable of properly expressing genes that consist of exons and introns. Thus, investigators will have to splice together the regions of the factor VIII:C gene that actually code for the protein in a bacterial expression vector in much the same way as were the cDNAs for albumin and interferon discussed earlier.

While a factor VIII:C gene spliced together from the separate gene segments may be necessary for expression of the gene by bacteria or yeast cells,

Table 44.—Companies Working on Cloning the Gene Coding for Factor VIII

1. Genentech, Inc., San Francisco, CA (in conjunction with Speywood Laboratories)
2. Genetics Institute, Boston, MA (in conjunction with Baxter-Travenol, Deerfield, IL)
3. Biogen, Cambridge, MA (in conjunction with Feijin in Japan and Kabi in Sweden)
4. Armour Pharmaceuticals, Kankakee, IL
5. Integrated Genetics, Boston, MA
6. Chiron Corp., Emeryville, CA

SOURCES: D. Clark, personal communication, 1984; Marketing Research Bureau, Inc. (1982); *Biotechnology Newswatch*, May 7, 1984.

an intact chromosomal gene with its exon/intron organization may be suitable for expression by mammalian cells. In fact, techniques exist for the efficient introduction of foreign DNA into a variety of cultured mammalian cell lines (585), and results from several studies have shown that the genetic information coded in a clone of human chromosomal DNA can be properly expressed by a mouse cell line. Because this approach may prove feasible, virtually all the rDNA companies working on cloning factor VIII:C are considering mammalian expression systems.

Several problems will be encountered in synthesizing factor VIII:C by rDNA methods. First, the molecule is fairly large in size (i.e., molecular weight of approximately 200,000). To date, the largest human protein efficiently made by bacteria has been albumin, which has a molecular weight about a third that of factor VIII:C (i.e., 68,000 vs. 200,000). But in the E. coli strain used to synthesize albumin as described by Lawn et al. (336), a significant proportion of the albumin made was smaller in size than the native molecule. These results suggest that when large recombinant proteins are produced by E. coli, incompletely synthesized proteins may also appear. Cloning the factor VIII:C gene in yeast or mouse cells may overcome this problem. In addition, it is possible that only a portion of the factor VIII:C molecule is required for the activity of the entire molecule, so DNA coding for the smaller fragment alone might be cloned and efficiently expressed in a bacterial system.

Another potential problem is that factor VIII:C is a glycoprotein, and it is still unclear whether or not the associated carbohydrate is important for procoagulant activity (600). If carbohydrate is important for coagulant activity, the factor VIII:C molecule synthesized by recombinant bacteria somehow has to be glycosylated before it is clinically effective. Alternatively, the factor VIII:C gene could be cloned and expressed using hosts capable of glycosylating proteins (e.g., yeast or mammalian cells).

One final problem to be faced by the rDNA industry in producing factor VIII:C will be the inherent instability of the molecule. Factor VIII:C is extremely sensitive to proteases (enzymes that degrade protein), and recombinant organisms synthesizing factor VIII:C will have to be engineered to have low levels of protease. Furthermore, since disrupting virtually any cell results in the release of proteases, it would be desirable for the recombinant organism to secrete the molecule into the medium.

Because of our lack of knowledge regarding the precise molecular biology of factor VIII:C, it is unclear how difficult or cumbersome it will be to produce the recombinant-made product. Thus, it is impossible to estimate its potential costs. But availability of the product and its safety with regard to infectious diseases are also important, and recombinant factor VIII:C should be a far better product than the plasma derivative. Since the worldwide market for factor VIII:C has been estimated at only 280 grams, recombinant organisms synthesizing factor VIII:C, even inefficiently, should have little problem producing this amount.

Several rDNA companies have publicly announced that recombinant factor VIII:C will soon be available. Genetics Institute, for example, has claimed that it hopes to begin testing recombinant factor VIII:C in about 2 years (216). Genentech has announced that it had cloned the entire Factor VIII:C gene and inserted it into mammalian cells, which then made and secreted Factor VIII:C into the culture medium. The gene was found to consist of 26 exons separated by introns and consisted of about 200,000 nucleotides, of which about 9,000 comprised the exon segments. Laboratory experiments showed that the product, about 4 times larger than albumin, was biologically active (484). These findings were published in November 1984 (226,536,570,592). The next steps to be undertaken include increasing the amount of Factor VIII:C produced by the cell line, scale-up, purification and producing a homogenous product, and pre-clinical and clinical testing.

Factor IX.—Factor IX is another plasma coagulation factor whose congenital deficiency results in the bleeding disorder known as hemophilia B (148,287). Although less common than hemophilia A, hemophilia B can be equally severe, and treatment is by infusion of Factor IX complex (404). Factor IX complex actually consists of several procoagulant proteins, including Factors II, VII, IX and X. Thus, it can be used for treatment of the congenital deficiency for each of these factors as well as for other hemorrhagic conditions (404). Like plasma-derived Factor VIII, however, treatment with Factor IX complex presents an increased risk of infectious disease.

The market for Factor IX is fairly limited because of the relative rarity of hemophilia B and an ample supply of Factor IX from plasma fractionation (78). A recent survey showed the Factor IX market to be only approximately $13 million in 1982, and that reflected a 15 percent gain over 1981 (356). The Factor IX market is not as great as for Factor VIII ($13 million v. $51 million in the United States), and some analysts believe the synthesis of recombinant Factor IX is not financially practical at this time (78). Nonetheless, several rDNA companies as well as academic laboratories have actually cloned the gene coding for Factor IX (115,290,323).

Factor IX consists of a single polypeptide chain of approximately 55,000 molecular weight (148, 287), containing 26 percent carbohydrate (148). It is synthesized in the liver in an inactive form and subsequently modified by glycosylation and by conversion of 12 molecules of glutamic acid to gamma-carboxyglutamic acid, a vitamin K-dependent process (571).

Upon activation in the coagulation process, Factor IX is cleaved into three polypeptide chains of 29,000, 16,000 and 9,000 molecular weight (MW) (287). The 9,000-MW fragment contains most of the carbohydrate associated with the entire Factor IX molecule, while the 16,000-MW chain appears necessary for its activation. The site for Factor IX coagulation activity is located on the 29,000-MW species (287). Circulating concentration of Factor IX is approximately 2 to 4 mg/ml (115).

The Factor IX gene clone was identified from a cDNA library generated by using mRNA extracted from human liver. An oligonucleotide probe was chemically synthesized based upon the known amino acid sequence of Factor IX. These oligonucleotides were subsequently radioactively labeled and used as specific hybridization probes against the liver cDNA library (115,290,323). The cDNA clone isolated by Kurachi and Davie (323) contained the entire coding sequence for Factor IX. In addition to the identification of cDNA clones, Choo et al. (115) have cloned the actual chromosomal DNA coding for Factor IX.

Production of recombinant Factor IX protein should be less difficult than making Factor VIII:C. The size of the polypeptide (i.e., 55,000 MW) is within the current limits of commonly used expression vectors. Furthermore, a report detailing the cloning of the Factor IX gene has already been published (323) and other clones have been constructed by some rDNA companies (535). Finally, an organism producing even a moderate amount of Factor IX should be capable of yielding sufficient amounts to meet market demands. However, the limited market and the availability of an ample supply of Factor IX fractionated from plasma, have together slowed the impetus to develop a recombinant Factor IX in favor of the more profitable Factor VIII:C molecule.

Production of recombinant Factor IX will not, however, be an altogether easy task. In the first place, the molecule is a glycoprotein, and it is not yet known how the activity of Factor IX is influenced by the associated carbohydrate. As with Factor VIII:C, it may be necessary to clone the Factor IX gene in a yeast or mammalian host capable of correctly glycosylating the protein. However, a large part of the carbohydrate associated with Factor IX is attached to the 9,000-MW fragment, which is cleaved from the molecule as it is activated (323). Thus, the carbohydrate portion of Factor IX may not function in coagulation. If this is the case, glycosylation of recombinant Factor IX may not be necessary to obtain a useful molecule.

A second, more challenging, obstacle to the production of functional recombinant Factor IX will involve the other major post-translational modification of the protein that normally occurs in the liver, the conversion of several N-terminal glutamic acid molecules of Factor IX to gamma-carboxyglutamate residues by a vitamin K-dependent enzyme system (416). This enzyme system is lacking in bacterial and yeast hosts (571). It may therefore be necessary to modify these glutamic acids by chemical means in order to produce a functional Factor IX molecule.

In summary, it does not appear that a great deal of industrial interest has been generated toward production of recombinant Factor IX. The lack of interest appears to result from the smaller market for the product as well as an abundant supply of Factor IX concentrate from plasma fractionation. Thus, development of recombinant Factor IX is likely to occur after the development of recombinant Factor VIII:C. Although the production of recombinant Factor IX will probably require some post-expression modification, chemical rather than enzymatic reactions may be used to accomplish that goal.

Other Coagulation Factors.—There is currently a great deal of scientific and medical interest in all of the other protein factors that participate in coagulation. As a result, virtually all of the coagulation factors have attracted the attention of rDNA companies. Should a market for these proteins develop, the genes for these additional factors will probably be identified using oligonucleotide probes synthesized from known stretches of the amino acid sequence of these proteins. Industrial development of these products is likely to occur after development of Factor VIII:C and Factor IX.

Plasma Enzyme Inhibitors.—There are numerous proteins in plasma whose physiological role is to inhibit proteases. Although these inhibitors are not currently fractionated from plasma on a commercial basis, they have gained widespread attention for their potential as therapeutic agents. The plasma proteins of interest are alpha 1-antitrypsin, anti-thrombin III, and C1-esterase inhibitor (496).

Alpha 1-antitrypsin. Alpha 1-antitrypsin inhibits the enzyme, neutrophil elastase, a potent protease that degrades structural proteins (335). In addition to inhibiting elastase, alpha 1-antitrypsin is capable of inhibiting a number of other proteases, including trypsin, chymotrypsin, collagenase, thrombin, kallikrein and plasmin (335). The inhibitor appears to act by combining with the protease to form a stable, inactive complex consisting of equal amounts of protease and inhibitor.

Alpha 1-antitrypsin is a glycoprotein and is synthesized in the liver. The protein consists of a single polypeptide chain of approximately 50,000 MW (139) with three carbohydrate side chains (370). Its normal plasma concentration is about 2 mg/ml, and a low circulating level of the protein is often associated with chronic obstructive pulmonary emphysema and infantile cirrhosis of the liver (335). In essence, the continuous action of proteases on structural tissues, particularly in the lung and liver, results in autodigestion of the tissue. Alpha 1-antitrypsin inhibits this self-destructive process. At present more than 30 genetic variants of alpha 1-antitrypsin have been identified (138).

Preparations of alpha 1-antitrypsin are not currently available for routine use but are being evaluated in certain experimental protocols. The protein can be prepared from plasma using one of several methods. Polyethylene glycol precipitation has been used to prepare a crude concentrate of alpha 1-antitrypsin which retains some biological activity (210). Alpha 1-antitrypsin concentrates have also been made by further processing of the remaining plasma after the usual plasma fractions have been extracted (102). The product can be pasteurized to inactivate potential infectious contaminants.

The potential market for alpha 1-antitrypsin is uncertain. As of 1982, only 2.5 percent of the plasma fractionated in the United States was devoted to preparation of all inhibitor products (i.e., alpha 1-antitrypsin, anti-thrombin III, Cl-esterase inhibitor, etc.) (356). Patients suffering from a deficiency of the inhibitor require maintenance therapy, but the deficient condition is fairly uncommon. It is possible, however, that alpha 1-antitrypsin may play a role in the pathophysiology of other diseases, such as acute respiratory distress syndrome. Alpha 1-antitrypsin therapy is currently being evaluated for its effect on such patients. Should the inhibitor be of benefit for this disease, its use could become quite common (496).

The gene coding for alpha 1-antitrypsin has been cloned by at least one laboratory (323). This group synthesized an oligonucleotide probe based upon the known amino acid sequence of the molecule and used the oligonucleotide probe to screen a cDNA library prepared from liver mRNA. A cDNA clone was identified that coded for the C-terminal region of the molecule (323). Given that Kurachi and co-workers reported on their work in 1981, a full length cDNA clone has most likely been isolated, and one company, Chiron Corp., reportedly has the entire gene coding for alpha 1-antitrypsin cloned in both yeast and *E. coli* (569).

In the yeast system, 20 percent of the total protein inside the cell during fermentation is alpha 1-antitrypsin. By performing a simple calculation, one can deduce that every liter of ferment of this yeast strain would yield almost 1 gram of alpha 1-antitrypsin, which is the concentration of the molecule in approximately one unit of whole blood. While the Chiron Corp. claims to have a strain of yeast synthesizing the protein, the company would not provide information regarding the efficacy of the recombinant product. Alpha-1-antitrypsin has been given "orphan drug status" by the FDA (193), and this designation will hasten the FDA review process and provide manufacturers with tax credits to offset development costs.

Since alpha 1-antitrypsin is a glycoprotein, it is possible that the associated carbohydrate is necessary for activity. The yeast host should be capable of glycosylation, but Chiron Corp. would not divulge whether or not its yeast expression system glycosylated the molecule correctly, if at all. Therefore, many of the glycosylation problems discussed earlier for the coagulation proteins may also be relevant to the synthesis of functional alpha 1-antitrypsin.

Antithrombin III. Among members of a family of plasma proteins with antithrombin activity, anti-thrombin III (ATIII) is the most potent and physiologically relevant inhibitor of the procoagulant protease, thrombin. In addition to inhibiting thrombin, ATIII significantly inhibits many other proteases involved in coagulation (496). The mechanism of ATIII inhibition, like that of alpha 1-antitrypsin, involves the binding of protease to inhibitor to form an inactive complex (114,448). The rate of inactive complex formation is greatly enhanced by heparin. This finding has led to successful use of ATIII in conjunction with low doses of heparin to prevent post-operative thrombosis (304).

Increasing awareness of the clinical importance of ATIII has also come from descriptions of hereditary deficiencies of the molecule. The frequency of congenital ATIII deficiency is approximately 1:3500 (410). Most cases of the inherited disorder are characterized by ATIII levels at approximately 50 percent of normal; levels less than 25 percent of normal are rare. Yet, families with even 50 percent of normal ATIII levels have a hyperactive clotting system.

A transient deficiency in ATIII levels can also be acquired, especially in patients with venous thrombosis from a number of causes, including chronic liver or kidney disease. ATIII depression also occurs in women taking oral contraceptives (496). Such women have an increased propensity for thrombosis, and the ATIII deficiency is felt by many to be the underlying cause. However, this theory is not firmly established.

Several varieties of ATIII concentrates are available commercially, but as was mentioned in the discussion for alpha 1-antitrypsin, 1982 plasma fractionation statistics indicate that production of inhibitor concentrates constituted only about 2.5 percent of the total plasma fractionated (356). But in reviewing the literature concerning ATIII, it becomes apparent that a much more significant market may exist for the product.

ATIII is a glycoprotein and member of the alpha-globulin family of plasma proteins. It has a molecular weight of 55,000 to 60,000 (1,114, 512). Much of the amino acid sequence of the protein is known (426). As a result, an oligonucleotide probe to identify the ATIII gene has now been prepared in several laboratories, with both the cDNA coding for the entire protein sequence and the entire chromosomal gene having been cloned in *E. coli* (114,448,512). The ATIII gene has not yet been cloned in any host other than *E. coli*.

Although there has been no report of a recombinant cell that synthesizes ATIII, it should not be difficult to engineer such a cell, and several rDNA companies including Genex and Genentech have expressed interest (119,280). ATIII activity is present in stored blood (279), which suggests that the ATIII protein is a relatively stable molecule. Problems associated with production of recombinant ATIII should not present any unique challenge, other than the potential need for glycosylation of the protein.

C1 Esterase Inhibitor. C1 esterase inhibitor is a protein that inhibits the enzyme of the same name. Deficiency of the inhibitor results in prolonged esterase activity, with swelling of the surrounding tissue (496). The most serious consequences of C1 esterase deficiency can be angioedema of the upper respiratory tract, with the potential for suffocation.

The inhibitor can be extracted from fresh-frozen plasma and is effective in treating acute episodes of angioedema (496). Androgen (male hormone) analogs are also successful in stimulation C1 esterase levels in deficient patients, and therefore the widespread use of C1 esterase inhibitor concentrates will probably never be realized. The gene coding for C1-esterase inhibitor has not yet attracted the attention of the rDNA industry and has probably not been cloned.

Plasminogen Activators.—Plasma contains an enzyme system capable of digesting the fibrin in blood clots, thus leading to clot dissolution. One component of the system consists of a family of proteins collectively known as plasminogen activators (116). Plasminogen activator (PA) converts plasminogen to plasmin, which then degrades the fibrin network of the clot to form soluble products (130). The system is elegantly specific in that the activating effect of PA on conversion of plasminogen to plasmin is dependent upon the presence of fibrin. Thus, the anticoagulant effect of the system is limited to the immediate site of a clot. This is in contrast to the more widespread effects of other clot dissolution agents such as streptokinase and urokinase, which are widely used clinically. In some cases the nonspecificity of these drugs can cause serious bleeding problems due to the digestion of fibrinogen as well as fibrin (7).

Because of the site specificity of PA, production of the protein by recombinant methods has received considerable attention. Recent commercial interest in PA has come as a result of advances in two areas of research. First, it was shown that the infusion of 7.5 mg of a purified PA induced the dissolution of a 6-week-old thrombus without concomitant bleeding problems (580). Second, the PA used in this study was harvested from a melanoma cell line that overproduces PA and secretes it into the medium (461). This PA was found to be identical to the PA isolated from normal tissue (461). The 7.5 mg of PA used to treat this patient (at a cost of about $2,000) was harvested from about 75 liters of spent culture medium from the melanoma cell line (7).

PA is composed of a single polypeptide chain (578), and has a molecular weight of 70,000 (170,422). It is presumed that PA is the normal vascular regulator of clot dissolution and is synthesized and released into the circulation by vascular endothelial cells in response to the proper stimuli. The amino acid sequence of much of the molecule has been determined (578). Research on PA has been hampered by its extremely low concentration in blood, tissue extracts, and cell culture medium. However, since the amino acid sequence of the protein was known, it was relatively easy to synthesize an oligonucleotide probe for screening a cDNA library prepared from mRNA extracted from the melanoma cell line that overproduces PA (170,422).

Furthermore, Pennica et al. (1983) of Genentech, Inc. have cloned the entire coding sequence for PA and have engineered an *E. coli* cell to produce recombinant PA. In addition to Genentech, Inc., Integrated Genetics, Abbott Laboratories, Biogen, Collaborative Research and HEM Research have all been involved in PA research and gene cloning (119). Currently, Collaborative Research and Abbott Labs market PA synthesized by the melanoma cell culture method (582). It is likely that both companies have the gene sequences for PA cloned as well. It has been estimated that recombinant PA can be synthesized at 1/200 to 1/500 the cost of the product secreted by the melanoma cell line (7).

The future market for PA in the United States is estimated to be 400 million to 2 billion dollars (215). Because of the clinical potential of PA, and the difficulty incurred in purifying it from natural sources, recombinant PA is likely to have little competition for a potentially expanding clinical market. Initial results of Pennica et al. (422) suggest that a biologically active recombinant product can be produced by *E. coli* and optimizing the level of expression in the recombinant strain should be straightforward.

Immunoglobulin. The plasma fractionation industry currently isolates immunoglobulin fractions from plasma of donors hyperimmunized against known antigens. In 1970, production of immunoglobulins was significant, accounting for some 10,000 kg of total production (404). Of this, approximately 900 kg was immune globulin of known titer and specificity. As of 1982, the market for immune globulin had not expanded and, in fact, may have decreased slightly. Immunoglobulins are used for therapy and prophylaxis of tetanus, poliomyelitus, and other viral agents, including hepatitis (356,404).

Production of immunoglobulin using methods other than plasma fractionation will probably not utilize recombinant DNA technology. Instead, cell fusion techniques, originally described by Kohler and Milstein (318), will enable hybrid cell lines to be constructed that secrete antibodies of known specificity. A clonal population of such hybrid cells is known as a hybridoma, and the antibody product of the cell is said to be "monoclonal" because the antibodies are identical in structure and reactivity. Antibody-secreting cell lines (hybridomas) are routinely prepared in numerous academic and industrial laboratories. In fact, the number of new companies founded to produce and market hybridoma technology is almost equal to the number specializing in gene cloning. However, the major focus of the industry to date has been in the development of monoclonal antibodies as diagnostic reagents.

Construction of a hybridoma that secretes a useful antibody essentially involves the physical fusion of an antibody secreting lymphocyte isolated from an immunized host with a myeloma tumor cell line that multiplies rapidly in cell culture. The fusion process can occur simply by mixing the cell types, but is greatly facilitated in the presence of the chemical, polyethylene glycol. The resulting hybrid cells exhibit the properties of the two parents; namely, secretion of a specific antibody from the lymphocyte and capacity for unlimited growth from the myeloma. A mixture of hybridomas resulting from a fusion can be screened to select the hybrid that secretes the desired antibody. Once identified, the hybridoma is capable of providing an inexhaustible amount of the antibody.

To date, essentially all hybridomas are constructed using mouse or rat lymphocytes and mouse myeloma cells. The limited application of hybridoma technology to development of diagnostic reagents has resulted from this fact, since administration of a rodent antibody to humans would result in potent immunization against that antibody. The use of hybridomas employing human lymphocytes and human myeloma cells has been slow to develop. However, several reports have appeared claiming to have produced human hybridomas (321,414a,431), and human monoclonal antibodies reacting with tetanus toxoid have been produced using the cell fusion technique (223,332,414a). Unfortunately, a human myeloma cell line capable of producing stable hybridomas has not yet emerged. Therefore, human hybridoma technology has not yet developed sufficiently for the isolation of a wide variety of clinically suitable monoclonal antibodies.

Human hybridomas have also been produced through viral transformation of peripheral blood lymphocytes with Epstein-Barr virus (EBV) (515). The antibody-secreting lymphocytes are converted to leukemia cells with EBV, and therefore grow in culture yet still secrete their antibody product. Although viral transformation has been used to construct hybridomas, those produced using this technique reportedly do not secrete large amounts of antibody, and production is unstable (98,414a).

Replacement of plasma fractionation by hybridoma technology as a source of immunoglobulin is not likely to occur in the next few years. Although some useful human hybridomas have been developed, the industrial scale-up of antibody production is still in its infancy. One company, Celltech in Great Britain, has pioneered the scale-up of monoclonal antibody production, but their experience is primarily with diagnostic antibodies used for tissue typing or imaging of tumors.

Although most hybridoma companies are concentrating on the mass production of mouse antibodies, their experience should prove valuable to the scale-up of human antibody production, once the techniques for routine production of human hybridomas have been developed. Although thousands of kilograms of human immunoglobulins are fractionated from plasma, production of a monoclonal antibody need never approach that magnitude. The immune globulin fractionated from plasma represents a heterogeneous mixture of antibodies in which only a small percentage actually recognize a given viral or bacterial target. In contrast, in a preparation of monoclonal antibodies, every antibody molecule reacts with the target. Thus, it should be possible to produce much smaller amounts of monoclonal antibody to effectively replace those currently obtained from plasma.

Another problem facing monoclonal antibodies as therapeutic drugs will be to ensure that a product derived from a cancerous cell line is free of all carcinogenic agents. Since it has recently been shown that some types of human leukemia result from viral infections, there is an underlying threat that administration of a monoclonal antibody might also expose the patient to cancer-causing viruses.

Other Plasma Proteins of Potential Commercial Value.—In addition to the plasma proteins with a demonstrated therapeutic market, several plasma proteins exist that have potential as therapeutic agents. Two such proteins are fibrinogen and fibronectin. In the case of fibrinogen, its involvement in the terminal phases of blood coagulation made it an important protein even though it had no large therapeutic market. Fibrinogen was indicated for replacement therapy only in rare cases of congenital deficiency and for diagnostic procedures (404). But seriously limiting the therapeutic use of fibrinogen obtained as a fraction of plasma was the inherent risk of hepatitis transmission accompanying infusion. This risk was so high that FDA removed the product from the market in the late 1970s. An rDNA product would avoid this hazard.

Fibronectin also has no current demonstrated therapeutic need, but the protein has been shown to play a diversity of roles, ranging from cell adhesion to enhancing the phagocytic clearance of particulate contaminants from the body (496). In addition, fibronectin has been found inside platelets and is released following stimulation with thrombin (225). Thus, a potential role for fibronectin in hemostasis has been suggested.

Both proteins are very large in size, synthesized in the liver, and have molecular weights of approximately 400,000 (462,497). Fibronectin consists of two very large and similar protein subunits linked together, while fibrinogen is composed of three different subunits of moderate size. In addition, both are glycoproteins. Fibrinogen contains one further chemical modification to the protein after it is synthesized. The modification involves the conversion of several glutamic acid molecules to gamma carboxyglutamic acid (462). It should be recalled that coagulation Factor IX undergoes a similar modification during its synthesis.

Because of their large size, both fibrinogen and fibronectin contain distinct domains (or regions) of the protein that are responsible for a particular function. For example, fibronectin contains separate protein domains that are responsible for binding collagen and heparin (496).

The DNA sequences coding for regions of both molecules have been isolated. In the case of fibronectin, Fagan et al. (174) isolated a cDNA that coded for a small segment of the fibronectin gene. With fibrinogen, complete cDNA sequences coding for its three distinct protein subunits have been isolated (117,118,462).

Should a market for these proteins become apparent, industrial production would face many of the problems already discussed. Since fibronectin is composed of protein subunits that are very large, recombinant organisms will probably synthesize the protein inefficiently. However, it is possible that small domains of the larger molecules may be therapeutically effective and therefore recombinant clones synthesizing small fragments of the protein might prove valuable. Fibrinogen, consisting of three moderately sized subunits, may not pose a major problem for bacteria to synthesize, but the proper association and alignment of the subunits to produce a functional molecule may not occur spontaneously. These problems and the lack of a commercial market have resulted in only a limited industrial interest in these proteins.

Other Applications of Recombinant DNA Technology

A potential use for gene cloning in the more distant future will be to produce proteins for use in manufacture of artificial blood cells or blood substitutes. It will be important at that time to have a supply of the proteins that perform the primary function of the blood cell. For example, it is likely that a large supply of hemoglobin will be needed for use in artificial red blood cell production. In addition to hemoglobin, it may be necessary to prepare selected red cell membrane proteins for incorporation into liposomes if this approach proves worthwhile. If liposomes are used as artificial platelets, those membrane proteins involved in platelet aggregation and activation will have to be obtained in large quantity. Cloning technology may provide a source of these proteins.

It should be noted, however, that biotechnology companies are not as yet pursuing the isolation of the genes coding for these proteins. This is because the market for such products is in the distant future. As should be apparent from the earlier discussion on artificial blood cells and blood substitutes, major technical accomplishments must occur in several scientific areas before substitutes for red cells or platelets in transfusion therapy are at hand. Nevertheless, potentially useful cellular proteins have been, or could easily be, cloned.

The one obvious protein that immediately comes to mind in a discussion of artificial blood is hemoglobin. In fact, the genes coding for hemoglobin chains have been cloned by a number of laboratories. Furthermore, since the hemoglobin chains are small in size and not glycosylated, synthesis of the hemoglobin polypeptide chains by recombinant bacteria should present no unusual problem for scale-up. Purification of large amounts of hemoglobin will likely present the same technical problems that were outlined previously for the production of albumin.

In contrast, if a market for cell membrane proteins arises, it will be some time before recombinant organisms can supply a product. Very little information regarding the molecular structure of these proteins is known. Research and development is limited in this area and is essentially in academic laboratories at the basic research level. Thus, when an important membrane protein is identified, isolation of the gene sequence will require much work. While there may be a delay in obtaining these gene sequences, it is very likely that they can be obtained using standard techniques.

7.
Future Directions

Contents

	Page
Part 1: Voluntary v. Commercial Approaches	175
Introduction	175
Voluntary Efforts in the Plasma Sector	176
Prospects for Further Voluntary Sector Involvement in Plasma Operations	179
Part 2: Organ and Tissue Banking	181
Introduction	181
The Current Scene	182
The Procurement System	183
Supply and Demand	184
Compatibility	186
The American Council on Transplantation	187

TABLE

Table No.	Page
45. A Comparison of U.S. and Canadian Plasma Management	180

7.
Future Directions

PART 1: VOLUNTARY V. COMMERCIAL APPROACHES

Introduction

Federal policy attention in the past has concentrated on the whole blood collection process, spurred by differences in the safety of whole blood from voluntary v. paid donors. Currently, the distinction between voluntary and paid whole blood or blood component collections has been maintained through their labeling as being derived from a "paid donor" or "voluntary donor." This labeling is applicable to whole blood, red cells, platelets, single-donor plasma, and cryoprecipitate (21 CFR pt. 640), but does not apply to source plasma or plasma derivatives (21 CFR pt. 606.120).

Assurances of the safety of plasma and plasma derivatives have been pursued through regulatory policies of the Food and Drug Administration (FDA), which has spelled out donor screening and laboratory testing requirements (21 CFR, pts. 640.60-640.76). Pooling of large amounts of plasma from individual donors is necessary for the efficient processing of plasma into plasma derivatives. Together with the donor and laboratory screening tests that have been applied, these technologies have resulted in the situation where there are no substantial differences in the safety of plasma derivatives whether they are derived from voluntary or commercial sources of blood/plasma.

But the availability of products derived from human tissues may also be influenced by criteria other than whether the market has resulted in a safe, readily available product, as witnessed in current legislative efforts to prohibit profit-making in systems for collecting and distributing organs (e.g., kidneys, livers and hearts) and other tissues (e.g., bone, skin and corneas). Thus, another viewpoint on the issue of voluntary v. commercial sources is, regardless of how well the present dual system is working, whether or not public policy should steer blood resources to an all-volunteer supply.

An additional consideration in analyzing the adoption of this type of public policy is whether or not the United States and other countries should be self-sufficient in resources that depend on human sources. Much of the self-sufficiency argument has been made in the context of exploitation of donors in developing nations, whose plasma was then used by fractionation companies for products used in the developed nations (250). In 1975, at the Twenty-Eighth World Health Assembly, the World Health Organization issued a resolution urging its member States "to promote the development of national blood services based on voluntary nonremunerated donation of blood," and "to further study the practice of commercial plasmapheresis including the health hazards and ethical implications, especially in developing countries" (595).

Currently, however, at least as far as U.S. plasma fractionation and use of plasma derivatives are concerned, the situation is such that U.S. plasma sources constitute the world's single largest source of raw plasma and plasma derivatives, and the primary issue among nations that use U.S. fractionated derivatives seems to be self-sufficiency per se, regardless of the source of the plasma derivatives. In addition, these importing nations seem more concerned now with the safety of U.S. plasma derivatives (because of AIDS, see below) than with the ethical implications of importing these blood products.

A strict self-sufficiency policy would also mean that international trade in voluntary blood products, as well as in commercially obtained products, would be discouraged. Thus, for example, the sale of excess red cells accumulated by some European countries in collecting whole blood for plasma-derivative production to the New York Blood Center (and commonly referred to as "Euroblood") would also be discouraged.

On the issue of self-sufficiency, one possible outcome of the AIDS controversy is that it is forcing nations currently dependent on U.S. plasma to look into the question of whether or not they should and could be self-sufficient. Currently, only the United Kingdom officially prohibits the import of U.S. plasma, but several western European countries have recently investigated their imports of U.S. plasma and have urged their own fractionators to show cause why they must continue such importation. Since an immediate ban on U.S. imports would seriously curtail the availability of Factor VIII concentrates, these countries have not taken any official action (466).

Voluntary Efforts in the Plasma Sector

There have been some forays into plasma collection and fractionation by the voluntary sector. In the mid-1970s, at least one voluntary blood bank conducted a small-scale plasmapheresis program for over 4 years, and although it was not economically feasible to continue, it was found that people would donate plasma voluntarily on a regular basis (402).

Some plasma fractionation activities also exist in the voluntary sector, and a few years ago the Red Cross attempted to build a fractionation plant with one of the commercial fractionators. The States of Michigan and Massachusetts maintain plants with capacities to fractionate 50,000 liters of plasma a year, and the Massachusetts plant is currently the sole source of herpes zoster immune globulin in the United States (see ch. 3, pt. 2). The New York Blood Center also maintains its own 350,000 liter/year plasma fractionation plant to fractionate its own and some Red Cross plasma, which required an investment of approximately $12.5 million (306).

In 1978, the American Red Cross negotiated an agreement with Baxter-Travenol to jointly fund the construction of a fractionation plant for plasma products. The cost of the plant was estimated at $45 million (406). Under the agreement, each organization would have been entitled to half the production capacity of the plant, but each organization would have handled its own acquisition of plasma and distribution of the plasma products. The plant was to have an annual fractionation capacity of 1 million liters, and industry sources estimated that the joint venture would have resulted in control of 30 to 44 percent of the U.S. plasma fractionation business (103,134).

The American Red Cross had requested a business review in April 1978 by the antitrust division of the Justice Department in regard to the legality of the joint venture's effect on substantially lessening competition in the plasma fractionation industry. In May 1978, the American Blood Resources Association submitted comments arguing that the joint venture would violate the antitrust laws by eliminating actual and future competition between the Red Cross and Baxter-Travenol (328), but the Justice Department announced in October 1978 that it would not challenge the proposed venture.

The Justice Department discounted the lessening of potential competition on the grounds that the Red Cross lacked the requisite technological ability to enter the fractionation business alone. It also dismissed the notion of a lessening of actual competition because: 1) Red Cross and Baxter-Travenol were clearly not actual competitors in fractionation at the time the venture was being considered, and 2) although the market shares of the Red Cross and Baxter-Travenol would have been significant enough to violate the Court's interpretation of "reasonable," the structure of the joint venture clearly delineated plasma collection and product marketing as separate responsibilities of each organization (328,391). Thus, the department concluded that competition in the plasma industry would continue and that the joint venture should be allowed to proceed.

In March 1979, the Red Cross and Baxter-Travenol announced the agreement (406).

During June-December 1979, West Germany began a procedure to remove the German Red Cross's tax-exempt status on income from manufacture and sale of plasma derivatives through its blood donor service (317,329). In June 1981, the German Minister of Finance concluded that such income should be taxed and treated as a profitable business activity because of the competitive nature of the industry, distinguishing between blood collection and the "secondary step of fractionation" (438). The decision was made retroactive to January 1, 1981 (320).

Although no official statement to the effect was made, the joint venture may have raised similar issues for the American Red Cross. The issue would have been "whether plasma collection, fractionation, sale and other distribution constitute a trade or business which is sufficiently related to the Red Cross's exempt purposes that that business does not generate unrelated business income" (329). Traditionally, the provision of blood to health care facilities at the lowest possible price has been regarded as a charitable service to the public, and plasma has been included. The joint venture may have provided a new answer to one of the Internal Revenue Service's standard tests for taxable activities; i.e., whether or not the activities in question were "of a kind regularly carried on for profit" (Rev. Rul. 66-323).

In late 1979, the Red Cross and Baxter-Travenol terminated their agreement, citing general economic conditions as the cause. The Red Cross' public relations office gave increases in construction costs of one-third over the budgeted amounts, inflation, and the increase in interest rates, as the relevant factors in the decision to shelve the project. Today, the Red Cross continues to contract with independent fractionators for the necessary service. Recently, the Red Cross entered into an agreement with Travenol Laboratories for the fractionation of Red Cross-provided plasma by Travenol's Hyland Therapeutics Division. Under the agreement, Hyland will increase its fractionation for the Red Cross on a fee-for-service basis to four times the volume of plasma fractionated for the Red Cross under current agreements, and Hyland will provide the Red Cross with a pilot plant facility for research on new orphan products, to be developed by the Red Cross under Travenol's FDA license.

In Canada, all blood and most plasma, with the exception of a small amount of plasma collected for production of plasma products, are collected by the Canadian Red Cross (CRC) from volunteer donors. Although the Canadian national blood policy is still under development, all activities related to the blood program are guided by principles which have been followed since the early 1970s. The current version of the principles was adopted by the Ministers of Health (one Federal, ten provincial, and two territorial) in November 1980. As health services are the constitutional responsibility of the Provinces, their endorsement has considerable authority. The policy, however, is not incorporated in either Federal or Provincial law.

Further, the Ministers of Health have conferred on the Canadian Blood Committee (CBC) the responsibility to "direct the Canadian blood system on their behalf" in accordance with the four guiding principles. The members of the CBC are representatives of 13 governments (Federal, Provincial, and Territorial), and are funded equally by the Federal government and the Provincial and Territorial governments (337).

The "Four Principles" approved by the Provincial Ministers of Health are (106):

1. to protect the voluntary donor system by enhancing the opportunities of Canadians to voluntarily donate a gift for society's general benefit and by responsibly managing that resource;
2. to ensure self-sufficiency of blood products by reducing Canada's dependence on foreign sources of blood products supply, particularly those that rely on purchased plasma for raw material;
3. to ensure gratuity of blood products by reinforcing the Canadian tradition whereby no payment is made for a donation of blood and/or plasma and no specific charge is made to recipients of blood and blood products; and
4. that a Canadian nonprofit policy be maintained and that any charge to recover more than the real cost of producing a blood fractionation product for Canadians in Canada should be considered profit.

The first three principles were articulated in 1973, and the fourth was added in 1980 after Connaught Laboratories, one of the two fractionators serving the CRC, changed its status from nonprofit to commercial. The reason given for adding the fourth principle was that "it was considered that the Canadian public would not accept the 'exploitation' of plasma donated voluntarily to the CRC" (147).

The second principle was based on a national goal of self-sufficiency, especially with respect to plasma fractions. The third principle, which denies any specific charge for blood, means that patients or their insurers are not billed by CRC for any cost of providing blood products. They may, however, be billed for the service of crossmatching if provided by an institution (hospital or private laboratory) other than the CRC. (The Canadian Blood Committee sets the prices of blood fractions.) The CRC views the blood program as an expenditure. The Blood Transfusion Service recovers the costs of recruitment, processing, etc., through direct grants from the Provinces and funding from the Canadian Red Cross Society. (See subsequent discussion on finances of the Blood Programme.)

The nonprofit/no-charge principles apply to human products for therapeutic use, not to diagnostics. However, CRC itself produces diagnostic reagents for its own use and distributes some histocompatibility trays to other Canadian laboratories free of charge. (The human leukocyte antigen (HLA) trays distributed in 1982 at no charge had an estimated market value of $556,140 at average U.S. prices.)

Currently, there are two Canadian firms which pay donors for plasma. Their products are commercially marketed. The first is The Winnipeg RH Institute, Inc., which is associated with the University of Manitoba. It is a nonprofit organization which primarily produces immune globulins and is also licensed by the U.S. FDA as a source plasma location. The second is BioResources, Ltd., of Halifax, Nova Scotia, which collects plasma principally for manufacture of diagnostic reagents, some immune globulin products, etc.

Plasma is fractionated for the CRC by Connaught Laboratories Ltd., of Toronto, Ontario, and Cutter Laboratories, of Clayton, NC. Each receives 70,000 to 75,000 liters per year. New facilities in Winnipeg (RH Institute) and Montreal (Institute Armand Frappier) will allow fractionation of all CRC plasma in Canada; each will process 50,000 to 60,000 liters annually.

The blood collection system in Canada is administered by the Blood Transfusion Service (BTS) of the Canadian National Red Cross and is coordinated from a national (blood transfusion service) office in Toronto. The BTS includes 17 regional transfusion centers within 10 provincial divisions. The technical operations are directed nationally, but blood donor recruitment is the responsibility of each division. There is a national Blood Donor Recruitment Program which provides information, resources, etc., but the national division is not responsible for regional recruitment. The regional transfusion centers collect and distribute blood and blood products.

In addition, the BTS operates the National Reference Laboratory (NRL), which also functions as the World Health Organization's National Blood Group Reference Laboratory. The NRL's activities include reagent production and quality control, hepatitis testing, HLA typing tray production and distribution, and a variety of reference and investigational testing.

In 1982, there were 8,928 clinics throughout Canada. In the Canadian system, "blood donor clinics" (bloodmobiles, blood drives, blood collection sites, etc.) are divided into three types:

- **Region 1:** clinics are permanent sites at or close to a regional transfusion center. These represent 48 percent of the total number of clinics.
- **Region 2:** clinics are mobile clinics close enough for blood to be collected, delivered to a center, and processed within 12 hours of collection. These constitute 42 percent of all clinics.
- **Region 3:** clinics are mobile clinics beyond 12 hours of a regional center, and make up the remaining 10 percent of clinics. Blood collected from Region 3 clinics is used for the extraction of those components whose shelf life before processing exceeds 12 hours.

In 1982, the Blood Transfusion Service of the CRC collected 1,129,159 units of blood. Of these, 855,765 units were transfused as whole blood or red cell concentrates (There was a 24.2 percent national outdate rate for collected whole blood and red cells in 1982.) Ninety percent of the whole blood collected was processed into components.

Plasma recovered from whole blood equaled 797,922 units, or approximately 160,000 liters. In addition, 7,831 voluntary plasmapheresis donations yielded over 3,900 liters of plasma. About 51,600 liters of plasma were transfused, and 153,650 liters (including 113,267 liters of fresh-frozen plasma) were available for fractionation (107).

The CRC meets all Canadian requirements for blood and blood components, other than plasma fractions. The only major import is Factor VIII concentrate, which is imported at the rate of 20 million to 22 million activity units per year at a value of approximately $2 million in Canadian dollars. Other products imported in relatively small amounts are specific immunoglobulins to varicella zoster, hepatitis B, tetanus and rabies, and the activated Factor IX Complex. CRC plasma sources supply all albumin, normal Factor IX Complex and pooled immune serum globins, and about 20 million units of Factor VIII (147).

Both Canada and the United States collect approximately the same amount of whole blood from voluntary donations per capita. Both countries separate the majority of whole blood into components, although Canada processes a higher percentage (90 v. 77 percent) of the blood available after whole blood transfusions. Perhaps the most significant difference is the percentage of plasma which is prepared as fresh-frozen plasma (FFP). Plasma must be in the fresh-frozen state to be useful for Factor VIII preparation. Of the plasma prepared from whole blood donations, the United States prepared only 33 percent in the fresh-frozen state (in 1980, the last year for which national statistics are available), while Canada prepared 72 percent as fresh-frozen plasma (for 1982). A comparison of U.S. and Canadian plasma management by the voluntary sector is summarized in table 45.

The Blood Transfusion Service of the Canadian Red Cross Society is supported in part by the government and in part by CRC fundraising efforts. The Provinces fund the blood program directly by grants for operating budgets and also by payment per item for fractionation products supplied to hospitals. In addition, the Canadian Red Cross funds the blood program along with its other charitable activities, such as international disaster relief, veterans' services, and safety services. The Canadian Red Cross Society programs and budget are subject to the review and approval of the Canadian Blood Committee.

About 60 percent, or $80,959,000, of the Canadian Red Cross's total expenditures ($135,249,000) for 1982 was spent on the blood program. These expenditures include all aspects of the blood program; i.e., all 10 regions, the National Reference Laboratory, national BTS offices, and the Blood Donor Recruitment Program. There was a deficit of $451,000 in 1982 (108).

In 1983, the Canadian Red Cross instituted a revised system of accounting in order to provide for the large amount of working capital needed for operating the blood program. The new system provides for separate financial reporting for the activities of the BTS, the national BTS office and fractionation operations. Each dollar is budgeted in the following proportions:

$0.33 for collections
0.24 for processing
0.14 for administration of centers
0.11 for donor recruitment
0.07 for the national office
0.07 for distribution
0.04 for the National Reference Laboratory
$1.00   Total

Prospects for Further Voluntary Sector Involvement in Plasma Operations

Voluntary sources for all products made from human blood and plasma remain as the ideal goal for many, and volunteers are relatively untapped sources of plasma, perhaps even on the sustained basis that is the norm for the commercial source plasma industry. Furthermore, volunteers need not be the exclusive source of plasma for national policies that stress the voluntary approach, as witnessed by Canada's experience. However, other factors make it unlikely that a policy will be pursued to make the voluntary sector the exclusive or even dominant collector of plasma as well as whole blood in the United States.

Table 45.—A Comparision of U.S. and Canadian Plasma Management

	United States—1980	Canada—1982
Voluntary whole blood donation per 1,000 population[a]	47 units	46 units
Whole blood collected	10,863,442 units[b]	1,129,159 units
Paid donations	233,127	0
Voluntarily donated blood	10,630,315	1,129,159
Whole blood transfused	1,930,081	77,517
Units available whole blood	8,700,234 units	1,051,642 units
Percent whole blood processed into components[c]	77%	90%
Percent whole blood transfused[d]	18%	7%
Maximum recoverable plasma from volunteer donor blood left after whole blood transfusions[e]	1,740,047 liters	210,328 liters
Estimated plasma available from separated whole blood[f]	1,631,780 liters	202,585 liters
Fresh-frozen plasma produced[g]	440,377 liters	143,433 liters
Other plasma produced	878,536	56,151
Total plasma produced	1,320,510 liters	199,584 liters
Percent plasma prepared as FFP[h]	33%	72%
Donated source plasma[i]	21,722 liters	3,900 liters
Voluntarily donated source plasma per 1,000 population	96 ml.	160 ml.

[a]Calculated as units whole blood voluntarily donated/population:
U.S. population (1980) 227,020,000
Canada (1982) 24,438,000
Source: U.S. Bureau of the Census, World Population 1979, Recent Demographic Estimates for the Countries and Regions of the World, 1980; Demographic estimates for countries with 10 million or more, 1981; and unpublished data.
[b]Whole blood figure does not include Euroblood.
[c]Calculated as units RBC processed/units whole blood voluntarily donated; units RBC processed U.S.: 8,158,898 units, Canada: 1,012,926 units.
[d]Calculated as units whole blood transfused/units whole blood donated.
[e]200 ml (or 0.2 liters) of plasma is the industrywide standard for plasma recovered from a unit of whole blood. Source: R. Reilly, personal communication, Jan. 5, 1984.
[f]Calculated as (units RBC processed) x (0.2 liters/units).
[g]Recovered plasma must be in the fresh-frozen state to be useful for Factor VIII production. Source: AABB, *Plasma Products: Use and Management*, p. 17, 1982.
[h]Calculated as liters fresh-frozen plasma produced/liters plasma produced.
[i]Recovered plasma: plasma obtained as derivatives of whole blood donation. Source plasma: plasma obtained from plasmapheresis procedure (yield: approximately 600 ml/donation); U.S. figure does not include the approximately 6 million liters of source plasma collected annually by commercial organizations.
SOURCES: **U.S. data source:** Surgenor and Schnitzer/ABC, 1982. **Canada data source:** Canadian Red Cross Society Blood Transfusion Service, *1982 Statistical Report*.

One consideration is whether the voluntary sector could meet the U.S. demand for plasma derivatives. Drees has estimated that an additional 20 million whole blood donations would have to be made to replace the 5 million liters of plasma collected by commercial collectors (at the time of his estimate), assuming a 250 ml plasma yield per volunteer donation of 500 ml of whole blood (165). This would have required tripling the approximately 10 million units of whole blood collected at the time of his estimates. An equivalent amount of plasma collected by plasmapheresis would need approximately 8.34 million collections, based on a yield of 600 ml of plasma per procedure.

U.S. plasma sources, however, also supply a large part of the world market, and not as much plasma would be needed for the U.S. market alone. However, it has been argued that U.S. sales abroad at prices as high as three times the U.S. price for Factor VIII help keep domestic prices down (7), and a self-sufficiency policy that would discourage international sales of U.S.-derived plasma products might reduce this beneficial impact on U.S. prices. It could be argued that this salutary effect on U.S. prices is due to "price gouging" abroad, but the other side of the coin is that these other users are paying the "market price" for products they do not produce in sufficient quantities themselves.

There obviously is no resolution of these conflicting opinions on the "morality" of selling plasma products at prices which can be obtained in the market. Of interest to this essentially unresolvable debate is that, once plasma is processed into derivatives, they are treated as commodities, or perhaps more accurately, are treated in much the same way as prescription drugs by both manufacturers and purchasers. This is true especially for albumin (whose marketing is similar to that for generic drugs) and increasingly true even for Factor VIII concentrates, and nonprofit organizations are commonly involved in marketing both nationally and internationally (see ch. 3 on the plasma sector).

Marketing of plasma derivatives by both profit and nonprofit organizations in direct competition with each other also points to the fact that, once past the stage of plasma or whole blood collections, the profit and nonprofit sectors have become more intertwined over the past decade. This is largely due to the increasing use of component therapy and the excess plasma that has become available from the voluntary sector. So any fundamental changes that occur in the plasma derivatives industry will cause problems for the voluntary sector as well.

Voluntary organizations may also be unwilling to become the major suppliers of plasma and plasma derivatives. Aside from the problems of establishing and maintaining an adequate donor supply, costs for starting up or retooling plants for plasma fractionation are substantial, as witnessed by the abandoned Red Cross/Baxter-Travenol proposed joint venture.

Even if present commercial fractionators continued to fractionate plasma that would come primarily from voluntary sources, there is still the question of the medium- and long-range health of the plasma derivatives industry. Albumin is no longer the driving force in the derivatives market and sales are very competitive. As noted earlier (see ch. 3), the market is not large compared to other industrial sectors, and major companies have left the industry in recent years.

The major factor, however, in determining the future of the plasma derivatives industry is the real chance that, by the end of the century, plasma as a source of current biological proteins will be (largely) replaced by recombinant DNA and hybridoma technologies (see ch. 6). These developments would affect not only the source plasma industry, but also plasma fractionators, some of whom are sponsoring biotechnology R&D in anticipation of these events. Thus, biotechnology currently has two major impacts on the issue of voluntary v. commercial supplies of source plasma and plasma derivatives. First, it makes the future prospects of this sector of the blood services complex sufficiently doubtful so that no planned movement toward a voluntary system can be expected. Second, however, biotechnology shows sufficient promise that, for the first time, there are real prospects that the longstanding controversy over commercial plasma donors may be solved, not through implementation of a deliberate, contested public policy, but through advances in technology which could make the voluntary v. commercial policy debate moot.

PART 2: ORGAN AND TISSUE BANKING

Introduction

In a recent volume on the role of blood bankers in tissue and organ preservation, one conclusion was that: "Within a decade after the end of this century, it is unlikely that there will remain more than a few vestiges of conventional blood banking as it exists today. There are a number of health service areas into which blood centers can diversify, but one of the most obvious is tissue banking" (376).

The idea that blood bankers are particularly well-suited to have a central role in preservation and distribution of organs and tissues other than blood is not entirely novel. In its first paragraph, the decade-old National Blood Policy speaks not only of "improvement in the quality of blood and blood products," but also of "development of an appropriate ethical climate for the increasing use of *human tissues for therapeutic medical pur-*

poses" ((179); emphasis added). A year later, in 1975, an editorial in *Transfusion* (299) asked: "Are blood banks to become tissue banks?"

Advances in surgical techniques and development of more sophisticated immunological agents to combat rejection problems have made it possible to transplant a host of solid organs and tissues, including the heart, lungs, kidney, liver and pancreas. Some transplantable substances, like bone marrow, are akin to blood and its components because they are renewable substances which can be provided by living donors. Organs such as hearts, livers, and lungs are procured from the bodies of people who have been declared dead on the basis of total and irreversible loss of all brain functions, but whose heart and lungs continue to be supported by artificial means, allowing the organs to be perfused. For tissues, including corneas, skin, and bone, potential donors include almost any dead body. Clinically, tissue donors are unlike organ donors in that tissues can be taken after the donor's heart has stopped beating and the actual retrieval is technically less rigorous.

Although the nature of the donor and the techniques and methods used to arrange for collection, storage, and distribution vary among the different types of organs and tissues, many features of the process have much in common with the blood banking enterprise. Finding donors, storing and inventorying products, assuring safety through a variety of screening tests, distributing the product, and recovering costs are all features common to blood banking and tissue and organ banking.

The blood bank's traditional role is also a key element in many transplant procedures. One dramatic example of the need for blood is in the area of liver transplants. At the University of Pittsburgh, where this procedure was pioneered by Dr. Thomas Starzl, liver transplants require about 3,000 to 4,000 units of blood from the hospital blood bank's annual dispersal of about 130,000 units (229). The strain on the blood bank is not so much the volume of blood needed (open heart procedures at the same center account for five times as much blood usage) but rather the unpredictable nature of the need. When a liver from a brain-dead donor is found, blood must be available within 4 to 6 hours—on occasion as much as 100 units.

While the need for this much blood is the exception, routine requirements for a range of blood products are nevertheless rather substantial. One study of 60 adult first-time liver transplant recipients revealed the following mean intraoperative and postoperative requirements per patient: red blood cells, 42 units; fresh-frozen plasma, 39 units; platelets, 19 units; cryoprecipitate, 8 units (283). According to Richard Crout, the director of the Office of Medical Applications of Research of the National Institutes of Health: "The amount of blood required is much greater than most people realize. It is an important limitation on expansion of this new technology—a major reason why local hospitals aren't about to get into transplanting livers" (229).

The Current Scene

The modern era of transplantation began in the 1950s with the first attempts at kidney transplantation. These initial procedures were limited to identical twins, whose common genotype obviated the problem of rejection. With the development of immunosuppressive drugs to combat such problems, surgeons were soon able to utilize less closely related living donors and eventually, cadaver donors. In 1963 the first liver transplant was performed, and in 1967, the first heart transplant (389). To date, there have been approximately 500 heart transplants performed in the United States and about 600 liver transplants worldwide, most of them in this country (278). In 1983 alone there were 6,138 kidneys, 163 livers, 172 hearts, 37 heart-lung combinations, and 150 pancreatic transplants performed in the United States.

With burgeoning interest in transplantation in the late 1960s, it became apparent that the law was lagging behind medical advances. Law reform bodies and professional associations drafted a model statute to clarify the legal status of organ donation and transplantation, codifying the common-law powers of an individual to donate body parts for use after death. By 1971, all State jurisdictions save one had adopted the Uniform Anatomical Gifts Act (UAGA) as recommended by the National Conference of Commissioners on State Laws (Kentucky joined the rest in 1977) (362).

The UAGA allows people to make known their intention to become organ donors by signing wallet-sized documents they can carry with them. In addition a number of States have made similar provisions to provide evidence of such intent on drivers' licenses. The UAGA also allows family members, in the absence of any contrary intent, to consent to organ removal on behalf of their relatives who have been declared brain-dead. The act, in addition to specifying who may give third-party consent for organ donation, also spells out an important division of labor: in order to avoid any conflict of interest, physicians responsible for declaring that the donor is dead may not be the same ones involved in the transplant procedure.

The Procurement System

A network of approximately 110 independent and hospital-based procurement agencies exists to coordinate distribution of organs. There are about 360 people in the country whose full-time work involves coordinating organ donation (278). The procurement centers have also been grouped into regional networks and have established computer and phone links. For example, the Southeast Organ Procurement Foundation is one such network, consisting of 30 centers. In addition to transplant coordinators, surgical transplant teams, intensive care unit personnel, patients, and the families of donors are also involved. To date this patchwork system has worked remarkably well, but many predict that without further refinements it will be unable to meet the increasing demand for organs suitable for transplantation (152).

One key actor in the transplant process is the transplant coordinator. This person, often a nurse or social worker, is responsible for maintaining a liaison between the transplant team and the family and caregivers of the potential donor. Most often the potential donor is identified by a neurosurgeon or neurologist upon declaration of brain death or by a nurse in the intensive care unit. The coordinator is often the person who must broach the sensitive issue of organ donation to a grieving family, explaining the ofttimes disconcerting concept of "brain death." It has been estimated that only 1.6 to 3.5 percent of people dying in acute care settings are potential organ donors; most often these are people who have sustained traumatic injury (64). Since many fewer actually become donors, it is difficult to build ongoing relationships among the professionals involved. The situation can be further complicated when there are a number of teams involved seeking multiple organs from the same body (243).

The transplant coordinator's role in motivating the families of potential organ donors is critical. Studies have shown that when the situation presents itself, between 70 and 80 percent of families will consent to donation on behalf of their deceased relatives. But, as in the blood donation context, misunderstandings can confound the situation. A Gallup poll showed that willingness to donate one's own organs after death is linked to perceptions about the success of the procedure. Of the 49 percent who agreed that kidney transplantation would "extend a person's life substantially," 60 percent were willing to donate; but of the 42 percent who were uncertain and believed that a transplant "might or might not extend that person's life," only 36 percent were willing to donate (460). And in a further parallel to blood donor motivation, there are apparent cultural barriers to donation; for example, blacks are substantially less likely than whites to agree to donation.

Another group in need of education about transplantation possibilities are the physicians and nurses on the "front lines" in community hospitals or trauma centers. As one student of the procurement system put it: "The 'keys to the kingdom' are held, in organ procurement, by the nurses and neurosurgeons (sometimes neurologists) in nontransplant hospitals" (451). It is often complained that this is the weakest link in the system. Physicians and nurses are often understandably reticent about broaching the possibilities of organ donation with grief-stricken and vulnerable families.

There has been criticism of the current system's overreliance on single individuals as transplant coordinators. Critics of the practice describe the coordinator's role as inherently stressful because of the simultaneous dual allegiance to the donor's family and to the recipient and transplant team. These stressful and conflicting functions are often undertaken on a 24-hour-a-day, on-call basis. Red Cross spokespersons have argued that their cadre of volunteer and professional staff, experienced in motivating blood donors, would be well suited to the task of coordinating procurement and counseling the families of prospective donors (376).

The Red Cross first embarked on pilot programs in St. Louis, MO, and St. Paul, MN. In Minnesota, the opportunity for some Red Cross blood bankers long interested in tissue preservation and storage to get involved in organ and tissue procurement came about when the transplant coordinator at the University of Minnesota left and the Red Cross agreed to fill the gap. A March 1984 survey conducted by the Red Cross of its 57 regions revealed 6 with at least one active program in organ or tissue banking (or definite plans to begin within 6 months).

Thirteen regions are actively planning or investigating the need for a number of specific services: seven in the area of public and professional education, seven in bone banking, three in cornea retrieval, and one in skin banking. Thirty-two regions expressed some interest but were still in the investigatory stages of contacting other agencies, hospitals, and professional groups to assess possible roles for the Red Cross. Finally, representatives of six regions stated they were not planning to become involved in organ or tissue banking in the foreseeable future (51).

Upon reviewing the pilot programs in the Midwest and the survey of its regional centers, the Red Cross Board of Governors in 1984 adopted a policy statement, pledging to:

1. Participate in a national effort to increase the supply of tissues and organs for transplantation through a program of public and professional education and counseling.
2. Develop and coordinate systems for tissue donor identification, retrieval, distribution, and use that are equitable and meet high professional standards.
3. Provide tissue services to meet community needs as is feasible and appropriate.
4. Assess the need for, and when appropriate, develop programs in support of organ donation services.

In April 1984, the American Association of Blood Banks (AABB) also adopted policies relating to organ transplantation. It was agreed that the "AABB will promote, among its members, histocompatibility testing, organ procurement, tissue banking and organ exchange among members and non-members." The AABB also opposes the buying and selling of organs. In its policy statement, it also argued against any "operational" role for the Federal Government, instead urging it to increase public awareness about organ donation and encourage development of private sector organ procurement agencies. According to the AABB, the Federal Government should also explore mechanisms to pay the medical bills of transplant patients (27).

Supply and Demand

The number of brain-dead bodies available and suitable for the procurement of organs for transplantation is estimated by the Centers for Disease Control to be approximately 20,000 annually; yet only 2,000 are actually used as donors. In a recent 2-year period at the University of Pittsburgh, 71 candidates for liver transplantation died while awaiting transplants. Of the 58,000 patients who are maintained on dialysis under the federally funded End-Stage Renal Disease Program, there are 8,000 listed on formal recipient registries, awaiting compatible donors (52). The AMA's Council on Scientific Affairs estimates that up to half of those on dialysis may be eligible for transplant (37).

An additional supply issue involves organ preservation. Organs, once removed, must be transplanted quickly; hearts within 8 hours, kidneys within 30 to 50 hours (depending on the method of preservation), and livers within 4 hours. The "wastage" rate is quite high for a number of organs; e.g., about 20 to 25 percent of kidneys procured annually are wasted (460). (This contrasts with a wastage rate for kidneys of about 5 percent in Western Europe, which some have attributed to better typing and crossmatching capabilities.)

Recently, attention has been focused on the propriety of buying and selling human organs as a way to alleviate shortages. Much of this controversy can be traced to a proposal by a Virginia physician to open a brokerage service which would pay living kidney donors in the United States and the Third World (463). The hue and cry that greeted this proposal was considerable. The experience with the risk of blood from paid, "skid row" donors in the late 1960s and early 1970s has been frequently cited as a reason to be wary of embarking on commercial ventures in transplantation (231). Others have expressed concerns, often raised in the blood donation context, that the impact of payment will be to make it less likely for people to donate voluntarily.

The Uniform Anatomical Gifts Act and related Federal and State laws and regulations have not addressed the question of whether financial reimbursement could be provided to an organ donor or the donor's estate for the organ itself (as opposed to compensation for lost wages or medical expenses associated with the donation procedure). A number of groups, including the National Association of Patients on Hemodialysis and Transplantation and the International Transplantation Society, have issued statements opposing commercialism in organ transplantation. The Executive Council of the American Society of Transplant Surgeons (which includes virtually all of the organ transplant surgeons in the country) went so far as to agree to expel any member participating in a transplant "under proprietary conditions." A number of States have considered or adopted legislation to ban the buying and selling of organs. All of these statutes have explicitly excepted blood and blood components, because they are "self-replicating fluids" (374).

Increasing attention has been given to making the most use of each individual donor by procuring multiple organs from each body. Yet the 110 aforementioned procurement agencies are ostensibly funded by the Federal Government for the sole purpose of kidney procurement. As one comentator has observed (450):

> Legally speaking, however, they are "kidney" procurement agencies. With trivial exceptions, each is totally funded by the End-Stage Renal Disease Program, a program that only pays for kidney acquisition. In practice, however, they have already exceeded that limitation. Almost all organ procurement agencies routinely attempt to retrieve corneas and, frequently, skin and bone as well. The added costs of such efforts are minimal as the tissue-specific banks usually do the actual excision themselves. All the agency does is ask the permission of the family, make arrangements in the hospital, and contact the eye, skin, or bone bank. Government ignorance or benign neglect has simply allowed these organ procurement efforts to "piggy-back" on kidney procurement without cost.
>
> As the number of liver and heart transplants has increased in the last few years, "kidney" procurement agencies have taken responsibility for locating these organs as well. The transplant centers needing such organs have reimbursed the agencies for the additional costs. So long as the number of non-renal transplants is 2 or 3 percent of the number of kidney transplants, there is little problem with this informal, ad hoc approach. But what will occur when the percent is 10 percent, or 30 percent, or even 60 percent!

Thus, one of the reasons why blood bankers have been interested in organ banking is the need to develop "full-service" organ banks.

There are also a number of tissues of use in transplantation which do not have to be maintained in a "living" state and which carry no risk of rejection because of immunological barriers. Some of these, such as nerves, arteries, dura, and fascia, have been collected and stored (either freeze-dried or frozen) by individual surgeons for later use. Other tissues such as bone and corneas have been collected and distributed by banks established for these specific purposes (491).

One commentator has suggested that blood banks aggressively explore possibilities in bone transplantation, by undertaking the initial step of contacting medical and dental schools and societies (especially departments of neurosurgery and orthopedics) to find potential clients. Because of recent breakthroughs and new uses, there may be needs going unmet in the absence of an adequate supply (296).

Bone harvesting must take place within 24 hours of the time of death. It is recommended that procurement take place in a sterile environment, such as an operating suite or under a laminar-flow hood, so that there is no need to sterilize the material prior to transplantation. Although there are obvious logistical and cost considerations in the use of such facilities, it may also be preferable to retrieval in a funeral home or blood collection center because of "psychological concerns" (296).

Bones can be stored in a variety of forms and used in many ways. They can be freeze-dried and kept in a vacuum; stored in this way they have been kept for up to 15 years without any diminution in clinical quality. Bones can also be deep frozen below $-80°$ C for future use. Transplants of freeze-dried bone can be used to treat fractures, to reconstruct limbs after surgical removal of tumors, and to fill in bone cysts after cervical spinal fusions. Freeze-dried, crushed cortical bone has been especially useful in periodontal therapy and in maxilofacial surgery (473).

There are a number of uses for human skin, which can be procured from dead bodies and stored in a frozen state. Transplanted skin is especially critical in the treatment of severely burned patients and can be used to cover open wounds to ward off infection and guard against loss of water, electrolytes, protein, and heat—usually as an interim measure until the patient's own skin can be transplanted in an autograft procedure.

As with the establishment of bone banks, it has been suggested that blood banks interested in diversifying into skin banking first contact local trauma centers, plastic and reconstructive surgeons, burn treatment centers, and geriatricians to gauge the need for banked skin. The donor pool and economies of scale are such that it has been suggested that large metropolitan or regional blood banks are best suited for this enterprise. It has been estimated that investment in the equipment necessary for cryopreservation and microbiological screening and staffing costs make it inefficient to operate a skin bank using less than 50 donors per year (which would involve screening approximately 2,500 potential donors) (151).

Compatibility

Many in the blood banking field have considerable experience in doing the kinds of tests necessary to ensure immunologic compatibility. The use of donor-specific blood components for therapeutic procedures has led to the establishment of registries of donors, organized not only by ABO/Rh blood groups, but also by HLA types.

The Red Cross markets an HLA tissue typing tray, and also maintains files of donors with rare blood characteristics or needs. The AABB maintains a similar file, and there also is a similar file on an international basis. Since 1970, the American Association of Blood Banks has had a Committee on Organ Transplantation and Tissue Typing. Upon the recommendation of this Committee, the AABB recently established a Bone Marrow Transplantation Information Service, "designed to speed the flow of information between the various centers while insuring individual rights to privacy and avoiding the expense and encumbrance of maintaining a registry" (249). The AABB collects information about potential recipients provided by transplant centers, including the name of a staff contact person, a coded identifier for the recipient and the recipient's HLA type, ABO/Rh type, and relevant diagnostic information. This information is compiled and distributed at regular intervals.

According to the former chair of the AABB Committee on Organ Transplantation and Tissue Typing: "The 'matching' and subsequent considerations are carried on directly between the centers involved; the AABB is not a party to these, nor indeed, will it even know when such negotiations are going on." The AABB does, however, anticipate conducting retrospective evalations to judge the success of the procedures (249).

Use of such registries has not only raised hopes about increased ease of matching, but also has occasioned concerns about confidentiality of donor records and the integrity of the consent process

(110). These issues will be of increasing concern to blood bankers as they come under pressure to maintain such registries and share information in already existing registries. (On occasion in the past blood banks have been asked to turn over lists of blood donors to organ procurement officials, who have regarded the donors as potential organ donors. Blood bankers have generally not cooperated in such efforts.)

Although the Uniform Anatomical Gifts Act does not address this issue, a convention has developed among those in the transplant field to prevent, insofar as possible, the families of brain-dead donors from identifying actual or potential recipients of their loved one's organs (194). This convention has taken root because of concerns that the added pressures on the family to donate could reduce the informed consent process to a sham and the establishment of a bond between potential donors and recipients could make possible sub rosa payments for organs.

A recent case from Iowa illustrates some of the problems which might arise with the enhanced abilities to match up individual donors and recipients. A 28-year-old leukemia patient learned of the existence of a compatible bone marrow donor from a University of Iowa laboratory technician. The potential donor had originally been screened to determine whether or not she would be a suitable match for her daughter. When her daughter died the woman's tissue typing records remained on file. The potential recipient, through the university's institutional review board (IRB), attempted to contact the woman to apprise her of his plight and of her unique ability to come to his aid. When approached by intermediaries by letter and phone the potential donor balked, saying she would only consider donating for a member of her family.

The potential recipient went back to the IRB and eventually to the courts for permission to further press and personalize his plea. The IRB and the Iowa Supreme Court both refused to accede to his request. The IRB reasoned that however compelling, allowing such requests could set a dangerous precedent by allowing highly coercive forces into the decision to donate an organ (110). The Iowa Supreme Court, in denying the request, held that the HLA tissue typing data was a medical record within the meaning of the State law, and thus subject to confidentiality strictures which would preclude the potential recipient's request (254).

The American Council on Transplantation

In response to numerous and increasing pleas in the media for transplantable organs (especially livers for infants suffering from biliary atresia), which were garnering the attention of the White House and Capitol Hill, U.S. Surgeon General Koop sponsored two conferences in 1983. These meetings brought together families, physicians and other health care personnel, financing experts, and others to grapple with questions related to transplantation. The result of these sessions was the creation of the American Council on Transplantation (ACT) (248). With seed money from the Federal Government ($100,000) this group opened a Washington, DC, office and had its first annual meeting in January 1984. The meeting was attended by almost 400 people, including scores of representatives of the blood banking community. Although the group was begun with Federal funding, it is a private organization. Business and foundation contributions are expected to make up the bulk of its operating expenses. Gary Friedlaender, an orthopedic surgeon and President of the American Association of Tissue Banks, has been elected as the group's president.

Originally, both the AABB and the ARC had planned to propose nominees to ACT's board of directors. At a meeting of representatives of the AABB, ARC, CCBC, and ABC prior to the meeting of the transplantation council, it was noted that blood banking was only one of ACT's many constituencies, and it was agreed that attempting to elect more than one representative of the blood banking community to the ACT board would dilute its influence. CCBC and ARC agreed to this proposal; the AABB "neither concurred nor opposed the effort to consolidate representation and did not pursue a nomination from the floor" (13). Dr. William Miller, current chairman of the American Blood Commission, was elected to be the single representative of the blood banking community on the ACT board of directors.

The future of the American Council on Transplantation will depend on its ability to stake out a role for itself and solicit continued funding and private support. Whether already existing groups will see ACT as a useful umbrella group or an unnecessary interloper remains to be seen. At an early meeting of the ACT, Oscar Salvatierra, president of the American Society of Transplant Surgeons and originally a member of ACT's steering committee, resigned from ACT's interim executive committee because the organization was "appearing to increasingly assume a politically partisan position" regarding proposed Federal legislation (278).

The role most frequently suggested for such a group is as a forum for discussion and a source of public policy pronouncements and commentary. Friedlaender has specifically eschewed any interest in ACT's actually coordinating transplantation or directly supporting clinical research (200).

The parallels between the American Council on Transplantation, even in its embryonic stage, and the American Blood Commission are inescapable (383). Each is a private group, created by Federal seed money as a way to allay controversy and accommodate discordant interest groups and other factions without direct Federal intervention. Just as the AABB, CCBC, ARC, and ABRA represent the range of interests of blood bankers and their clients, the organ transplant enterprise has a similar array of actors. And not unlike the American Blood Commission, the formation of ACT has been surrounded by controversy.

Appendixes

Appendix A.—The Blood Resources Program, Division of Blood Diseases and Resources, National Heart, Lung, and Blood Institute[1]

The National Heart, Lung, and Blood Institute through its Division of Blood Diseases and Resources (DBDR) supports research to improve the quality, safety and availability of blood and blood products for therapeutic uses. The DBDR in collaboration with members of the scientific community recently completed a planning study in which research needs and opportunities in the field of blood resources were delineated. A summary of the recommendations that emerged from this study are underscored below. Immediately following each recommendation are brief descriptions of related research projects currently supported by the DBDR.

BLOOD BANK MANAGEMENT

<u>Better methods of collecting, separating, transferring, and preserving the cellular and liquid portions of blood are needed. These achievements depend upon developments in instrumentation, techniques, and automation.</u>

° A platelet harvesting device is being developed to separate platelet-rich plasma from blood, based upon a centrifugal elutriation technique. This device should improve the amount of platelets recovered and reduce the contamination of platelet-rich plasma by erythrocytes and leukocytes.

   (R43 HL-31873)

° Investigators are employing counter-current distribution techniques to separate cells and membranes in a two-polymer aqueous phase systems. This technique has been shown to be a sensitive, versatile method for characterizing and fractionating cell subpopulations based upon their surface or membrane properties.

   (R01 HL-24374)

° Studies are being performed to test the feasibility of using pressure, generated by ultrasonic waves, to separate cellular elements of blood from plasma.

   (R43 HL-31890)

° A regional blood distribution system, using computer bar codes to identify all products, is being developed and tested at a large metropolitan blood center. Results indicate that a uniform supply of blood could be maintained at all hospitals while reducing regional outdating.

   (P01 HL-09011)

---

[1] Provided by George Nemo, Ph.D., Chief, Blood Resources Branch, DBDR, NHLBI

More effective data collection on blood and blood resource usage would help guide the development of predoctoral and postdoctoral education programs and provide a basis for exploring the need for autotransfusion, blood substitutes, and related issues of blood management.

° In June, 1984, the NHLBI will initiate a study to determine future blood data collection, analysis, and reporting activities. The study will be conducted over a period of nine months. Technical support will be provided by a contractor experienced with medical records, medical abstracts, and standard coding and reporting systems. The study will involve a number of Federal agencies including the National Center for Health Statistics, the Food and Drug Administration, and the Department of Defense as well as major blood banking organizations.

CELLULAR ELEMENTS

An improved ability to reduce damage to the cellular elements from storage will depend on a better understanding of the factors responsible for the loss of viability and function of these cells. Basic research to understand the metabolic processes involved, the function of the cellular membrane in these activities, and how external forces interact with these features is critical to progress in this area.

° Biochemical and ultrastructural studies are being performed to characterize the structure of the platelet cytoskeleton. These studies are expected to provide basic information relevant to the practical aspects of separating, storing and preserving platelets for transfusion.

 (P01 HL-29583)

° Studies of the relationship between surface saccharides and senescence in normal red blood cells have shown that the glycoconjugates of the cell membrane play a significant role in aging and sequestration of old erythrocytes.

 (R01 HL-17881)

° A blood bag is being developed of semipermeable membrane material that will permit glycerolization and deglycerolization of blood cells without entry into the blood bag and thus insure sterility.

 (R01 HL-24466)

° Studies are being performed to define the morphologic, metabolic, and functional changes that occur during storage of platelets in the liquid state. Information gained from these studies will be used to develop techniques to permit storage of platelets for one week or more with minimal loss of viability and function.

 (R01 HL-20818)

° Baseline studies of changes in lipids and proteins of red cell membranes have demonstrated that improved methods of erythrocyte preservation result in a significant reduction of lipid loss. These studies have also shown that red blood cells lose pieces of membranes in vivo, supporting the finding that the membranes of older cells contain less lipid than membranes of younger cells.

(R01 HL-25867)

Frozen preservation of blood cells, including bone marrow and stem cells, would expand the range of therapeutic modalities available to the clinician in many conditions for which there is limited therapy at present. In addition, culture techniques for growing bone marrow, stem cells, and other cellular elements should be developed that permit the exploration of new therapeutic approaches.

° Research is being performed on the cryopreservation of human platelets and granulocytes. Studies are focusing on the use of varying concentrations of cryoprotectants to achieve good recovery of functioning cells.

(R01 HL-27537)

Immunologic characteristics of the cellular elements have long been recognized as important aspects of their viability and function. Better methods to identify important immunologic features of cells and a better understanding of the clinical function of specific antigenic determinants will aid greatly in providing matched cells for therapeutic use. HLA registries, particularly for platelet and for bone marrow donors, are already required, and this need will undoubtedly extend to the other cellular elements as well.

° Efforts are underway to determine the role of the HLA complex in the control of immune responses. Initial studies are focusing on the in vitro association of HLA phenotypes with cellular responses to artificial antigens.

(P01 HL-09011)

° A study of the membrane biochemistry of Rh antigens is providing information suggesting that the Rh antigen is associated with the main glycoprotein, band 3, of the red cell membrane.

(R01 HL-23108)

° Investigators are developing and applying immunochemical methods to detect and characterize structural variations on HLA Class I and Class II cell-surface glycoproteins. Specific HLA gene products will be isolated and defined on the basis of molecular weight. Attempts will be made to relate the newly identified structural components to specific HLA-D region genes.

(P01 HL-29583)

° Investigators are determining molecular weights of Rh antigens, as well as other antigens in the red cell membrane. These studies have shown that the molecular weight of solubilized Rh antigen is over 500,000 daltons.

(R01 HL-24009)

° Investigators are attempting to produce human monoclonal antiplatelet antibodies using spleen cells obtained from patients with immune platelet disorders. If monoclonal antibodies can be produced, useful reagents will be obtained that will enable investigators to identify antigen expression during the clinical course of immune platelet disorders.

(R01 HL-29513)

° Using allospecific hybridoma antibodies, investigators have shown that spondyloarthropathy is associated with the presense of HLA B27 antigens in the cells of patients. These data are significant because they demonstrate that the use of allospecific monoclonal antibodies may improve identification of susceptibility markers of inherited diseases.

(R01 HL-29572)

° An International Bone Marrow Transplant Registry has been established for the purpose of collecting, analyzing and disseminating data on bone marrow transplantation performed at medical centers throughout the world. This registry is concerned with the identification of factors that affect graft and patient survival. These factors include pre-transplant transfusion, donor compatibility, granulocyte transfusion, and infection.

(Intra-agency Agreement with NIAID)

<u>A large number of substances are actively transported on, or secreted by, cellular elements. Some are recognized to be of significant physiologic importance. The myriad of potentially useful agents found in association with these cells, including the lymphokines, mediators of several varieties, enzymes, and other biologically active chemicals, must be isolated, identified, and studied. When important functions are identified, isolation and purification using monospecific antibodies and other techniques.</u>

° A research project is focusing on the physiological functions of platelet-derived factors in the regulation of cellular growth, migration, and metabolism of specific target cells in culture. This project involves studies of platelet-derived growth factor, platelet factor 4, beta-thromboglobulin, serotonin and thrombin.

(P01 HL-29583)

° In an ongoing project, platelet-activating factor (PAF), a low molecular weight substance released by white blood cells, is being studied along with an inhibitor of PAF. Studies are focusing on the role of these molecules in several diseases, notably asthma and immunologically mediated lung diseases.

(R01 HL-25220)

PLASMA AND PLASMA DERIVATIVES

Perhaps the greatest immediate challenge in the area of plasma derivatives is related to the development of techniques that utilize existing or new methods of separation to isolate, purify, and prepare safe products for research and therapeutic use. Such advances in technology will not only lead to better, more abundant, and less costly products, but will also provide opportunities to isolate and study trace agents of the plasma that have important functions in relation to coagulation, inflammation, the complement system, and other important response mechanisms of the body.

° In an ongoing study, arginal peptides are being synthesized for use in the affinity chromatographic purification of serine proteases. Arginal peptides attached to agarose resins will serve as a general affinity chromatography procedure in plasma protease purification, and the procedure may have therapeutic importance in the isolation of proteases for the treatment of hemophilia and thrombolytic disorders.

(R01 HL-249100)

° Work is continuing on the combined use of polyethylene glycol precipitation and Cibacron Blue Sepharose in the purification of several plasma proteins.

(R01 HL-26887)

° A study is being conducted to determine the feasibility of purifying alpha-1-antitrypsin from the plasma of normal donors for supplementation in infants with alpha-1-antitrypsin deficiency who have early symptoms of liver disease.

(R01 HL-29731)

Specifically needed in this area (plasma and plasma derivatives) is the development of disease-free products, particularly reagents free of hepatitis virus, that can be used safely in clinical situations. There is also a need to identify the etiology of other adverse reactions caused by transfusion of plasma derivatives, such as those that occur with some clotting fractions and immune globulins.

° A variety of chemical and physical inactivation methods are being employed to reduce the infectivity of non-A,non-B hepatitis viruses (NANB) in labile blood derivatives. The efficacy of the inactivation process is being evaluated by inoculating treated material into chimpanzees.

(N01-HB-37009)

° Research is continuing on the development of new plasma derivatives which have existing or potential clinical use. A factor IX concentrate preparation has been developed that is non-thrombogenic. Methods are also being developed to reduce viral infectivity in factor VIII concentrates and similar methods are being applied to the production of factor X and Protein C concentrates.

(R01 HL-24944)

SAFETY

With the virtual elimination of posttransfusion hepatitis caused by hepatitis B virus, more attention must be focused on identifying, isolating, and developing suitable antibodies and vaccines against non-A,non-B virus (NANB), which is now the prime cause of this disease. Efforts to minimize the occurrence of cytomegalo- virus (CMV) and other less common agents as a cause of hepatitis, particularly in certain specialized patient populations, must be continued.

° Investigators are attempting to identify and to characterize NANB hepatitis agents or antigens in the sera, liver extracts and tissues of infected humans and chimpanzees. If successful, new tests for NANB agents would be developed; immunization with purified NANB antigens would be evaluated in chimpanzees; in vitro cultivation of the agents would be attempted; and the epidemiology and natural history of NANB hepatitis would be studied.

(P01-HL-09011-18A1)

° Attempts are being made to modify hepatitis B surface antigen (HBsAg) by chemical means in order to induce or amplify an immune response in nonresponder mice. If successful, these studies will be extended to humans and include HBsAg carriers and vaccinated individuals. In addition, interferon, which decreases the concentration of Dane particles and HBsAg in human carriers, will be encapsulated in polysomes or covalently linked to polysaccharides in an effort to direct the lymphokine to liver tissue. A separate project entails introduction of the HBV genome into eukaryotic cells in order to study viral expression.

(P01 HL-09011)

° A computerized serum and data bank, established in 1969, is projected to contain approximately 300,000 samples by 1985. Long-term surveillance studies continue to be performed with these serum samples to explore epidemiological patterns of NANB hepatitis.

(P01 HL-09011)

° Studies are focusing on the relationship of HLA-linked genes to immune responses that include vaccination with HBsAg or natural infection with HBV.

(P01 HL-09011)

° A repository of coded, frozen serum samples from the Transfusion-Transmitted Viruses Study is being maintained. These samples are available to investigators for hepatitis research, with approval of the National Heart, Lung, and Blood Institute.

(N01 HB-27000)

- A breeding colony of chimpanzees, presently consisting of 43 animals, is being maintained for hepatitis research.

  (N01 HB-27004)

- A prospective investigation is being conducted to identify the agent(s) of NANB hepatitis. A rapid screening procedure, initially developed to detect anti-HBsAg, is being applied to the detection of the agent(s) of NANB hepatitis. Serum samples from NANB patients and liver homogenates from infected chimpanzees are being evaluated with this method.

  (N01 HB-37010)

- A blood donor survey and serum sample analysis is being performed to correlate clinical manifestations of hepatitis with concentrations of liver enzymes in the blood. Studies also include the development of methods for detecting and isolating DNA in serum with elevated concentrations of alanine aminotransferase (ALT), and of methods for molecular cloning of the nucleic acid isolates.

  (N01 HB-37011)

- The transmission of Epstein-Barr virus (EBV) by blood transfusion is being studied. Investigations are concerned with the frequency of EBV transmission, the frequency of clinical illness in infected individuals, antibody responses to parenterally derived infections, and the role of passive immunity and transfusion volume in the development of infection.

  (R01 HL-30311)

- A prospective study is being performed to determine the incidence of transfusion-associated cytomegalovirus (CMV) infections, including primary, reinfection, and reactivated latent infection in immunocompetant and immunodeficient blood recipients. Investigators will determine the clinical significance of CMV infection in these patients and will attempt to develop tests for determining which blood donors are capable of transmitting CMV.

  (R01 HL-30329)

- A longitudinal study is being performed to determine the prevalence of immunologic abnormalities in patients with hemophilia. These abnormalities may be induced by factor VIII treatment and are similar to the severe dysfunction of the immune system observed in patients with acquired immunodeficiency syndrome (AIDS).

  (R01 HL-31015)

- A study is underway to investigate the possible causative and contributing factors and their interactions in the pathogenesis of AIDS. A large population of healthy, but at-risk, homosexual men will be followed prospectively, using a variety of serologic and immunologic markers to define the sequence of events leading from good health, to altered immunity, to AIDS.

  (P01 HL-09011)

° A study has been initiated to demonstrate whether an AIDS-inducing infectious agent is present in the plasma of patients with this syndrome. Plasma samples have been inoculated into chimpanzees that are being monitored for a variety of immune functions as well as clinical manifestations of the disease.

(Y02-HB-30006)

° Investigators are attempting to determine whether patients with hemophilia A display immune function changes similar to those observed in patients with AIDS. In addition to hemophilia patients, the immunological status of patients with sickle cell anemia and thalassemia major will be evaluated, since both groups repeatedly receive substantial quantities of cellular blood products.

(Y01-HB-30034)

° An outbreak of an acquired immunodeficiency disorder, which resembles human AIDS, has been observed in rhesus monkeys at the University of California Davis Primate Center. The disorder is referred to as Simian Acquired Immunodeficiency Syndrome or SAIDS. Recently, it was found that SAIDS could be experimentally transmitted to monkeys. A project is currently in progress to determine the role of blood and blood components in the transmission of this disease in monkeys.

(Y02-HB-30018)

° Methods are being developed to detect circulating antigen-antibody complexes containing the putative agent of AIDS. A variety of laboratory procedures will be used to detect and characterize specific antigens and antibodies found in the sera of patients with AIDS.

(R01 HL-32434)

° A study is being performed to quantitate specific breakdown products of nucleic acid metabolism, including purine and pyrimidine bases, in the serum and urine of several study groups including patients with AIDS. It is hoped that this study will lead to the development of a laboratory test to detect asymptomatic carriers of AIDS.

(R01 HL-32432)

° A study is being performed to determine the functional role and significance of human CMV, human T-cell leukemia virus (HTLV), and other agents associated with AIDS. Several experimental approaches, including transmission experiments in non-human primates, will be tried.

(R01 HL-32505)

° A research program is underway to assess the value of a battery of assays to detect the carrier state of AIDS. These include tests for T-cell subsets using 10 diverse monoclonal antibodies, measurement of antibodies to the three known types of HTLV, and measurement of immune complexes. Study groups will be followed prospectively for a three year period.

(R01 HL-32453)

° A number of tests are being conducted that include serological assays (thymosin, microglobulin, alpha interferon, anti-HTLV, anti-HB core antigen and anti-CMV) and cell marker assays (helper T cells, suppressor T cells, B cells, natural killer cells, monocytes, DR-antigen-positive cells, and surface immunoglobulin positive cells) in an attempt to discriminate between healthy individuals and those who are asymptomatic carriers of AIDS.

(R01 HL-32477)

° Methods are being developed that would make biological assays of human alpha interferon feasible for mass screening procedures. Studies will specifically focus on the ability of these assays to detect asymptomatic carriers of AIDS.

(R01 HL-32473)

° DNA hybridization procedures are being applied to the detection of viral nucleic acid in lymphocytes of patients with AIDS, AIDS-related complex, homosexuals with immune abnormalities, and controls. Viruses to be studied include CMV, EBV, and HTLV.

(R01 HL-32471)

Donor safety is only now being viewed with any degree of interest. Because of the proliferation of apheresis techniques and the increasing use of single donors to provide large quantities of a reagent, more information must be developed on the threat that accompanies the loss of cellular or plasma constituents and the hazards posed by the repeated introduction of steroids and colloids into the circulation of the donor.

° A project concerned with the effects of cytapheresis on the lymphoid system of donors is underway. This study deals with the short and long-term effects of repeated cytapheresis, particularly on the number, distribution, and function of lymphocyte subpopulations.

(P01 HL-09011)

APHERESIS

The technique of apheresis is being applied to many diverse clinical conditions. Research in the immediate future must deal with the development of new instrumentation, new immunoabsorbents, hazards to the donor, the clinical efficacy of newly emerging treatment strategies, and cost-benefit ratios of its large-scale use.

° In a study of methods to reverse platelet alloimmunization, therapeutic apheresis and immunoabsorbant columns are being used to remove platelet alloantibodies.

(R01 HL-28880)

IMMUNOLOGY

Although immunologic investigation is important in many of the topics already mentioned, new concepts are being associated with transfusions and specific blood cell antigens in organ transplantation. In addition, further work is needed on the use of extracorporeal systems to treat blood and bone marrow tissues with monoclonal antibodies.

BLOOD SUBSTITUTES

The clinical evaluation of existing and newly formulated perfluorochemicals represents an immediate challenge for the blood transfusion specialist. Although additional perfluorochemical reagents are being developed and new surfactants are being devised, research with other oxygen-carrying solutions should be pursued.

° In an ongoing study, investigators are testing hemosomes, which are stroma-free hemoglobin solutions encapsulated in artificial phospholipid membranes, as red cell substitutes. Sterile hemosomes are being produced in sufficient quantities for safety and efficacy tests in laboratory animals.

(R01 HL-28595)

° New red cell substitutes, utilizing hemoglobin bound to polymeric compounds, are being synthesized and tested for safety and efficacy in laboratory animals. The polymeric compounds such as hydroxyethyl starch or dextran are coupled to hemoglobin to increase the circulatory dwell time of the oxygen-carrier in the circulation.

(R01 HL-25955)

° Investigators are determining oxidation-reduction equilibria of hemoglobin covalently modified with various organic phosphates. These studies will provide new information on modified hemoglobins which are of potential importance as red cell substitutes.

(R01 HL-30850)

° Investigators are exploring the use of tetrameric and polymerized hemoglobin solutions and perfluorochemical red cell substitutes in the treatment of moderate and severe anemia.

(R01 HL 30113)

° A perfluorochemical emulsion is being used to obtain hemoglobin-free rat neural tissue preparations that will permit characterization of cerebral intramitochondrial respiratory chain function in situ. The long-term objective of this project is to evaluate the potential therapeutic effectiveness of perfluorochemicals to prevent or reduce central nervous system metabolic damage caused by cerebrovascular pathology.

(R01 HL 30100)

° Investigators are using perfluorochemical emulsions of defined particle size as models of platelets and chylomicra in order to determine their distribution near the wall of microcirculatory vessels. This work combines methods of rheology, transport phenomena, and circulatory physiology. Its aim is to obtain a comprehensive rheologic picture of blood cell effects in flowing blood.

(R01 HL 30087)

° Investigators are studying the nuclear magnetic resonance (NMR) spectral characteristics of new and promising perfluorochemicals. It is hypothesized that perfluorochemical emulsions can accelerate the restoration of myocardial function following coronary flow reduction and that imaging could be used to monitor this process.

(R01 HL 30104)

° The efficacy of a number of selected perfluorochemicals in the in vitro perfusion of mammalian testis is being explored to determine the effect of on these artificial oxygen carriers testosterone secretion.

(R01 HL 30083)

CLINICAL TRIALS

Throughout the entire range of subjects in the blood resources area, the need for controlled, statistically significant clinical trials repeatedly surfaces. Clinical indications for the use of the various blood fractions must be better delineated, and the appropriate use of the resource must be ascertained. Timely development of indications for the use of a product will not only assure the rapid application of techniques but also limit the use of costly, ineffective treatment modalities popularized by anecdotal reports and inadequate trials.

° A multi-institutional clinical study is underway to evaluate the capacity of intravenously administered CMV immune globulin to protect high risk premature infants against CMV infection acquired by blood transfusion.

(R01 HL-29883)

EDUCATION

The authors of this report make frequent reference to the need to develop appropriate educational opportunities for users of blood fractions. In this summary, the importance of this plea to provide proper training for those who administer blood is reemphasized, since both the success of clinical care and the control of health care costs are intimately related to the appropriate use of this vital resource. In addition, the factors that motivate or inhibit blood donors should be investigated, inasmuch as an understanding and sympathetic public is necessary for an adequate supply of blood.

° In September, 1984, the NHLBI and the FDA will cosponsor an NIH Consensus Development Conference entitled, "Fresh Frozen Plasma: Indications and Risks."

° In 1983, the NHLBI implemented the Transfusion Medicine Academic Award. This program provides for the integration of educational programs in transfusion medicine into the medical school curriculum. The program will be announced each year until needs in transfusion medicine are fulfilled. "Transfusion Medicine" is defined as a multidisciplinary area concerned with the proper use or removal of blood and its components in the treatment or prevention of disease states (other than in renal hemodialysis).

K07 HL-01252
K07 HL-01253
K07 HL-01258
K07 HL-01270
K07 HL-01274

Appendix B.—Glossary of Acronyms and Terms

Glossary of Acronyms

AABB	—	American Association of Blood Banks
ABC	—	American Blood Commission
ABRA	—	American Blood Resources Association
ACT	—	American Council on Transplantation
ADP	—	Adenosine Triphosphate
AHF	—	Antihemophilic Factor
AIDS	—	Acquired Immunodeficiency Syndrome
ALT	—	Alanine Aminotransferase
AMA	—	American Medical Association
AMS	—	Automated Microplate Systems
ARC	—	American Red Cross
ASCP	—	American Society of Clinical Pathologists
ATIII	—	Antithrombin III
ATP	—	Adenosine Triphosphate
BTS	—	Blood Transfusion Service
CBC	—	Canadian Blood Committee
CCBC	—	Council of Community Blood Centers
cDNA	—	Complementary DNA
CDC	—	Centers for Disease Control
CFR	—	Code of Federal Regulations
CMV	—	Cytomegalovirus
CPDA-1	—	Citrate Phosphate Dextrose Adenine-1
CRC	—	Canadian Red Cross
DBDR	—	Division of Blood Diseases and Resources (Division of NHLBI)
DHEW	—	(See USDHEW)
DHHS	—	(See USDHHS)
DNA	—	Deoxyribonucleic Acid
DRG	—	Diagnosis-Related Group
EBV	—	Epstein-Barr Virus
EIA	—	Enzyme Immunoassays
ELISA	—	Enzyme-linked Immunosorbent Assay
FDA	—	Food and Drug Administration
FFP	—	Fresh-Frozen Plasma
GAO	—	General Accounting Office
HBIG	—	Hepatitis B Immune Globulin
HBcAg	—	Hepatitis B Core Antigen
HBsAg	—	Hepatitis B Surface Antigen
HCFA	—	Health Care Financing Administration
HLA	—	Human Leukocyte Antigen
HTLV	—	Human T-cell Lymphotropic Virus
IATC	—	Interagency Technical Committee
IRB	—	Institutional Review Board
ISBT	—	International Society of Blood Transfusion
ISG	—	Immune Serum Globulin
IVGG	—	Intravenous Gamma Globulin
JCAH	—	Joint Commission on the Accreditation of Hospitals
KS	—	Kaposi's Sarcoma
mRNA	—	Messenger RNA
MWBB	—	Metropolitan Washington Blood Bank
MW	—	Molecular Weight
NANB	—	Non-A, Non-B Hepatitis
NBP	—	National Blood Policy
NCI	—	National Cancer Institute
NHF	—	National Hemophilia Foundation
NHLBI	—	National Heart, Lung, and Blood Institute
NIAID	—	National Institute of Allergies and Infectious Diseases
NIH	—	National Institutes of Health
NRDC	—	National Research and Demonstration Center
NSA	—	Normal Serum Albumin
NTIS	—	National Technical Information Service
NYBC	—	New York Blood Center
OoB	—	Office of Biologics Research and Review
OTA	—	Office of Technology Assessment
PA	—	Plasminogen Activator
PAF	—	Platelet Activating Factor
PCP	—	*Pneumocystis Carinii* Pneumonia
PFC	—	Perfluorochemicals
PPF	—	Plasma Protein Fraction
PTC	—	Prothrombin Complex
RBC	—	Red Blood Cells
RES	—	Reticuloendothelial System
RHo(D)	—	Anti-Rh Antigen Immune Globulin
RIA	—	Radioimmunoassays
RNA	—	Ribonucleic Acid
RSA	—	Resource Sharing Agreement
SBB	—	Specialist in Blood Banking
SFBS	—	South Florida Blood Service
STS	—	Serological Test for Syphilis
T&S	—	Type-and-Screen
UAGA	—	Uniform Anatomical Gifts Act
USDHEW	—	U.S. Department of Health, Education and Welfare
USDHHS	—	U.S. Department of Health and Human Services
VZIG	—	Varicella Zoster Immune Globulin
WHO	—	World Health Organization

Glossary of Terms

ABO blood group: The major human blood type determined by the presence or absence of two antigenic structures, A and B, on red blood cells, consisting of four blood types (A, B, AB, and O).

Acquired immunodeficiency syndrome (AIDS): A disease believed to be of viral origin (human T-cell lymphotropic virus, type III) and characterized by a deficiency of the immune system, that is complicated by infections caused by organisms that usually do not produce infections in individuals with normal immunity and/or by the development of a rare type of cancer (Kaposi's sarcoma) usually seen in the elderly or in individuals who are severely immunocompromised from other causes.

Agglutination: A reaction in which particles (e.g., red blood cells or bacteria) suspended in a liquid collect into clumps and which occurs especially as a serologic response to a specific antibody.

Albumin: A small protein, synthesized in the liver, which is the principal protein in plasma and is important in maintaining plasma volume through maintenance of an osmotic gradient between plasma in the blood vessels and fluids in the surrounding tissues. Albumin also serves as the carrier molecule for fatty acids and other small molecules in plasma.

Allogeneic: Refers to individuals of the same species who are sufficiently unlike genetically to interact antigenically.

Alloimmunity: Development of immunity by one individual against the antigens of another individual of the same species; for example, development of anti-Rh antibodies in a Rh negative individual upon infusion of R(h) positive blood.

Antibiotic: A chemical substance used against bacterial infections which is produced by a micro-organism and has the capacity to inhibit the growth of or to kill other micro-organisms.

Antibody: A protein component of the immune system in mammals found in blood.

Antigen: A large molecule, usually a protein or carbohydrate, which when introduced into the body stimulates the production of an antibody that will react specifically with the antigen.

Antihemophilic factor (AHF) (or Factor VIII): A plasma coagulation factor whose congenital deficiency results in the bleeding disorder known as hemophilia A.

Anti-inhibitor complex: An "activated" form of Factor IX concentrate, which is used in the treatment of hemophilia A patients with inhibitors to Factor VIII. (See also "Factor IX concentrate" and "concentrate.")

Apheresis: A method of collecting individual components of blood instead of whole blood from the donor; e.g., plasmapheresis, plateletapheresis.

Autologous donation: A blood donation that is stored and reserved for return to the donor as needed, usually in elective surgery.

Bacillus subtilis: A common nonpathogenic, anaerobic soil bacterium that has been used industrially for the large-scale production of proteins used in detergents and in the processing of corn starch and has attracted the attention of the recombinant DNA industry because of its great biosynthetic capability.

Bacteria: Any of a group of microscopic organisms having round, rodlike, spiral, or filamentous single cell or noncellular bodies that are often aggregated into colonies or motile by means of flagella, living in soil, water, organic matter, or in the bodies of plants and animals.

Bacteriophage: Any of various viruses that multiply in bacteria. The bacteriophage, lambda, is commonly used as a vector in recombinant DNA processes.

Biologics: Vaccines, therapeutic serums, toxoids, antitoxins, and analogous biological products used against the agents of infectious diseases or their harmful byproducts.

Biotechnology: Techniques that use living organisms, or substances from such organisms, to make or modify a product.

Blood: A complex liquid mixture of specialized cells (white cells, red cells, and platelets), proteins and other molecules, among whose functions are the transport of oxygen and nutrients to body tissues, removal of carbon dioxide and other wastes, transfer of hormonal messages between organs, prevention of bleeding, and transport of antibodies and infection fighting cells to sites of infection.

Blood bank: General name for a facility or part of a facility (e.g., a hospital) that stores blood and blood components and which also may collect and process blood.

Blood cells: Erythrocytes (red blood cells), leukocytes (white blood cells), or thrombocytes (platelets).

Blood center: A facility that provides a full range of blood services, including the collection, testing, processing, and distribution of blood and blood products, to a particular geographic area (e.g., community or regional).

Blood components: Products separated from whole blood; i.e., red cells, white cells, platelets and plasma. Compare with "plasma derivatives."

Bone marrow: A highly vascular, modified connective tissue found in the long bones and certain flat bones of vertebrates that is the origin of blood cells.

Cell line: Living cells obtained from humans and other animals and which are cultured under special conditions so that they can multiply indefinitely in vitro.

Centrifugation: The rapid whirling of fluids in a machine known as a centrifuge to separate substances of different densities by centrifugal force.

Clone: A group of genetically identical cells or organisms produced asexually from a common ancestor. (See also "recombinant DNA techniques.")

Coagulation: The process of blood clotting, in which the plasma protein prothrombin (Factor II) is converted to thrombin, which in turn converts the soluble plasma fibrinogen (Factor I) to insoluble fibrin.

Coagulation concentrates or complexes: Products obtained through selective precipitation of the proteins in plasma, resulting in concentrated forms of the plasma proteins that are needed for blood to coagulate (clot). Immune globulins and albumin are also obtained in this manner. See also "cold ethanol precipitation technique."

Coagulation factors or proteins: Naturally occurring proteins in plasma (e.g., Factor VIII, Factor IX) that aid in the coagulation of blood. See also "Factors I-XII."

Cold ethanol precipitation technique: The principal method used to separate plasma into its major protein groups. A three-variable system (temperature, ionic strength, and ethanol concentration (pH)) is used to precipitate different proteins in the following order: Fraction I (chiefly Factor VIII and fibrinogen); Fraction II (the immune globulins); Fractions III and IV (other coagulation proteins and trace components); Fraction V (the albumins); and Fraction VI (the remaining residue).

Complementary DNA (cDNA): DNA that is complementary to messenger RNA; used for cloning or as a probe in DNA hybridization studies.

Components: See "blood components."

Concentrates: In general, refers to blood cells or proteins that have been separated from the rest of blood or plasma in concentrated form. For example, preparations of platelets that are separated from whole blood after donation are called "platelet concentrates" (see also "coagulation concentrates").

Cosmids: Genetic hybrids constructed from plasmids and the bacteriophage, lambda, and used as vectors in DNA cloning.

Crossmatching: Testing to determine compatibility of blood types between donor and recipient.

Cryoprecipitate: A precipitate that remains after blood plasma has been frozen and then thawed. This precipitate is rich in Factor VIII (antihemophilic factor), fibrinogen, and fibronectin.

Cytomegalovirus (CMV): One of a group of highly host-specific herpes virus that infect man, monkeys, or rodents, with the production of unique large cells bearing intranuclear inclusions.

Diagnosis-related groups (DRGs): A classification system that groups patients according to principal diagnosis, presence or absence of a surgical procedure, presence or absence of significant comorbidities or complications, age, and other criteria; used as the basis for Medicare's current hospital payment system.

DNA: Deoxyribonucleic acid.

Directed donations: Donations from identified individuals, such as family and friends, intended to be used as the sole source of blood for the patient for whom the donations were made.

Enzyme: Any of a group of catalytic proteins that are produced by living cells and that mediate and promote the chemical processes of life without themselves being altered or destroyed.

Erythrocytes: Red blood cells.

Escherichia coli **(E. coli):** A species of bacteria that inhabits the intestinal tract of most vertebrates. Some strains are pathogenic to humans and animals. Many nonpathogenic strains are used as hosts in recombinant DNA technologies.

Eukaryote: A cell or organism with membrane-bound, structurally discrete nuclei and well-developed cell organelles. Eukaryotes include all organisms except viruses, bacteria, and blue-green algae. (Compare with "prokaryote.")

Exons: Fragments of eukaryotic genes which contain the coding regions of DNA for gene expression. (See also "introns.")

Factors I-XII: Refers to a classification of the multiple factors involved in coagulation. For example, hemophilia A is a result of a deficiency in Factor VIII, while hemophilia B is a deficiency in Factor IX.

Fibrinogen: Factor I; a plasma protein, synthesized in the liver, which is involved in coagulation as the precursor of fibrin.

Fibronectin: A plasma protein, synthesized in the liver, which plays a variety of roles ranging from cell adhesion to enhancing the phagocytic clearance of particulate contaminants from the body.

Fractionation: See "plasma fractionation."

Fresh frozen plasma (FFP): Plasma that has been frozen soon after collection to preserve the activity of the coagulation proteins.

Gene: The basic unit of heredity; an ordered sequence of nucleotide bases, comprising a segment of DNA. A gene contains the sequence of DNA that encodes one polypeptide chain (via RNA).

Gene expression: The mechanisms through which

directions contained within the genes that code for the cell's products are transferred and used to direct the production process.

Genome: The genetic material of an organism.

Glycosylation: The attachment of a carbohydrate molecule (glycogen) to another molecule such as a protein.

Granulocytes: White blood cells (leukocytes) containing neutrophilic, basophilic, or eosinophilic granules in their cytoplasm; a term used to identify a particular subset of white blood cells in one of several methods of classification.

Hemagglutination: Visual clumping of red blood cells; refers to compatibility testing between donor and recipient and observation of clumping from antibodies against the red blood cells. (See also "agglutination.")

Hematocrit: The volume occupied by the cellular elements of blood in relation to the total volume.

Hematology: The science of blood, its nature, function, and diseases.

Hematopoiesis: The process by which the cellular elements of blood are formed.

Hemoglobin: The iron-containing, oxygen-carrying proteins within red blood cells.

Hemolysis: The lysis, or destruction, of erythrocytes.

Hemolytic transfusion reaction: An antigen-antibody reaction in the recipient of a blood transfusion that results in the destruction of red blood cells.

Hemophilia: A rare, hereditary bleeding disorder caused by a deficiency in the ability to synthesize one or more of the coagulation proteins; e.g., Factor VIII (hemophilia A) or Factor IX (hemophilia B).

Hemorrhage: The escape of blood from the vascular system.

Hemostasis: The arrest of a flow of blood or hemorrhage; stopping or slowing of blood circulation.

Hepatitis: Inflammation of the liver; may be due to many causes, including viruses, several of which are transmissible through blood transfusions.

Histocompatibility: The extent to which individuals (or their tissues) are immunologically similar.

Hybridoma: Product of fusion between a myeloma cell (which divides continuously in culture and is "immortal") and a lymphocyte (antibody-producing cell). Such cells are used to produce monoclonal antibodies.

Hyperimmune globulins: Immune globulin products, derived from the plasma of donors hyperimmunized against known antigens. An example is hyperimmune anti-Rh globulin for the prevention of hemolytic disease of newborns.

Immune globulins (immunoglobulins): A type of plasma protein that comprises the antibodies.

Interferon: A class of glycoproteins (proteins with carbohydrate groups attached at specific locations) important in immune function and thought to inhibit viral infections.

Introns: Fragments of eukaryotic genes that contain the noncoding regions of DNA for gene expression. In prokaryotes such as bacteria, genes do not consist of exons and introns but rather consist of a single coding sequence of DNA.

In vitro: Literally, in glass; pertaining to a biological reaction taking place in an artificial apparatus; sometimes used to include the growth of cells from multicellular organisms under cell culture conditions.

In vivo: Literally, in life; pertaining to a biological reaction taking place in a living cell or organism.

Lambda: A bacterial virus that infects *E. coli;* used as a vector in gene cloning.

Leukocytes: White blood cells. Lymphocytes and granulocytes are particular types of leukocytes.

Liposomes: Closed spheroidal vesicles composed of lipid molecules arranged in a bilayer structure as in a normal cell membrane and enclosing an aqueous internal compartment.

Lymphocytes: Specialized white blood cells involved in the immune response.

Lymphokines: Proteins that mediate interactions among lymphocytes and are vital to proper immune function.

Lyophilized: Freeze-dried.

Megakaryocytes: Precursors of platelets.

Messenger RNA (mRNA): RNA (ribonucleic acid) that serves as the template for protein synthesis in living organisms; it carries the transcribed genetic code from the DNA to the protein synthesizing complex to direct protein synthesis.

Monoclonal antibodies: Homogeneous antibodies derived from clones of a single cell. Monoclonal antibodies recognize only one chemical structure and thus have remarkable specificity. They are easily produced in large quantities and have a variety of industrial and medical uses.

Nonreplacement fee: An additional fee that may be charged to users of whole blood or red cells if no replacement donations are made.

Normal serum albumin: Concentrates of albumin obtained through plasma fractionation and used to maintain or restore plasma volume. The appropriateness of using albumin preparations instead of other fluids is under examination. (See also "plasma protein fraction.")

Oligonucleotides: Short segments of DNA or RNA.

Oncotic (osmotic) pressure: The maximum pressure that develops in a solution separated from a solvent by a membrane permeable only to the solvent.

Perfluorochemicals (PFCs): Organic compounds in

which all the hydrogen atoms have been replaced by fluorine atoms and which are chemically inert and not metabolized by the body.

Plasma: The liquid portion of blood, excluding the cellular elements but including the proteins. (See also "serum.")

Plasma derivatives: Products derived from the fractionation of plasma to concentrate selected proteins. Compare with "blood components."

Plasma fractionation: The separation of plasma into its major proteins. (See also "cold ethanol precipitation techniques.")

Plasma protein fraction (PPF): A product of plasma fractionation that is at least 85 percent albumin and used interchangeably with albumin preparations. (See also "normal serum albumin.")

Plasmapheresis: Collection of plasma. (See also "apheresis.")

Plasmid: An extrachromosomal, self-replicating, circular segment of DNA found in the cytoplasm of various strains of *E. coli* and other bacteria; used as a vector in gene cloning in bacterial "host" cells.

Plasminogen activator: A substance that converts plasminogen to plasmin, a proteolytic enzyme in plasma which degrades the fibrin network in a blood clot, leading to clot dissolution.

Platelets (thrombocytes): Cells (minute protoplasmic disks) in blood which are involved in blood clotting.

Prokaryote: A cell or organism lacking membrane-bound, structurally discrete nuclei and organelles, such as bacteria. (Compare with "eukaryote.")

Proteins: Polypeptides consisting of amino acids. In their biologically active states, they function as catalysts in metabolism and as structural elements of cells and tissues.

Prothrombin: Factor II; an inactive plasma protein precursor of thrombin.

Prothrombin complex (PTC): A product of plasma fractionation consisting of Factors II, VII, IX, and X, but mostly Factor IX; also known as Factor IX complex (concentrate). Used in the treatment of hemophilia B. An "activated" form of this concentrate is used in the treatment of hemophilia A patients with inhibitor to Factor VIII. (See also "anti-inhibitor complex.")

Recombinant DNA (rDNA): The hybrid DNA produced by joining pieces of DNA from different organisms.

Recombinant DNA techniques: Techniques that allow specific segments of DNA to be isolated and inserted into a bacterium or other host (e.g., yeast, mammalian cells) in a form that will allow the DNA segment to be replicated and expressed as the cellular host multiplies. The DNA segment is said to be "cloned" because it exists free of the rest of the DNA of the organism from which it was derived. (See also "cloned.")

Recovered plasma: Plasma removed from outdated blood or remaining after the cells have been removed but not frozen in time to preserve the coagulation proteins; it is fractionated for the remaining proteins.

Red blood cells: The oxygen-carbon dioxide transporting cells of blood; erythrocytes.

Restriction enzymes (endonucleases): Enzymes that cut DNA at specific nucleotide sequences.

Reticuloendothelial system (RES): A diffuse system of cells arising from mesenchyme and comprising all the phagocytic cells of the body except the circulating leukocytes.

Rh blood group: A major blood group consisting of genetically determined substances present on the red blood cells of most persons and of higher animals and capable of inducing intense antigenic reactions. (See also "ABO blood group.")

Serum: The liquid portion of blood that remains when blood clots, removing the cells and coagulation proteins.

Source plasma: Plasma collected directly by plasmapheresis for fractionation into plasma derivatives.

Stem cells: Undifferentiated cells in the bone marrow with the ability both to replicate and to differentiate into specific hematopoietic cell lines.

Thrombin: An enzyme which induces clotting by converting fibrinogen to fibrin; precursor form in blood is prothrombin.

Thrombocytes: Platelets.

Typing and screening (T&S): Determining ABO and Rh blood groups and screening of blood for unexpected antibodies prior to transfusion.

Vector: In recombinant DNA technology, refers to the DNA molecule used to introduce foreign DNA into host cells. Vectors include plasmids, bacteriophages (viruses), and other forms of DNA. A vector must be capable of replicating autonomously and must have cloning sites for the introduction of foreign DNA.

Viruses: A large group of submicroscopic agents capable of infecting plants, animals, and bacteria, and characterized by a total dependence on living cells for reproduction and by a lack of independent metabolism.

White blood cells: General description of specialized cells involved in defending the body against invasion by organisms and chemical substances and including the circulating white blood cells and the cells of the reticuloendothelial system; defenses mediated through phagocytosis and immune responses; leukocytes.

Appendix C.—Acknowledgments and Health Program Advisory Committee

The staff would like to express its appreciation to the following people for providing information and assistance.

Amoz Chernoff
National Institutes of Health
Bethesda, MD

Gilbert Clark
American Association of Blood Banks
Arlington, VA

Paul Cumming
American Red Cross
Washington, DC

Martin Davey
Canadian Red Cross
Toronto, Canada

Dennis Donohue
U.S. Food and Drug Administration
Bethesda, MD

Bernice Hemphill
Irwin Memorial Blood Bank
San Francisco, CA

Nancy Holland
American Blood Commission
Arlington, VA

Robert Huitt
Council of Community Blood Centers
Falls Church, VA

Joan Maher
American Association of Blood Banks
Arlington, VA

Stephen Paik
Claremont College
Claremont, CA

Robert Reilly
American Blood Resources Association
Annapolis, MD

Joel Solomon
National Institutes of Health
Bethesda, MD

Chester Somerville
American Red Cross
Washington, DC

Jane Starkey
Council of Community Blood Centers
Falls Church, VA

HEALTH PROGRAM ADVISORY COMMITTEE

Sidney S. Lee, (Committee Chair)
President, Milbank Memorial Fund
New York, NY

H. David Banta
Deputy Director
Pan American Health Organization
Washington, DC

Carroll L. Estes**
Chair
Department of Social and Behavioral Sciences
School of Nursing
University of California, San Francisco
San Francisco, CA

Robert Evans
Professor
Department of Economics
University of British Columbia
Vancover, BC

Rashi Fein
Professor
Department of Social Medicine and Health Policy
Harvard Medical School
Boston, MA

Harvey V. Fineberg
Dean
School of Public Health
Harvard University
Boston, MA

Melvin A. Glasser*
Director
Health Security Action Council
Committee for National Health Insurance
Washington, DC

Patricia King
Professor
Georgetown Law Center
Washington, DC

Joyce C. Lashof
Dean
School of Public Health
University of California, Berkeley
Berkeley, CA

Frederick Mosteller
Professor and Chair
Department of Health Policy and Management
School of Public Health
Harvard University
Boston, MA

Norton Nelson, Ph.D.
Professor
Department of Environmental Medicine
New York University Medical School
New York, NY

Nora Piore
Senior Advisor
The Commonwealth Fund
New York, NY

Dorothy P. Rice
Regents Lecturer
Department of Social and Behavioral Sciences
School of Nursing
University of California, San Francisco
San Francisco, CA

Richard K. Riegelman
Associate Professor
George Washington University
School of Medicine
Washington, DC

Walter L. Robb
Vice President and General Manager
Medical Systems Operations
General Electric Co.
Milwaukee, WI

Frederick C. Robbins
President
Institute of Medicine
Washington, DC

Rosemary Stevens
Professor
Department of History and Sociology of Science
University of Pennsylvania
Philadelphia, PA

---

*Until October 1983.
**Until March 1984.

References

References

1. Abildgaard, U., "Purification of Two Progressive Antithrombins of Human Plasma," *Scand. J. Clin. Lab Invest.* 19:190-195, 1967.
2. Abramowitz, K., "Economics of Automation," *Plasma Quarterly* 1(2):41,61-62, 1979.
3. Acker, Loren, Engineering aand Research Associates, Inc., Tucson, AZ, personal communication, Feb. 23, 1984.
4. Adams, D. M., Joyce, G., Richardson, V. J., et al., "Liposome Toxicity in the Mouse Central Nervous System," *J. Neurol. Sci.* 31:173-180, 1977.
5. Aledort, L. M., "AIDS: An Update," *Hospital Practice* 18(9):159-171, 1982.
6. Aledort, L. M., "Lessons From Hemophilia," *N. Engl. J. Med.* 306:607-608, 1982.
7. Aledort, L. M., Pannekoek, H., Vehar, G. A., and Veltkamp, J. J., "What Is the Prospective Impact of Recombinant DNA Technique on the Production of Human Plasma Derivatives? Which Are the Derivatives Where Donor Plasma Could Be Replaced?" *Vox Sang.* 44:390-395, 1983.
8. Alexander, M. R., Ambre, J. J., Liskow, B. I., and Trost, D. C. "Therapeutic Use of Albumin," *J.A.M.A.*, 241:2527-2529, 1979.
9. Almog, J., Baldwin, J. E., and Huff, J., "Reversible Oxygenation and Antioxidation of a "Capped" Porphyrin Iron (II) Complex," *J. Am. Chem. Soc.* 97:227-228, 1975.
10. Amberson, W. R., Jennings, J. J., and Rhode, C. N., "Clinical Experience With Hemoglobin-Saline Solutions," *J. Appl. Physiol.* 1:469-489, 1949.
11. Ambler, R. P., and Scott, G. K., "The Partial Amino Acid Sequence of the Penicillinase Coded by *E. coli* Plasmid pR6K," *Proc. Natl. Acad. Sci.* 75:3732-3936, 1978.
12. American Association of Blood Banks, "AABB Members Comment on the Medicare Prospective Payment System," American Association of Blood Banks, Arlington, VA, no date.
13. American Association of Blood Banks, press release on ACT representation, Arlington, VA, January 1984.
14. American Association of Blood Banks, American Red Cross and Council of Community Blood Centers, "Joint Statement on Acquired Immune Deficiency Syndrome (AIDS) Related to Transfusion" (Jan. 13, 1983), *Transfusion* 23(2):87-88, March-April 1983.
15. *American Association of Blood Banks Clearinghouse Transaction Reports* (Arlington, VA: American Association of Blood Banks, 1973-83).
16. American Association of Blood Banks, *Blood Clearinghouse Lifeline Information Sheet* (Arlington, VA: American Association of Blood Banks, May 1984).
17. American Association of Blood Banks, *Blood Transfusion Therapy: A Physician's Handbook* (Arlington, VA: American Association of Blood Banks, 1983).
18. American Association of Blood Banks, *Guide for the National Clearinghouse Lifeline Program of the American Association of Blood Banks, Third Edition* (Arlington, VA: American Association of Blood Banks, July 1984).
19. American Association of Blood Banks, Hospital Transfusion Committee Meeting, Arlington, VA, Apr. 20, 1984.
20. American Association of Blood Banks, *Interim Annual Report: 1982-1983* (Arlington, VA: American Association of Blood Banks, 1983).
21. *American Association of Blood Banks Newsletter* (Arlington, VA: American Association of Blood Banks, January 1984).
22. American Association of Blood Banks, "Plasma Products: Use and Management" (Arlington, VA: American Association of Blood Banks, 1982).
23. American Association of Blood Banks, "Plasma Products: Use and Management," Educational program at Annual Meeting of the American Association of Blood Banks, New York, NY, 1983.
24. American Association of Blood Banks, Seminar on Prospective Payment at Annual Meeting of the American Association of Blood Banks, New York, NY, 1983.
25. *American Association of Blood Banks Newsbriefs*, "AABB AIDS Survey Completed" 7(4):1-2, April, 1984.
26. *American Association of Blood Banks Newsbriefs*, "AABB Announces New Physician Self-Assessment Program" 7(4):12, April, 1984.
27. *American Association of Blood Banks Newsbriefs*, "AABB Takes Stand on Organ Procurement and Transplantation" 7(4):1,8, April 1984.
28. American Association of Blood Banks, *Untitled* [Information Sheet] (Arlington, VA: American Association of Blood Banks, 1982).
29. American Association of Blood Banks, *Untitled*

[1981 American Association of Blood Banks, American Red Cross, and Council of Community Blood Banks Blood Data], 1983.
30. American Blood Commission Annual Meeting, Washington, DC, Dec. 13, 1983.
31a. American Blood Commission, *Blood Facts: Answers to Some Often Asked Questions* (Arlington, VA: September, 1981).
31b. American Blood Commission Board of Directors Meeting, *Report by Regionalization Committee* (Washington, DC: March, 1983).
32. American Blood Commission, *Final Report: Regional Association of Blood Service Units Program, Contract NO1-HB-6-2967 SA #2: Operating Relationship and Resource Sharing (of Blood Banking Services) on a Regional Basis* (Washington, DC: Jan. 31, 1980).
33. American Blood Commission, *Financial Statements as of March 31, 1983* (Arlington, VA: 1983).
34. American Blood Commission, *Regionalization Program Information Sheet* (Washington, DC: September, 1983).
35. American Blood Commission, *Summary Report of the Task Force on Donor Recruitment* (Arlington, VA: American Blood Commission, 1977).
36. *American College of Surgeons 69th Annual Clinical Congress October 16-21, 1983, Postgraduate Course 1: Pre- and Post-Operative Care: Blood and How to Use It*, G. S. Moss, Chair, American College of Surgeons, Chicago, IL, 1983.
37. American Medical Association, Council on Scientific Affairs: Organ Donor Recruitment *J.A.M.A.* 246:2157, 1981.
38. American Medical Association House of Delegates, "AIDS and Blood Donations," Resolution 39 (A-84), Chicago, IL, June 20, 1984.
39. American Medical Association, *General Principles of Blood Transfusion* (Monroe, WI: American Medical Association, 1977).
40. American Red Cross, *Annual Report 1980* (Washington, DC: 1980).
41. American Red Cross, *Annual Report 1981* (Washington, DC: 1981).
42. American Red Cross, *Annual Report 1982*, (Washington DC: 1982).
43. American Red Cross, *Annual Report 1983* (Washington, DC: 1983).
44. American Red Cross, *Blood Services Directive 1.57* (Washington, DC: American Red Cross, Revised, 1982).
45. American Red Cross, *Blood Services Operations Report: 1979-1980*, ARC 591 (Washington, DC: 1980).
46. American Red Cross, *Blood Services Operations Report: 1980-1981*, ARC 591 (Washington, DC: 1981).
47. American Red Cross, *Blood Services Operations Report: 1981-1982*, ARC 591 (Washington, DC: 1982).
48. American Red Cross, *Blood Services Operations Report: 1982-1983*, ARC 591 (Washington, DC, 1983).
49. American Red Cross, *Red Cross Blood Donor Inquiry*, Blood Services, Mid-American Region, Survey conducted by J. Walter Thompson Co., Chicago, IL, 1978.
50. American Red Cross, *Report 1982: Blood Research and Development*, ARC 2729, Washington, DC, October 1982.
51. American Red Cross, "Summary-Blood Service Regions" (activities related to organ and tissue services), attachment N, Mar. 8, 1984.
52. Aroesty, J., and Rettig, R. A., *The Cost Effects of Improved Kidney Transplantation* (Santa Monica, CA: The Rand Corp., 1984).
53. Aronson, D. L., Director, Coagulation Branch, Division of Blood and Blood Products, Center for Drugs and Biologics, U.S. Food and Drug Administration, personal communication, June 1984.
54. Aronstam, A., Arblaster, P. G., Rainsford, S. G., et al., "Prophylaxis in Haemophilia: A Double-Blind Controlled Trial," *Brit. J. Haemat.* 33:81-90, 1976.
55. Aster, R., "Clinical Use of Platelet Concentrates," *Transfusion and Immunology: Plenary Session Lectures of the XIV Congress of the International Society of Blood Transfusion and the X Congress of the World Federation of Hemophilia*, E. Ikkala and A. Nykanen (eds.) 1975.
56. Baker, S. B., and Dawes, R. L. F., "Experimental Hemoglobinuric Nephrosis," *J. Pathol. Bacteriol.* 87:49-56, 1964.
57. Baldassare, J. J., Knipp, M. A., and Kahn, R. A., "Reconstitution of Platelet Proteins Into Phospholipid Vesicles: Functional Proteoliposomes," unpublished.
58. Baldwin, J. E., and Huff, J., "Binding of Dioxygen to Iron (II). Reversible Behaviour in Solution," *J. Am. Chem. Soc.* 95:5757-5759, 1973.
59. Baldwin, J. E., "Recent Researches Towards Oxygen Carrying Chelates as Blood Substitutes,"

Advances in Blood Substitute Research, R. B. Bolin, G. P. Geyer, and G. J. Nemo (eds.) (New York: Alan R. Liss, Inc., 1983), pp. 149-156.
60. Baltimore, D., "Viral RNA-Dependent DNA Polymerase," *Nature* 226:1209-1211, 1970.
61. Barker, L., and Hoofnagle, J., "Transmission of Viral Hepatitis, Type B, By Plasma Derivatives," *Develop. Biol. Standard.* 27:178, 1974.
62. Barker, L., "World Blood Resources: The Relationship of Medical Needs for Whole Blood, Red Cells, and Plasma Derivatives to Blood Collection, Plasmapheresis and Fractionation Practises," Report for the World Blood Resources Subcommittee of the Council of the International Society of Blood Transfusion, Montreal, Canada, August 1980.
63. Barrow, E. S., Reisner, H. M., and Graham, J. B., "The Separation of Willebrand Factor From Factor VIII-Related Antigen," *Brit. J. Haematol.* 42:455-468, 1979.
64. Bart, K. J., Macon, E. J., Whittier, F. C., et al., "Cadaveric Kidneys for Transplantation" *Transplantation* 31:379, 1981.
65. Baxter-Travenol Laboratories, Inc., "Annual Report and Form 10-K for Fiscal Year Ended December 31, 1982," Securitites and Exchange Commission, Commission File No. 1-4448.
66. Bayer, R., "Gays and the Stigma of 'Bad Blood'," *Hastings Center Report* 13(2):5-7, April 1983.
67. Benesch, R., and Benesch, R. E., "The Effect of Organic Phosphates From the Human Erythrocyte on the Allosteric Properties of Hemoglobin," *Biochem. Biophys. Res. Comm.* 26: 162-167, 1967.
68. Benesch, R. E., Yung, S., Suzuki, T., et al., "Pyridoxal Compounds as Specific Reagents for the Alpha and Beta N-termini of Hemoglobin," *Proc. Natl. Acad. Sci.* 70:2595-2599, 1973.
69. Benesch, R. E., Benesch, R., Renthal, R. D., et al., "Affinity Labeling of the Polyphosphate Binding Site of Hemoglobin," *Biochemistry* 64:3576-3581, 1972.
70. Bennett, J. S., and Vilaire, G., "Exposure of Platelet Fibrinogen Receptors by ADP and Epinephrine," *J. Clin. Invest.* 64:1393-1401, 1979.
71. Bettinghaus, E. P., and Milkowich, M. B., "Donors and Non-Donors: Communication and Information," *Transfusion* 15:165-180, 1975.
72. Billings, P. B., Allen, R. W., Jensen, F. C., et al., "Anti-RNP Monoclonal Antibodies Derived From a Mouse Strain With Lupus-Like Autoimmunity," *J. Immunol.* 128:1176-1180, 1982.

73. *Biotechnology Newswatch*, "Genentech Spurts in Secret Factor-VIII Cloning Race" 4(9):2-3, May 7, 1984.
74. Birndorf, N. I., Lopas, H. L., and Robboy, S., "Disseminated Intravascular Coagulation and Renal Failures," *Lab. Invest.* 25:314-319, 1971.
75. Birndorf, N. I., Lopas, H. L., and Robboy, S., "The Effects of Red Cell Stroma-Free Hemoglobin Solutions on Renal Function in Monkeys," *J. Appl. Physiol.* 20:573-578, 1970.
76. Blatt, P. M., White, G. C., II, McMillan, C. W., and Webster, W. P., "Failure of Activated Prothrombin Complex Concentrates in a Hemophiliac With an Anti-Factor VIII Antibody," *J.A.M.A.* 251(1):67, 1984.
77. Blattner, F. R., Williams, B. G., Blechl, A. E., et al., "Charon Phages: Safer Derivatives of Bacteriophage Lambda for DNA Cloning," *Science* 196:161-163, 1977.
78. Bloom, A. L., "Benefits of Cloning Genes for Clotting Factors," *Nature* 303:474-475, 1983.
79. Blue Cross & Blue Shield Association, "Statement on Voluntary Donation and Replacement of Blood" (Chicago, IL: Blue Cross & Blue Shield, 1972).
80. Blumberg, B. S., Alter, H. J., and Visnich, S., "A New Antigen in Leukemia Sera," *J.A.M.A.* 191:541, 1965.
81. Boggs, J. M., Clement, I. R., Moscarello, M. A., et al., "Antibody Precipitation of Lipid Vesicles Containing Myelin Proteins: Dependence on Lipid Composition," *J. Immunol.* 126: 1207-1211, 1981.
82. Bolin, R., Smith, D., Moore, G., et al., "Hematologic Effects of Hemoglobin Solutions in Animals," *Advances in Blood Substitute Research*, R. B. Bolin, R. P., Geyer, and G. J. Nemo (eds.) (New York: Alan R. Liss, Inc., 1983), pp. 117-126.
83. Bolin, R., Letterman Army Institute of Research, San Francisco, CA, personal communication, February 1984.
84. Bolivar, F., Rodriguez, R. L., Betlach, C., et al., "Construction and Characterization of New Cloning Vehicles: 1. Ampicillin-Resistant Derivatives of the Plasmid pMB9," *Gene* 27:75-79, 1977.
85. Bolivar, F., Betlach, M. C., Heyneker, H. L., et al., "Origin and Replication of pBR345 Plasmid DNA," *Proc. Natl. Acad. Sci.* 74:5265-5269, 1977.
86. Bolivar, F., Rodriguez, R. L., Green, J., et al., "Construction and Characterization of New

Cloning Vehicles: II. A Multi-Purpose Cloning System," *Gene* 2:95-100, 1977.
87. Bonhard, K., "Acute Oxygen Supply by Infusion of Hemoglobin Solutions," *Fed. Proc.* 34:1466-1467, 1975.
88. Bonhard, K., Biotest, Inc., Frankfurt, Germany, personal communication, March 1983.
89. Boswell, G., and Rodkey, W. G., "Pharmacokinetics of Hemoglobin Infusion," *Advances in Blood Substitute Research*, R. B. Bolin, R. P. Geyer, and G. J. Nemo (eds) (New York: Alan R. Liss, Inc., 1983), pp. 139-148.
90. Bove, J., "Improvements in Transfusion Safety: Past, Present, and Future" (abstract), CCBC 22d Annual Meeting, Feb. 26-29, 1984.
91. Boyer, H. L., Betlack, M. C., Bolivar, F., et al., "The Construction of Molecular Cloning Vectors," *Recombinant Molecules: Impact on Science and Society*, R. F. Beer and E. Bassett (eds.) (New York: Raven Press, 1977).
92. Bradley, T. R., and Metcalf, D., "The Growth of Mouse Bone Marrow Cells In Vitro," *Aust. J. Exp. Biol. Med. Sci.* 44:287-299, 1966.
93. Brandt, J. L., Frank, N. R., and Lichtman, H. C., "The Effects of Hemoglobin Solutions on Renal Functions in Man," *Blood* 6:1152-1158, 1951.
94. Broome, S., and Gilbert, W., "Immunological Screening Method to Detect Specific Translation Products," *Proc. Natl. Acad. Sci.* 75:2746-2749, 1978.
95. Browdie, D., and Smith, H., "'Stroma-free Hemoglobin: Simplified Preparation and In Vivo and In Vitro Effects on Coagulation in Rabbits," *Am. J. Surg.* 129:365-368, 1975.
96. Brown, J. R., "Structural Origins of Mammalian Albumin," *Fed. Proc.* 35:2141-2144, 1976.
97. Brown, M., and McCool, B. P. "Changes in the Ownership and Governance of America's Hospitals," unpublished contractor's report prepared for the Office of Technology Assessment, 1982.
98. Brown, N., and Miller, G., "Immunoglobulin Expression by Human B-Lymphocytes Clonally Transformed by Epstein-Barr Virus," *J. Immunol.* 128:24-29, 1982.
99. Brownstein, A., Executive Director, National Hemophilia Foundation, personal communication, Jan. 5, 1984.
100. Brummelhuis, H. G. J., Over, J., Duivis-Vorst, C. C., et al., "Contributions to the Optimal Use of Human Blood: IX. Elimination of Hepatitis B Transmission by (Potentially) Infectious Plasma Derivatives," *Vox Sang.* 45:205-216, 1983.
101a. Brunn, H. F., "Erythrocyte Destruction and Hemoglobin Catabolism," *Semin. Hematol.* 9:3-18, 1972.
101b. Bucala, R., Kawakami, M., and Cerami, A., "Cytotoxicity of a Perfluorocarbon Blood Substitute to Macrophages In Vitro," *Science* 220:965-967, 1983.
102. Busby, T. F., Atha, D. H., and Ingham, K. C., "Thermal Denaturation of Antithrombin III. Stabilization by Herapin and Lyotropic Agents," *J. Biol. Chem.* 256:12140-12147, 1981.
103. *Business Week*, "The Red Cross: Drawing Blood From Its Rivals," Sept. 11, 1978, pp. 113, 117, 119.
104. Bussion, R. W., and Wriston, J. C., Jr., "Influence of Incorporated Cerebrosides on the Interaction of Liposomes With Hela Cells," *Biochem. Biophys. Acta.* 471:336-340, 1977.
106. Canadian Blood Committee, "The Four Principles Approved by the Ministers of Health," 1980.
107. Canadian Red Cross Society Blood Transfusion Service, *1982 Statistical Report*, Toronto, Ontario, Canadian Red Cross Society, 1982.
108. Canadian Red Cross Society, *1982 Annual Report*, Toronto, Ontario, Canadian Red Cross Society, 1982.
109. Cannon, R. K., and Redish, J. R., "The Large Scale Production of Crystalline Human Hemoglobin: With Preliminary Observation on the Effect of Its Injection in Man," *Blood Substitutes and Blood Transfusion*, S. Mudd and W. Thallimer (eds.) (Springfield, IL: C. Thomas Publishers, 1942), pp. 147-155.
110. Caplan, A., Lidz, C. W., Meisel, A., and Roth, L. H., "Mrs. X and the Bone Marrow Transplant," *Hastings Center Report* 13:17-19, June 1983.
111. Caride, V. J., Waylor, W., Cramer, J. A., et al., "Evaluation of Liposome Entrapped Radioactive Tracers as Scanning Agents: 1. Organ Distribution of Liposome Technetium-99m Deithylenetramine Penta Acetic-Acid in Mice," *J. Nucl. Med.* 17:1067-1076, 1976.
112. Carlson, R. W., "Albumin and Resuscitation," *American College of Surgeons 69th Annual Clinical Congress October 16-21, 1983, Postgraduate Course 1: Pre- and Postoperative Care: Blood and How to Use It*, G. S. Moss, Chair, American College of Surgeons, Chicago, IL, 1983.

113. Cerney, L. C., Cerney, E. L., and Cerney, M. E., "Mixtures of Whole Blood and Hydroxyethyl Starch-Hemoglobin Polymers," *Crit. Care Med.* 11:739-743, 1983.
114. Chandra, T., Stackhouse, R., Ridd, V. J., and Woo, S. L. C., "Isolation and Sequence Characterization of a cDNA Clone of Human Antithrombin III," *Proc. Natl. Acad. Sci.* 80:1845-1848, 1983.
115. Choo, K. H., Gould, K. G., Rees, D. J. G., et al., "Molecular Cloning of the Gene for Human Anti-haemophiliac Factor IX," *Nature* 299:178-180, 1982.
116. Christman, J. K., Silverstein, S. C., and Acs, G., "Plasminogen Activators," *Proteinases in Mammalian Cells and Tissues*, A. J. Baret (ed.) (Amsterdam: Elsevier, 1977), p. 91.
117. Chung, D. W., Que, B. G., Rixon, M. W., et al., "Characterization of Complementary Deoxyribonucleic Acid and Genomic Deoxyribonucleic Acid for the Beta Chain of Human Fibrinogen," *Biochem.* 22:3244-3250, 1983.
118. Chung, D. W., Chan, W. Y., and Davie, E. W., "Characterization of a Complementary Deoxyribonucleic Acid Coding for the Gamma Chain of Human Fibrinogen," *Biochem.* 22: 3250-3257, 1983.
119. Clark, D. B., Plasma Derivatives Section, American Red Cross Blood Services Laboratory, Bethesda, MD, personal communication, February 1984.
120. Clark, G., Executive Director, American Association of Blood Banks, Arlington, VA, personal communication, 1984.
121. Clark, G., "Task Force to Study the Feasibility of a Public Education Program on AIDS and the Safety of Blood Donation and Transfusion," paper presented at the American Blood Commission Board of Directors Meeting, Washington, DC, Dec. 14, 1983.
122. Clark, L. C., Jr., and Becattini, F., "Physiology of Synthetic Blood," *J. Thorac. Cardiovasc. Surg.* 60:742-773, 1970.
123. Clark, L. C., Jr., Clark, E. W., Moore, R. E., et al., "Room Temperature-Stable Biocompatible Fluorocarbon Emulsions," *Advances in Blood Substitute Research*, R. B. Bolin, R. P. Geyer, and G. J. Nemo (eds.) (New York: Alan R. Liss, Inc., 1983), pp. 169-180.
124. Cline, M. J., and Golde, D. W., "Controlling the Production of Blood Cells," *Blood* 53:156-165, 1979.
125. Cochin, A., Das Gupta, T. K., De Voskin, R., et al., "Immunologenic Properties of Stroma vs. Stroma-free Hemoglobin Solution," *Surg. Forum.* 23:19-21, 1972.
126. Cohen, S., Chang, A., Boyer, H., and Helling, R., "Construction of Biologically Functional Bacterial Plasmids In Vitro," *Proc. Natl. Acad. Sci.* 70:3240-3244, 1973.
127. Cohn, E. J., Strong, L. E., Hughes, W. L., et al., "Preparation and Properties of Serum and Plasma Proteins: IV. A System for the Separation Into Fractions of the Protein and Lipoprotein Components of Biological Tissues and Fluids," *J. Am. Chem. Soc.* 68:459-475, 1946.
128. Cohn, E. J., Gurd, F. R. N., Surgenor, D. M., et al., "A System for the Separation of the Components of Human Blood: Quantitative Procedures for the Separation of the Protein Components of Human Plasma," *J. Am. Chem Soc.* 72:465-474, 1950.
129. College of American Pathologists, "Autologous and Directed Blood Donations," reprinted in *Council of Community Blood Centers Newsletter*, Apr. 6, 1984.
130. Collen, D., "On the Regulation and Control of Fibrinolysis," *Thromb. Haemostasis* 43:77-89, 1980.
131. Collins, J., and Hohn, B., "Cosmids: A Type of Plasmid Gene-Cloning Vector That Is Packageable In Vitro in Bacteriophage Lambda Heads," *Proc. Natl. Acad. Sci.* 75:4292-4245, 1978.
132. Condie, S., and Maxwell, N., "Social Psychology of Blood Donors," *Transfusion* 10:79-83, 1970.
133. Condie, S. J., Warner, W. K., and Gilman, DC, "Getting Blood From Collective Turnips: Volunteer Donation in Mass Blood Drives," *J. Appl. Psych.* 61:290-294, 1976.
134. Cook, J., "Blood and Money," *Forbes*, Dec. 11, 1978, pp. 37-38.
135. Coulombel, L., Eaves, A. C., and Eaves, C. J., "Enzymatic Treatment of Long-Term Human Marrow Cultures Reveals the Preferential Location of Primitive Hemopoietic Progenitors in the Adherent Layer," *Blood* 62:291-297, 1983.
136. Council of Community Blood Centers, *Audited Financial Statements* (Falls Church, VA: Mar. 31, 1983).
137. Council of Community Blood Banks, "San Francisco Bay Area Blood Centers Announce Anti-HBc Test Plans," *Council of Community Blood Centers Newsletter*, Apr. 6, 1984, pp. 1-2.
138. Cox, D. W., Johnson, A. M., and Fagerhol, M.

K., et al., "Report of Nomenclature Meeting for Alpha-1-Antitrypsin," *Hum. Genet.* 53: 429-433, 1980.
139. Crawford, I. P., "Purification and Properties of Normal Human Alpha-1-Antitrypsin," *Arch. Biochm. Biophys.* 156:215-222, 1973.
140. Crispen, J., Polyclinic Medical Center, Harrisburg, PA, personal communication, Feb. 24, 1984.
141. Cumming, P. D., Manager of Planning, Marketing, and Operations Research, Blood Services, American Red Cross, Washington, DC, personal communication, 1984.
142. Cumming, P. D., Wallace, E. L., Surgenor, D., et al., "Public Interest Pricing of Blood Services," *Medical Care* 12:743-753, 1974.
143. Curran, J. W., et al., "Acquired Immunodeficiency Syndrome (AIDS) Associated With Transfusions," *N. Engl. J. Med.* 310(2):69-75, 1984.
144. Dahlke, M. B., "Designated Blood Donations," *N. Engl. J. Med.* 310(18):1195, 1984.
145. Daly, P. A., "Platelet Transfusion—Clinical Applications in the Oncology Setting," *Am.J. Med. Sci.* 280(1):130-142, 1980.
146. Datta, N., and Kontomichalou, P., "Penicillinase Synthesis is Controlled by Infectious R Factors in Enterobacteriae," *Nature* 208:239-241, 1965.
147. Davey, M., Assistant National Director, Blood Transfusion Service, Canadian Red Cross Society, personal communication, Jan. 9, and May 31, 1984.
148. Davie, E. W., and Fujikawa, K., "Basic Mechanisms in Blood Coagulation," *Ann. Rev. Biochem.* 44:799-829, 1975.
149. Davis, T. A., and Asher, W. J., "Artificial Red Cells," United States Patent 4390521, June 28, 1983.
150. Dawson, R. B., Crispen, J., Gorsuch, C., et al., "Laboratory Findings on Long-Term Plasmapheresis Donors: Protein Levels," *Proceedings of the Plasma Forum III*, W. L. Warner (ed.) (Berkeley, CA, American Blood Resources Association, 1980).
151. DeClement, F. A., and May, S. R., "Procurement, Cryopreservation and Clinical Application of Skin," *Cryopreservation of Tissue and Solid Organs for Transplantation*, A. B. Glassman and J. Umlas (eds.) (Arlington, VA, American Association of Blood Banks, 1983), pp. 29-56.
152. Denny, D., "How Organs Are Distributed," *Hastings Center Report* 13(6):26-27, December 1983.
153. Derynck, R., Remaut, E., Saman, E., et al., "Expression of Human Fibroblast Interferon Gene in *E. coli*," *Nature* 287:192-197, 1980.
154. Devas, R., Cheroutre, H., Taya, Y., et al., "Molecular Cloning of Human Immune Interferon cDNA and Its Expression in Eukaryotic Cells," *Nucl. Acids Res.* 10:2487-2501, 1982.
155. DeVenuto, F., Zuck, T. F., Zegna, A. I., et al., "Characteristics of Stroma-Free Hemoglobin Prepared by Crystallization," *J. Lab Clin. Med.* 89:509-516, 1977.
156. DeVenuto, F., and Zegna, A.I., "Distinctive Characteristics of Pyridoxalated-Polymerized Hemoglobin," *Advances in Blood Substitute Research*, R. B. Bolin, R. P. Geyer, and G. J. Nemo (eds.) (New York: Alan R. Liss, Inc., 1983), pp. 29-40.
157. DeVenuto, F., Moores, W. Y., Zegna, A. I., et al., "Total and Partial Blood Exchange in the Rat With Hemoglobin Prepared by Crystallization," *Transfusion* 17:555-562, 1977.
158. Dexter, T. M., Allen, T. D., and Lojtha, L. G., "Conditions Controlling the Proliferation of Hemopoietic Stem Cells *In Vitro*," *J. Cell Physiol.* 91:335-344, 1977.
159. Dexter, T. M., Wright, E. G., Krizsa, F., et al., "Regulation of Haemopoietic Stem Cell Proliferation in Long-Term Bone Marrow Cultures," *Biomedicine* 27:344-352, 1977.
160. Djordjevich, L., and Miller, I. F., "Synthetic Erythrocytes From Lipid Encapsulated Hemoglobin," *Exp. Hemat.* 8:584-592, 1980.
161. Donohue, D., "Qualifications, Management, and Care of Blood Donors," *Clinical Practice of Blood Transfusion*, L. Petz and S. Swisher (eds.) (New York: Churchill Livingstone, 1981).
162. Donohue, D., Special Assistant to the Director, Center for Drugs and Biologics, U.S. Food and Drug Administration, personal communication, December 1983 and April 1984.
163. Drake, A. W., Finkelstein, S. M., and Sapolsky, H. M., *The American Blood Supply* (Cambridge: The MIT Press, 1982).
164. Drees, T. C., *Blood Plasma: The Promise and the Politics* (Port Washington, NY: Ashley Books, 1983).
165. Drees, T. C., "Can the Voluntary Blood System Replace the Paid Pheresis System?" *Plasma Quarterly* 2(1):7, March 1980.
166. Drees, T. C., "World Wide Plasma Supply and Demand," *Plasma Forum*, R. L. Couch (ed.) (Santa Barbara, CA: McNally & Loftin, West, 1979).
167. Drees, T. C., Downing, M., and Heldebrandt, C., "Biotechnology, Here Today or Tomor-

row," *Plasma Quarterly* 5(4):120-121, winter 1983.
168. Dugaicyzk, A., Law, S. W., and Dennison, O. E., "Nucleotide Sequence and the Encoded Amino Acids of Human Serum Albumin mRNA," *Proc. Natl. Acad. Sci.* 79:71-75, 1982.
169. Dunlap, E., Department of Biotechnology, Washington University, St. Louis, MO, personal communication, Feb. 23, 1984.
170. Edlund, T., Ny, T., Ranby, M., et al., "Isolation of cDNA Sequences Coding for a Part of Human Tissue Plasminogen Activator," *Proc. Natl. Acad. Sci.* 80:349-352, 1983.
171. Ervin, D. M., Christian, R. M., and Young, L. E., "Dangerous Universal Donors: II. Further Observations on the *In Vivo* and *In Vitro* Behavior of Isoantibodies of Immune Type Present in Group O Blood," *Blood* 5:553-567, 1950.
172. Esterley, Michael C., Assistant Manager, Group Claims, Medicare Unit, Travelers Insurance Co., Bloomington, MN, personal communications, March and April 1984.
173. Eyster, E., Co-Medical Director, National Hemophilia Foundation, personal communication, May, 1984.
174. Fagan, J. B., Sobel, M. E., Yamada, K. M., et al., "Effects of Transformation on Fibronectin Gene Expression Using Cloned Fibronectin cDNA," *J. Biol. Chem.* 256:520-525, 1981.
175. Fairley, N. H., "The Fate of Extracorpuscular Circulating Hemoglobin," *Brit. J. Med.* 2:213-217, 1940.
176. Fantus, B., "The Therapy of Cook County Hospital," *J.A.M.A.* 109:128-131, July 10, 1937.
177. Farmer, M. C., and Gaber, B. P., "Encapsulation of Hemoglobin in Phospholipid: Surrogate Red Cells *In Vitro* and *In Vivo*," *Biophysical Journal* 45:201a, 1984.
178. Fay, P. J., Chavin, S. I., Schroeder, D., et al. "Purification and Characterization of Highly Purified Human Factor VIII Consisting of a Single Type of Polypeptide Chain," *Proc. Natl. Acad. Sci.* 79:7200-7204, 1982.
179. *Federal Register*, 39(47):9326-9330, Mar. 8, 1974.
180. *Federal Register*, 39(176):32701-32711, Sept. 10, 1974.
181. *Federal Register*, 49 (87):18899-18900, May 3, 1984.
182. *Federal Register*, 45(213); Oct. 31, 1980.
183. Fendler, J. H., *Membrane Mimetic Chemistry* (New York, John Wiley & Sons, 1982).
184. Fendler, J. H., "Polymerized Surfactant Vesicles: Novel Membrane Mimetic Systems," *Science* 223:888-894, 1984.
185. Feola, M., *Advances in Blood Substitute Research*, R. B. Bolin, R. P. Geyer, and G. J. Nemo (eds.) (New York: Alan R. Liss, Inc., 1983).
186. Ferrari, E. F., Genentech, Inc., San Francisco, CA, personal communications, February and March 1984.
187. Firkin, B. G., Arimura, G., and Harrington, W. J., "A Method for Evaluating the Hemostatic Effect of Various Agents in Thrombocytopenic Rats and Mice," *Blood* 15:388-394, 1960.
188. Flood, A. B., Scott, W. R., and Ewy, W., "Does Practice Make Perfect? Part I: The Relation Between Hospital Volume and Outcomes for Selected Diagnostic Categories," *Medical Care* 22:98-114, 1984.
189. Flynn, Linda S., "The Hospital Blood Bank vs. the Regional Blood Center," paper presented at the 36th Annual Meeting of the American Association of Blood Banks, New York, NY, Oct. 28-Nov. 2, 1983.
190. Ford, J. M., Cullen, M. H., Roberts, M. M., et al., "Prophylactic Granulocyte Transfusions: Results of a Randomized Controlled Trial in Patients With Acute Myelogenous Leukemia," *Transfusion* 22:311-316, 1982.
191. Ford, J. M., Lucey, J. J., Cullen, M. H., et al., "Fatal Graft-versus-Host Disease Following Transfusion of Granulocytes From Normal Donors," *Lancet* ii:1167-1169, 1976.
192. Foss, R. D., "Using Social Psychology to Increase Altruistic Behavior: Will it Help?" *Advances in Applied Social Psychology*, vol. 3, M. Saks and L. Saxe (eds.) (Hillsdale, NJ: Erlbaum, 1984).
193. Fox, J. L., "Gene Splicing Protein to Have Orphan Drug Status," *Science* 223:914, 1984.
194. Fox, R. C., and Swazey, J. P., *The Courage to Fail: A Social View of Organ Transplants and Dialysis* (Chicago, IL: University of Chicago Press, 1974).
195. Frank, L., and Massaro, D., "Oxygen Toxicity," *Am. J. Med.* 69:117-126, 1980.
196. Frankl, J., Director, Administrative Services, Miller Memorial Blood Center, Bethlehem, PA, personal communication, March 1984.
197. Fratantoni, J., Center for Drugs and Biologics, U.S. Food and Drug Administration, Bethesda, MD, personal communication, April 1984.
198. Fratantoni, J., Office of Biologics Research and Review, U.S. Food and Drug Administration, Platelet Workshop, May 21-22, 1984.

199. Fried, W., "Platelets and White Blood Cells" *American College of Surgeons 69th Annual Clinical Congress October 16-21, 1983, Postgraduate Course 1: Pre- and Postoperative Care: Blood and How to Use It,* G. S. Moss, Chair, American College of Surgeons, Chicago, IL, 1983.
200. Friedlaender, G., Yale University, President, American Council on Transplantation, personal communication, Dec. 14, 1983.
201. Friedman, B. A., "Making Blood More Available," *American College of Surgeons 69th Annual Clinical Congress October 16-21, 1983, Postgraduate Course 1: Pre- and Postoperative Care: Blood and How to Use It,* G. S. Moss, Chair, American College of Surgeons, Chicago, IL, 1983.
202. Friedman, B. A., Burns, T. L., and Schork, M. A., "An Analysis of Blood Transfusion of Surgical Patients by Sex: A Quest for the Transfusion Trigger," *Transfusion* 20:179-188, 1980.
203. Friedman, B. A., Burns, T. L., and Schork, M. A., "A Study of Blood Utilization by Diagnosis, Month of Transfusion, and Geographic Region of the United States," *Transfusion* 19:511-525, 1979.
204. Friedman, B. A., Burns, T. L., and Schork, M. A., *A Study of National Trends in Transfusion Practice,* publication No. 1381125437 (Springfield, VA: National Technical Information Service, 1980).
205. Friedman, B. A., Burns, T. L., Schork, M. A., and Kalton, G., "A Description and Analysis of Current Blood Transfusion Practices in the United States With Applications for the Hospital Transfusion Committee," *Clinical Laboratory Annual, Volume 1,* Henry A. Homburger (ed.) (New York: Appleton-Century-Crofts, 1982).
206. Friedman, B. A., Schork, M. A., Mocniak, J. L., and Oberman, H. A., "Short-Term and Long-Term Effects of Plasmapheresis on Serum Proteins and Immunoglobulins," *Transfusion* 15(5):467-472, 1975.
207. Friedman, L. I., American Red Cross Blood Services Laboratory, Bethesda, MD, personal communication, 1983.
208. Friedman, L. I., "Status of Automated ABO/Rh Testing—A Cost Comparison," American Red Cross Internal Report, 1983.
209. Friedman, L. I., "Automation and Instrumentation," paper presented at the Mid-Atlantic Association of Blood Banks Annual Meeting, Baltimore, MD, Mar. 1-3, 1984.
210. Gadek, J. E., Klein, H. C., Holland, P. V., et al., "Replacement Therapy of Alpha-Antitrypsin Deficiency: Reversal of Protease-Antiprotease Imbalance Within the Alveolar Structures of PiZ Subjects," *J. Clin. Invest.* 68:1158-1165, 1981.
211. Gallo, R., Salahuddin, S. Z., Popovic, M., et al., "Frequent Detection and Isolation of Cytopathic Retroviruses (HTLV-III) From Patients With AIDS and at Risk for AIDS," *Science* 224:500-502, 1984.
212. Garby, L., and Noyes, W. D., "Studies on Hemoglobin Metabolism: 1. The Kinetic Properties of the Plasma Hemoglobin Pool in Normal Man," *J. Clin. Invest.* 38:1479-1483, 1959.
213. Gartner, S., and Kaplan, H., "Long-Term Culture of Human Bone Marrow Cells," *Proc. Natl. Acad. Sci.* 77:4756-4759, 1980.
214. *Genetic Engineering News,* "Chiron Develops Proprietary Hormone Process Using Yeast" 3(4):16, 1983.
215. *Genetic Engineering News,* "Integrated Genetics, Toyobo in TPA Research Contract" 3(3):24, 1983.
216. Genetics Institute, *Information Summary on the Factor VIII Project* (Boston, MA: Genetics Institute, Nov. 30, 1983).
217. Gerety, R., and Aronson, D., "Plasma Derivatives and Viral Hepatitis," *Transfusion* 22:347-351, 1982.
218. Geyer, R. P., "Whole Animal Perfusion With Fluorocarbon Suspensions," *Fed. Proc.* 29:1758-1763, 1970.
219. Geyer, R. P., Taylor, K., Duffett, E. B., et al., "Successful Complete Replacement of Blood of Living Rats With Artificial Substitutes," *Fed. Proc.* 32:927-929, 1973.
220. Giblett, E. R., "Blood Group Alloantibodies: An Assessment of Some Laboratory Practices," *Transfusion* 17:299-308, 1977.
221. Giblett, E. R., Executive Director, Puget Sound Blood Center and Program, personal communication, Feb. 10, 1984.
222. Gibson, R. M., Waldo, D. R., and Levit, K. R., "National Health Expenditures, 1982," *Health Care Financing Review* 5(1):1-31, fall 1983.
223. Gigliotti, F., and Insel, R., "Protective Human Hybridoma Antibody to Tetanus Toxin," *J. Clin. Invest.* 70:1306-1309, 1982.
224. Gilligan, D. R., Altshule, M. D., and Katersky, E. M., "Studies of Hemoglobinemia and Hemoglobinuria Produced in Man by Intravenous Injection of Hemoglobin Solutions," *J. Clin. Invest.* 20:177-187, 1941.

225. Ginsberg, M. H., Pointer, R., Forsyth, J., et al., "Thrombin Increases Expression of Fibronectin Antigen on the Platelet Surface," *Proc. Natl. Acad. Sci.* 77:1049-1053, 1980.
226. Gitschier, J., Wood, W., Goralka, T., et al., "Characterization of the Human Factor VIII Gene," *Nature* 312(5992):326-330, 1984.
227. Goeddel, D. W., Kleid, D. G., Bolivar, F., et al., "Expression in *E. Coli* of Chemically Synthesized Genes for Human Insulin," *Proc. Natl. Acad. Sci.* 76:106-110, 1979.
228. Goeddel, D., Yelverton, E., Ullrich, A., et al., "Human Leukocyte Interferon Produced by *E. Coli* is Biologically Active," *Nature* 287:411-416, 1980.
229. Goldsmith, M. F., "Liver Transplants: Big Business in Blood," *J.A.M.A.* 250(21):2905-6, Dec. 2, 1983.
230. Goodfield, J., "Vaccine on Trial," *Science 84* 5(2):78-83, March 1984.
231. Gore, A., Jr., Statement before Subcommittee on Health and the Environment, House Committee on Energy and Commerce, U.S. Congress, Hearing on H.R. 4080, The "National Organ Transplant Act," Oct. 17, 1983.
232. Gould, S. A., "Who Needs Blood," *American College of Surgeons 69th Annual Clinical Congress October 16-21, 1983, Postgraduate Course 1: Pre- and Postoperative Care: Blood and How to Use It*, G. S. Moss, Chair, American College of Surgeons, Chicago, IL, 1983.
233. Gould, S. A., Rosen, H. L., Sehgal, L. R., et al., "Assessment of a 35% Fluorocarbon Emulsion," *J. Trauma* 22:618, 1982.
234. Gould, S. A., Rosen, H. L., Sehgal, L. R., et al., "The Effect of Altered Hemoglobin-Oxygen Affinity on Oxygen Transport by Hemoglobin Solution," *J. Surg. Res.* 28:246-251, 1980.
235. Gould, S. A., Rosen, H. L., Sehgal, L. R., et al. "How Good Are Fluorocarbon Emulsions as O_2 Carriers?" *Surg. Forum* 32:299-301, 1981.
236. Grace, H. A., "Blood Donor Recruitment: A Case Study in the Psychology of Communication," *J. Soc. Psych.* 46:269-74, 1957.
237. Gray, P. W., Leung, D. W., Pennica, D. et al., "Expression of Human Immune Interferon cDNA in *E. Coli* and Monkey Cells," *Nature* 295:503-508, 1982.
238. Greenberg, A. G., Elia, C., Levine, B., et al., "Hemoglobin Solution and the Oxyhemoglobin Dissociation Curve," *J. Trauma* 15:943-950, 1975.
239. Greenberg, A. G., Newburger, P. E., and Parker, L. M., "Human Granulocytes Generated in Continuous Bone Marrow Culture Are Physiologically Normal," *Blood* 58:724-732, 1981.
240. Greenberg, A. G., Pearl, J., Balsha, J., et al., "An Improved Stroma-Free Hemoglobin Solution," *Surg. Forum* 26:53-55, 1976.
241. Greenberg, A. G., Schooley, M., and Peskin, G., "Improved Retention of Stroma-Free Hemoglobin by Chemical Modification," *J. Trauma* 17:501-504, 1977.
242. Greenwalt, T. J., Director, Paul I. Hoxworth Blood Center, University of Cincinnati Medical Center, Cincinnati, OH, personal communications, Nov. 22, Dec. 28, 1983, and Feb. 8, 1984.
243. Grenvik, A., et al., "Multiple Organ Procurement by Interhospital Transfer of Heartbeating Cadavers," G. Koostra, B. Husberg, and J. A. Vander Vliet (eds.), *Proceedings of the International Congress on Organ Procurement, Maastricht, Holland*, Apr. 14-16, 1983 (Orlando, FL: Grune & Stratton, 1984).
244. Grgicevic, D., Pistotnik, M., and Pende, B., "Observation of the Changes of Plasma Proteins After Long-Term Plasmapheresis," *Devel. Biol. Standard*, 48:279-286, 1981.
245. Grindon, A. J., Bergin, J. J., Klein, H. G., et al., "The Hospital Transfusion Committee Guidelines for Improving Practice," unpublished draft (Arlington, VA: American Association of Blood Banks Committee on Hospital Transfusion Practices, April 1984).
246. Grossman, J., and Schmitt, V., "The Plasma Derivative Market, An Overview," contract No. 433-5650.0, submitted to the Office of Technology Assessment, Washington, DC, May 1984.
247. Grunstein, M., and Hogness, D., "Colony Hybridization: A Method for the Isolation of Cloned DNAs That Contain a Specific Gene," *Proc. Natl. Acad. Sci.* 72:3961-3965, 1975.
248. Gunby, P., "Organ Transplant Group Formed," *J.A.M.A.* 250(16):2103, 1983.
249. Hackel, E., "New AABB BMTx Information Service," *American Association of Blood Banks Newsbriefs* 6(11):1-2, November/December 1983.
250. Hagen, P. J., *Blood: Gift or Merchandise* (New York: Alan R. Liss, Inc., 1982).
251. Hamilton, P. B., Huiller, H., and Van Slyke, D. D., "Renal Effects of Hemoglobin Infusions in Dogs in Hemmorrhagic Shock," *J. Exp. Med.*, 86:477-487, 1947.
252. Harfst, P., Acting Director, Division of Institu-

tional and Ambulatory Services, Office of Survey and Certification, Health Care Financing Administration, Department of Health and Human Services, Baltimore, MD, personal communication, June 1984.
253. Hayes, S. G., and Peetoom, F., *Regionalization of Blood Services: A Report on the Present Status and Future Direction*, contract No. 1-HB-6-2967, SA No. 10, submitted to the National Heart, Lung, and Blood Institute, Arlington, VA, June 30, 1981.
254. *Head v. Colloton*, 331 N.W. 2d 870 (Iowa, 1983).
255. Heath, D., "Genentech, Speywood Close Ranks in Move to Clone Factor VIII:C for $400 Million Antihemophilic Market," *Biotechnology Newswatch*, vol. 2, Nov. 15, 1982.
256. Heckler, M., Secretary, U.S. Department of Health and Human Services, Statement announcing the discovery of the possible etiologic agent for AIDS, Washington, DC, Apr. 23, 1984.
257. Hedlund, B., Carlsson, J., Condie, R., et al. "Aspects of Large Scale Production of a Hemoglobin Band Blood Substitute," *Advances in Blood Substitute Research*, R. B. Bolin, R. P. Geyer, and G. J. Nemo (eds.) (New York: Alan R. Liss, Inc., 1983), pp. 71-78.
258. Helfman, D. M., Feramisco, J., Jr., Fiddes, J. C., et al., "Identification of Clones That Encode Chicken Tropomyosin by Direct Immunological Screening of a cDNA Expression Library," *Proc. Natl. Acad. Sci.* 80:31-35, 1983.
259. Hemphill, B., Chairman, National Committee on Clearinghouse Lifeline Program, American Association of Blood Banks, San Francisco, CA, personal communication, Mar. 22, 1984.
260. Hennessen, W., "The Clinical Uses of Albumin: Report of an IABS Study," *Develop. Biol. Standard.* 48:49-52, 1981.
261. Hermetter, A., and Paltauf, F., "Interaction Between Ether Glycophospholipid Vesicles and Serum Proteins In Vitro," *Biochem. Biophys. Acta.* 752:444-450, 1983.
262. Hirsch, R. L., "Resources and Responsibility for Professional Education in Blood Transfusion Therapy," *Transfusion* 21:127-129, 1981.
263. Hjort, P. F., Perman, V., and Cronkite, E. P., "Fresh, Disintegrated Platelets in Radiation Thrombocytopenia: Correction of Prothrombin Consumption Without Correction of Bleeding," *Proc. Soc. Exp. Biol. Med.* 102:31-35, 1959.
264. Hoak, J. C., and Koepke, J. A. "Platelet Transfusions," *Clinical Practice of Blood Transfusion*, L. D. Petz and S. N. Swisher (eds.) (New York: Churchill Livingston, 1981).
265. Hoch, J. A., Department of Cellular Biology, Scripps Clinic and Research Foundation, La Jolla, CA, personal communications, February, March, and April 1984.
266. Hocking, W. G., and Golde, D. W., "Long-Term Human Bone Marrow Cultures," *Blood* 56:118-124, 1980.
267. Hogman, C. F., Akerblom, O., Hendlund, K., et al., "Red Cell Suspensions in SAGM Medium—Further Experience of In Vivo Survival of Red Cells, Clinical Usefulness and Plasma-Saving Effects," *Vox Sang.* 45:217-223, 1983.
268. Hohn, B., and Murray, K., "Packaging Recombinant DNA Molecules Into Bacteriophage Particles In Vitro," *Proc. Natl. Acad. Sci.* 74:3259-3263, 1977.
269. Hohn, B., and Collins, J., "A Small Cosmid for Efficient Cloning of Large DNA Fragments," *Gene* 11:291-299, 1980.
270. Holland, Nancy B., Executive Director, American Blood Commission, Arlington, VA, personal communication, February 1983.
271a. Hollinger, F. B., Mosley, J. W., Szmuness, R. D., et al., "Transfusion-Transmitted Viruses Study: Experimental Evidence for Two Non-A, Non-B Hepatitis Agents," *Journal of Infectious Diseases* 142(3):400-407, September 1980.
271b. Hollinger, J., Alter, H., Holland, P., Aach, R., "Non-A, Non-B Posttransfusion Hepatitis in the United States," *Non-A, Non-B Hepatitis*, R. Gerety (ed.) (New York: Academic Press, 1981), pp. 49-70.
272. Honda, K., Hoshimo, S., Shoji, M., et al., "Clinical Use of Blood Substitute," *N. Engl. J. Med.* 303:391-392, 1980.
273. Huestis, D. W., Bove, J. R., and Busch, S., *Practical Blood Transfusion*, 3d ed. (Boston: Little, Brown, & Co., 1981).
274. Huitt, R. E., Executive Director, Council of Community Blood Centers, Falls Church, VA, personal communications, Sept. 19, 1983, and Jan. 5, 1984.
275. Humes, J. J., "Hospital Laboratory Perspective," paper presented at the Annual Meeting of the American Association of Blood Banks, New York, Oct. 28-Nov. 2, 1983.
276. Hunt, C. A., and Burnette, R. R., "Neohemocytes," *Advances in Blood Substitute Research*, R. B. Bolin, R. P. Geyer, and G. J. Nemo (eds.) (New York: Alan R. Liss, Inc., 1983), pp. 71-78.

277. Hyman, L., "The Economics of Plasmapheresis by Automation: Revisited," *Plasma Quarterly* 6(1):23-24, spring 1984.
278. Igelhart, J. T., "The Politics of Transplantation," *N. Engl. J. Med.* 310(13):864-68, 1984.
279. Inkster, M., Sherman, L. A., Ahmed, P., et al., "Preservation of Antithrombin III Activity in Stored Whole Blood," *Transfusion* 24:57-59, 1984.
280. *International Blood/Plasma News*, "Pricing Trends," December 1983.
281. International Federation of Pharmeceutical Manufacturers Associations, *A Study of Commercial and Non-Commercial Plasma Procurement and Plasma Fractionation*, Zurich, Switzerland, IFPMA, 1980.
282. International Society of Blood Transfusion, *ISBT Guide 6. Blood Component Therapy*, Paris, France, International Society of Blood Transfusion, 1980.
283. Israel, L., "Staffing and Managing a Transfusion Service for Liver Transplantation," paper presented at the 36th Annual Meeting of the American Association of Blood Banks, New York, NY, Oct. 31, 1983.
284. Issitt, P. D., and Issit, C.H., *Applied Blood Group Serology*, 2d ed. (Oxnard, CA: Spectra Biol., 1977).
285. Ivankovich, L., and Djordjevich, L., "Synthetic Erythrocytes," *Advances in Blood Substitute Research*, R. B. Bolin, R. P. Geyer, and G. J. Nemo (eds.) (New York: Alan R. Liss, Inc., 1983).
286. Iverson, W., Department of Research, Anheuser-Busch, Inc., St. Louis, MO, personal communication, February 1984.
287. Jackson, C. M., and Nemerson, Y., "Blood Coagulation," *Ann. Rev. Biochem.* 49:765-811, 1980.
288. Jackson, D. P., Sorenson, D. K., Cronkite, E. P., et al., "Effectiveness of Transfusions of Fresh and Lyophilized Platelets in Controlling Bleeding Due to Thrombocytopenia," *J. Clin. Invest.* 38:1689-1694, 1959.
289. Jaffe, H. W., "Transfusion-Associated AIDS: Serologic Evidence of Human T-Cell Leukemia Virus Infection of Donors," *Science* 223:1309-11, Mar. 23, 1984.
290. Jaye, M., de la Salle, H., Schamber, F., et al., "Isolation of a Human Anti-haemophiliac Factor IX cDNA Clone Using a Unique 52-Base Synthetic Oligonucleotide Probe Deduced From the Amino Acid Sequence of Bovine Factor IX," *Nucl. Acid Res.* 11:2325-2335, 1983.
291. Johnson, D. B. (ed.), *Blood Policy: Issues and Alternatives*, papers presented at a Conference on Blood Policy sponsored by the American Enterprise Institute, Washington, DC, 1976.
292. Jonah, M. M., Carny, E. A., and Rahman, Y. E., "Tissue Distribution of EDTA Encapsulated Within Liposomes Containing Glyco Lipids or Brain Phospholipids," *Biochem. Biophys. Acta.* 541:321-329, 1978.
293. Jones, P., "Factor VIII Supply and Demand," *Brit. Med. J.* 280:1531-1532, 1980.
294. Kagawa, Y., "Reconstruction of the Energy Transformer Gate and Channel Subunit Reassembly Crystalline ATPase and ATP Synthesis," *Biochem. Biophys. Acta.* 505:45-52, 1978.
295. Kahn, R., "Remarks in Questions and Answers," in W. L. Warner (ed.), *Plasma Forum III* (Feb. 25-27, 1980) (Berkeley, CA: American Blood Resources Association, 1980), pp. 127-130.
296. Kahn, R., "Establishing a Tissue Bank in a Blood Collection Facility: An Introduction to Bone Banking," *Cryopreservation of Tissue and Solid Organs for Transplantation*, A. B. Glassman and J. Umlas (eds.) (Arlington, VA: American Association of Blood Banks, 1983).
297. Kahn, R., Allen, R., Baldassare, J., and Cheetham, P., *Alternate Sources and Substitues for Theraputic Blood Components* contract No. 433-2390.0, submitted to the Office of Technology Assessment, Mar. 6, 1984.
298. Kane, W. H., Lindhout, M. J., Jackson, C. M., et al., "Factor V: Dependent Binding of Factor Xa to Human Platelets," *J. Biol. Chem.* 255:1170-1174, 1980.
299. Karow, A. M., and Glassman, A. B., "Should Blood Banks Become Organ Banks," *Transfusion* 15:285-286, 1975.
300. Kasahara, M., and Hinkle, P. C., "Reconstitution of D-Glucose Transport Catalyzed by a Protein Fraction From Human Erythrocytes in Sonicated Liposomes," *Proc. Natl. Acad. Sci.* 73:376-400, 1977.
301. Katz, A. J., Genco, P. V., Blumberg, N., et al., "Platelet Collection and Transfusion Using the Fenwal CS-3000 Cell Separator," *Transfusion* 21:560-563, 1981.
302. Katz, A., American Red Cross National Headquarters, Information on Donation Trends presented to the AIDS Working Group; Division of Blood Diseases and Resources; National Heart, Lung, and Blood Institute, Bethesda, MD, Mar. 5, 1984.
303. Keefer, L. M., Piron, M. A., and De Meyto, P., "Human Insulin Prepared by Recombinant

DNA Techniques and Native Human Insulin Interact Identically With Insulin Receptors," *Proc. Natl. Acad. Sci.* 78:1391-1395, 1981.
304. Kekkar, V., "Low Dose Heparin in the Prevention of Venous Thromboembolism—Rationale and Results," *Thromb. Diath. Haemorrh.* 33:87-96, 1974.
305. Kelley, W., Biogen, Inc., Boston, MA, personal communication, February 1984.
306. Kellner, A., President, New York Blood Center, personal communication, 1984.
307. Kennedy, L., "Community Blood Banking in the United States From 1937-1975: Organizational Formation, Transformation and Reform in a Climate of Competing Ideologies," Ph.D. dissertation, New York University, 1978.
308. Kessler, C., Department of Hematology and Oncology, George Washington University Medical Center, Washington, DC, personal communication, Dec. 1, 1983.
309. Kimelberg, H. K., "Differential Distribution of Liposome-Entrapped (^{3}H) Methotrexate and Labelled Lipids After Intravenous Injection in a Primate," *Biophys. Acta.* 448:531-550, 1976.
310. Kimelberg, H. K., and Mayhew, E. G., "Properties and Biological Effects of Liposomes and Their Uses in Pharmacology and Toxicology," *CRC Crit. Res. Toxicol.* 6:25-103, 1978.
311. Kirby, C., Clarke, J., and Gregoriadis, G., "Effect of the Cholesterol Content of Small Unilamellar Liposomes on Their Stabillity *In Vivo* and *In Vitro*," *Biochem. J.* 186:591-598, 1980.
312. Kitazawa, M., and Ohnishi, Y., "Long Term Experiment of Perfluorochemicals Using Rabbits," *Virchows Arch. A.* 398:1-10, 1982.
313. Klein, E., Farber, S., Freeman, G., et al., "The Effects of Varying Concentrations of Human Platelets and Their Stored Derivatives on the Recalcification Time of Plasma," *Blood* 11:910-919, 1956.
314. Klein, E., Toch, R., Farber, S., et al., "Hemostasis in Thrombocytopenic Bleeding Following Infusion of Stored, Frozen Platelets," *Blood* 11:693-699, 1956.
315. Klein, H., "Problems and Perspectives in Blood Banking," paper presented to the Interagency Technical Committee Working Group on Blood and its Substitutes, National Institutes of Health, Bethesda, MD, Mar. 25, 1981.
316. Klein, S. J., Secretary, New York State Council on Human Blood and Transfusion Services, Center for Laboratories and Research, Department of Health, Albany, NY, personal communication, Apr. 18, 1984.

317. Klein, T., "The Politics of Plasma," *Plasma Quarterly* 2(1):6-7, 29, March 1980.
318. Kohler, G., and Milstein, C., "Continuous Cultures of Fused Cells Secreting Antibody of Predefined Specificity," *Nature* 256:495-497, 1975.
319. Kolins, J., Britten, A., and Silvergleid, A. J. (eds.), *Plasma Products: Use and Management* (Arlington, VA: American Association of Blood Banks, 1982).
320. Konig, J., First Secretary, Embassy of the Federal Republic of Germany, personal communication, Jan. 11, 1984.
321. Kozbor, D., Lagarde, A. E., and Roder, J. C., "Human Hybridomas Constructed With Antigen-specific Epstein-Barr Virus-Transformed Cell Lines," *Proc. Natl. Acad. Sci.* 79:6651-6655, 1982.
322. Krauthammer, C., "The Politics of a Plague," *The New Republic* 189(5):18-21, Aug. 1, 1983.
323. Kurachi, K., Chandra, T., Friezner Degen, S. J., et al., "Cloning and Sequence of cDNA Coding for Alpha-l-antitrypsin," *Proc. Natl. Acad. Sci.* 78:6826-6830, 1981.
324. Kushwaka, S. C., Kates, M., and Martin, W. G., "Characterization and Composition of the Purple and Red Membranes From *Halobacterium cutirubrum*," *Can. J. Biochem.* 53:284-291, 1975.
325. Kushnik, H., "A Mother Tells How a Blood Donation, The Gift of Life, Led to Her Young Son's Death From AIDS," *People* 21(22):62-68, June 4, 1984.
326. Lachs, J., "On Selling Organs," *Forum on Medicine* 2(11):746-7, November 1979.
327. Landfield, R., Brief of American Blood Resources Association and Florida Association of Plasmapheresis Establishments as *Amici Curiae*, in *Automated Medical Laboratories, Inc. v. Hillsborough County*, No. 83-3014, U.S. Court of Appeals, 11th Circuit, July 8, 1983, p. 9.
328. Landfield, R., "A Quick Look at the Joint Venture," *Plasma Quarterly* 1(1):11, 28-29, February 1979.
329. Landfield, R., "Red Cross Plasma Business and Federal Taxes," *Plasma Quarterly* 1(4):100-101, December 1979.
330. Landfield, R., General Counsel, American Blood Resources Association, and Partner, Landfield, Becker & Green, personal communication, Nov. 22, 1983.
331. Landsteiner, K., and Weiner, A. S., "An Agglutinable Factor in Human Blood Recognized by Immune Sera for Rhesus Blood," *Proc. Soc. Exp. Bio. Med.* 43:223, 1940.

332. Larrick, J. W., Truitt, K. E., Raubitschek, A. A., et al., "Characterization of Human Hybridomas Secreting Antibody to Tetanus Toxoid," *Proc. Natl. Acad. Sci.* 80:6376-6380, 1983.
333. Latham, W., "The Renal Excretion of Hemoglobin: Regulatory Mechanisms in the Differential Excretion of Free and Plasma-Bound Hemoglobin," *J. Clin. Invest.* 38:652-658, 1959.
334. Lau, P., Shankar, V. S., Mayer, L. L., et al., "Coagulation Defects After Infusion of Dispersed Fluorochemicals," *Transfusion* 15:432-438, 1975.
335. Laurell, C. B., and Jeppsson, J. O., in F. W. Putnam (ed.), *The Plasma Protein*, 2d ed., vol. 1 (New York: Academic Press, 1975), pp. 229-264.
336. Lawn, R. M., Adelman, J., Bock, S. C., et al., "The Sequence of Human Serum Albumin cDNA and Its Expression in *E. coli*," *Nucl. Acids. Pres.* 9:6103-6144, 1981.
337. Leclerc-Chevalier, D., Executive Director, Canadian Blood Committee, personal communication, June 1984.
338. Leder, P., Tiemeier, D., and Enquist, L., "EK2 Derivatives of Bacteriophage Lambda Useful in the Cloning of DNA From Higher Organisms: The Lambda gtWES System," *Science* 196:175-178, 1977.
339. Legaz, M. E., Schmer, G., Counts, R. G., et al., "Isolation and Characterization of Human Factor VIII (Antihemophiliac Factor)," *J. Biol. Chem.* 248:3926, 1973.
340. Lehninger, A. L., "Biochemistry: The Molecular Basis of Cell Structure and Function" (New York: Worth Publishers, 1970).
341. Levine, C., "Blood: Designated Gifts, Experimental Therapy, and Racial Labels," *Hastings Ctr. Rep.* 13(4):3-4, August 1983.
342. Levine, P., and Stetson, R., "An Unusual Case of Intra-Group Agglutination," *J.A.M.A.* 113:126-127, 1939.
343. Levy, S. B., McMurray, L., Onigman, P., and Saunders, R. M., "Plasmid-Mediated Tetracycline Resistance in *E. coli*," *Topics in Infectious Disease*, J. Drews and G. Hagnauer (eds.) (New York: Springer-Verlag, 1978).
344. Lewisohn, R., "Blood Transfusion by the Citrate Method," *Surg. Gynecol. Obstet.* 21:37-47, 1915.
345. Lovric, V. A., Schuller, M., Bryant, J., et al. "Better Erythrocyte Concentrates—More Plasma for Components," *Med. J. Australia* 1:635-637, 1981.
346. Lundsgaard-Hansen, P., "Donor Safety in Plasmapheresis," *Develop. Biol. Standard* 48:287-295, 1981.
347. Lundsgaard-Hansen, P., "Intensive Plasmapheresis," *Transfus. Int.* 21(2)1:(8-10), April 1980.
348. Lundsgaard-Hansen, P. "Impact of the Protein Content of Red Cell Concentrates on the Optimum Use of Blood," *Vox. Sang.* 37:65-72, 1979.
349. Lundsgaard-Hansen, P., Pappova, E., and Frei, E., "Clinical Indications for Human Serum Albumin," *Develop. Biol. Standard* 48:69-74, 1981.
350. Lutz, J., Barthal, U., and Metzenauer, P., "Variation in Toxicity of *E. coli* Endotoxin After Treatment With Perfluorated Blood Substitutes in Mice," *Circ. Shock* 9:99-106, 1982.
351. MacPherson, J., Assistant Director, Regional Hemophiliac Blood Services, National Headquarters, American Red Cross Blood Services, personal communication, Washington, DC, Feb. 6, 1984.
352. Malcolm, A. D. B., "The Use of Restriction Enzymes in Genetic Engineering." *Genetic Engineering*, vol. 2, R. Williamson (ed.) (New York: Academic Press, 1981), pp. 129-173.
353. Maniatis, T., Kee, S. G., Efstratiades, A., and Kafato, F. C., "Amplification and Characterization of a B-golbin Gene Synthesized *In Vitro*," *Cell* 8:163-182, 1976.
354. Maples, J., U.S. Naval Research Institute, Bethesda, MD, personal communication, March 1984.
355. Marguerie, G. A., Edgington, T. S., and Plow, E. F., "Interaction of Fibrinogen With Its Platelet Receptor as Part of a Multistep Reaction in ADP-Induced Platelet Aggregation," *J. Biol. Chem.* 255:154-161, 1980.
356. Marketing Research Bureau, Inc., "The Plasma Fractions Market in the United States, 1982," *The Marketing Research Bureau, Inc.*, Newport Beach, CA, 1983.
357. Marks, D., Letterman Army Institute of Research, San Francisco, CA, personal communication, February 1984.
358. Mauch, P., Greenberger, J. S., Botneck, L. E., et al., "Evidence for Structured Variation in the Self-Renewal Capacity of Hemopoietic Stem Cells Within Long-Term Bone Marrow Cultures," *Proc. Natl. Acad. Sci.* 77:2927-2930, 1980.
359. Mauk, M. R., Gamble, R. C., and Baldeschwiller, J. S., "Targeting of Lipid Vesicles: Specificity of Carbohydrate Receptor Analogues for Leukocytes in Mice," *Proc. Natl. Acad. Sci.* 77:4430-4434, 1980.
360. Mayer, K., Chair, Blood Services Committee, New York State Council on Human Blood and

Transfusion Services, Albany, NY, personal communications, Nov. 8, 1983, and Mar. 15, 1984.
361. Mayhew, E., and Papahadjopoulos, D., "Therapeutic Applications of Liposomes," *Liposomes*, M. J. Ostro (ed.) (New York: Marcel Dekker, Inc., 1983).
362. McCabe, J. M., Legislative Director, National Conference of Commissioners on Uniform State Laws, statement before Subcommittee on Investigations and Oversight, House Committee on Science and Technology, U.S. Congress, hearings on organ transplants, Apr. 5, 1983.
363. McCurdy, P., Chairman, Public Education Committee, American Red Cross Blood Services, Washington Region, personal communication, February 1984.
364. McCurdy, P. R., Alexandria, VA, personal communication, June 1984.
365. McGill, M., Fugman, D., and Vittorio, N., "Platelet Membrane Concentrates Stored for Six Months Decreased Bleeding Times in Thrombocytopenic Rabbits," *Transfusion* 23:414, 1983.
366. McGill, M., Associate Director for Scientific Development, Paul Hoxworth Blood Center, Cincinnati, OH, personal communication, April 1983.
367. McLaughlin, W. F., "Membrane Hemapheresis: A Cost Effective Approach to a Two Tiered Market," unpublished, 1983.
368. McShane, D. J., and Schram, N. R., "Cause of Acquired Immune Deficiency Syndrome" (letter), *J.A.M.A.* 251(3):341, 1984.
369. Medical and Technical Staff of the Aurora Area Blood Bank, *Circular of Information on the Use of Blood and Blood Components* (Aurora, IL: Aurora Area Blood Bank, 1983).
370. Mega, T., Lujan, E., and Yoshida, A., "Studies on the Oligosaccharide Chains of Human Alpha-1-proteinase Inhibitor," *J. Biol. Chem.* 255:4057-4061, 1980.
371. Meloun, B., Moravek, L., and Kosta, V., "Complete Amino Acid Sequence of Human Serum Albumin," *FEBS Letters* 58:134-137, 1975.
372. Memorial Sloan Kettering Cancer Center, "Blood Bank, Donor Room, Special Procedures, Hematology and Urinalysis Laboratories Annual Report, 1983," unpublished manuscript, 1983.
373. Menache-Aronson, D., Associate Director, Plasma and Plasma Derivative Services, Blood Services Laboratories, American Red Cross, personal communication, June 1984.

374. Merritt, R. A., "State Legislation Relating to Organ Transplantation," paper presented to meeting of the American Council on Transplantation, Arlington, VA, Jan. 23, 1984.
375. Mertz, J. E., and Davis, R.W., "Cleavage of DNA by R1 Restriction Endonuclease Generates Cohesive Ends," *Proc. Natl. Acad. Sci.* 69:3370-3374, 1972.
376. Meryman, H., American Red Cross, Washington, DC, personal communication, December 1983.
377. Messmer, K., Jesch, F., and Schaff, J., "Oxygen Supply by Stroma-Free Hemoglobin," *Prog. Clin. Biol. Res.* 19:175-190, 1978.
378. Meyer, D., McKee, P. A., Noyer, L. W., et al., "Molecular Biology of Factor VIII/von Willebrand Factor," *Thrombosis Haemostas* 40:245-251, 1978.
379. Meynell, E., and Datta, N., "Mutant Drug Resistance Factors of High Transmissibility," *Nature* 241:885-886, 1967.
380. Miletich, J. P., Jackson, C. M., and Majerus, P. W., "Properties of the Factor Xa Binding Site on Human Platelets," *J. Biol. Chem.* 253:6908-6916, 1978.
381. Miller, J. H., and Mcdonald, R. K., "The Effect of Hemoglobin on Renal Function in the Human," *J. Clin. Invest.* 30:1033-1040, 1951.
382. Miller, T., and Weikel, M. K., "Blood Donor Eligibility, Recruitment and Retention," in American Red Cross, *Selected Readings in Donor Motivation and Recruitment*, vol. 2 (Baltimore: Reese Press, 1974).
383. Miller, W. V., American Red Cross, St. Louis, MO, President, American Blood Commission, personal communications, March and April 1984.
384. Mitsuno, T., Okyanagi, H., and Naito, R., "Clinical Studies of a Perfluorochemical Whole Blood Substitute (Fluosol-DA)," *Ann. Surg.* 195:60-69, 1982.
385. Modrich, P., "Structures and Mechanisms of DNA Restriction and Modification Enzymes," *Q. Rev. Biophys.* 12:315-369, 1979.
386. Mok, W., Chen, D. E., and Mazur, A., "Cross-Linked Hemoglobins as Potential Protein Expanders," *Fed. Proc.* 34:1458-1460, 1975.
387. Mollison, P. L., *Blood Transfusion in Clinical Medicine*, 6th ed. (Oxford: Blackwell Scientific Publications, 1979).
388. Mollison, P. L., *Blood Transfusion in Clinical Medicine*, 7th ed. (Oxford: Blackwell Scientific Publications, 1983).
389. Moore, F. D., *Transplant: The Give and Take*

of Tissue Transplantation (New York: Simon & Schuster, 1972).

390. Moore, M. A. S., Sheridan, A. P. C., Allen, T. D., et al., "Prolonged Hermatopoiesis in a Primate Bone Marrow Culture System: Characteristics of Stem Cell Production and the Hematopoietic Microenvironment," *Blood* 54:775-793, 1979.

391. Morgan, Lewis & Bockius, Attorneys for American National Red Cross, *Memorandum Re: Joint Venture for the Construction, Ownership and Operation of a Fractionation Facility*, submitted to the Antitrust Division, U.S. Department of Justice, Apr. 25, 1978.

392. Moroff, G., and Dende, D., "The Additive Solution System Approach to Blood Preservation and Component Preparation," Technical Report for the American Red Cross, 1983.

393. Morrisett, J. D., Jackson, R. L., and Gotto, A. M., "Lipid Protein Interactions in the Plasma Lipoproteins," *Biochem. Biophys. Acta.* 472:93-133, 1977.

394. Moss, G. S., "Crystalloids and Resuscitation" *American College of Surgeons 69th Annual Clinical Congress October 16-21, 1983, Postgraduate Course 1: Pre- and Postoperative Care: Blood and How to Use It*, G. S. Moss, Chair, American College of Surgeons, Chicago, IL, 1983.

395. Moss, G. S., Letter in Questions and Answers Column, *J.A.M.A.*, 250:2211, 1983.

396. Moss, G. S., and DeWoskin, R., Rosen, A. L., et al., "Transport of Oxygen and Carbon Dioxide by Hemoglobin-Saline Solution in the Red Cell-Free Primate," *Surg. Gynecol. Obstet.* 142:357-362, 1976.

397. Murray, C., and Tishkoff, G. H., "Preparation of Components and Their Characteristics; Plasmapheresis and Cytapheresis," *Clinical Practice of Blood Transfusion*, L. D. Petz and S. N. Swisher (eds.) (New York: Churchill Livingston, 1981).

398. Nagata, S., Taira, H., Hall, A., et al., "Synthesis in *E. coli* of a Polypeptide With Human Leukocyte Interferon Activity," *Nature* 284:316-320, 1980.

399. National Hemophilia Foundation, Medical and Scientific Advisory Council, "Recommendations to Prevent AIDS in Patients With Hemophilia," *Medical Bulletin #9: Chapter Advisory #12* (New York: National Hemophilia Foundation, Oct. 22, 1983).

400. National Hemophilia Foundation, *State and Federal Resources Guide for Hemophiliacs* (New York: National Hemophilia Foundation, 1979).

401. National Hemophilia Foundation, *1982 Annual Report* (New York: National Hemophilia Foundation, 1982).

402. Navota, R., President, Mississippi Valley Regional Blood Center, personal communication, March 1984.

403. Nemo, G. J., Chief, Blood Resources Branch, Division of Blood and Blood Resources, National Heart, Lung, and Blood Institute, National Institutes of Health, Public Health Service, U.S. Department of Health and Human Services, personal communications, March and May 1984.

404. Ness, P. M., and Pennington, R. M., "Plasma Fractionation in the United States: A Review for Clinicians," *J.A.M.A.* 230;247-250, 1974.

405. New York Cytapheresis Task Force, "Cytapheresis Practise," *NY St. J. Med.* October 1982.

406. *New York Times*, "Red Cross and Laboratory Plan Blood Plasma Facility," Mar. 16, 1979, p. A14.

407. Nusbacher, J., "Transfusion of Red Blood Cell Products," *Clinical Practice of Blood Transfusion*, L. D. Petz and S. N. Swisher (eds.) (New York: Churchill Livingston, 1981).

408a. Nusbacher, J., and Bove, J., "Rh Immunoprophylaxis: Is Antepartum Therapy Desirable?" *N. Engl. J. Med.* 303:935, 1980.

408b. Oberman, H. A., Barnes, B. A., and Friedman, B. A., "The Risk of Abbreviating the Major Crossmatch in Urgent or Massive Transfusion," *Transfusion* 18:137-41, 1978.

409. Oborne, D. J., Bradley, S., and Lloyd-Griffiths, M., "The Anatomy of a Volunteer Blood Donation System," *Transfusion* 18(40):458-465, 1978.

410. Odegaard, O., and Abildgaard, U., "Antithrombin III: Critical Review of Assay Methods: Significance of Variation in Health and Disease," *Haemostasis* 7:127-134, 1978.

411. Ogawa, M., Porter, P. N., and Nakahata, T., "Renewal and Commitment to Differentiation of Hemopoietic Stem Cells (An Interpretive Review)," *Blood* 61:823-829, 1983.

412. O'Hara, John L., Jr., Associate Regional Administrator, Division of Program Operations, Health Care Financing Administration, Region IX, U.S. Department of Health and Human Services, personal communication, April 1984.

413. Ohyanagi, H., Toshima, K., Mitsuno, T., et al., "Clinical Studies of Perfluorochemical Whole Blood Substitutes: A Safety of Fluosol-DA in

Normal Human Volunteers," *Clin. Therap.* 2:306-312, 1979.
414a. Olsson, L., and Kaplan, H., "Human-Human Hybridomas Producing Monoclonal Antibodies of Predefined Antigenic Specificity," *Proc. Natl. Acad. Sci.* 77:5429-5431, 1980.
414b. *On Center* 1:2 (Emeryville, CA: Cutter Biological, 1983).
415. O'Shaughnessy, L., Mansell, H. E., and Slome, D., "Hemoglobin Solution as a Blood Substitute," *Lancet* ii:1068-1069, 1939.
416. Osterud, B., Bouma, B. N., and Griffin, J. H., "Human Blood Coagulation Factor IX: Purification, Properties and Mechanism of Activation by Activated Factor XI," *J. Biol. Chem.* 253:5946-5951, 1978.
417. Oswalt, R. M., "A Review of Blood Donor Motivation and Recruitment," *Transfusion* 17(2):123-35, March/April 1977.
418. Ottenberg, R., and Fox, C. L., "The Rate of Removal of Hemoglobin From the Circulation and Its Renal Threshold in Human Beings," *Am. J. Physiol.* 123:516-525, 1938.
419. Over, J., Oh, J., Henrichs, H., et al., "The Effects of the Cooling Rate During Freezing of Plasma on Solute Concentration and Factor VIII Recovery in Cryoprecipitates," *Abstracts of the International Society of Thrombosis and Haemostasis*, Abstract No. 0320 (Stockholm, Sweden: July 5, 1983).
420. Page, P., American Red Cross Blood Services, Northeast Region, Boston, MA, personal communication, June 1984.
421. Parise, L. V., and Phillips, D. R., "Reconstitution of Platelet Membrane Glycoproteins IIb and IIIa Into Phospholipid Vesicles," abstract #961 presented at the American Society of Hematology Meeting, San Francisco, 1983, *Blood* 62: 264a, 1983.
422. Pennica, D., Holmes, W., Kohr, W. J., et al., "Cloning and Expression of Human-Tissue Type Plasminogen Activator cDNA in *E. coli*," *Nature* 301:214-221, 1983.
423. Perutz, M. F., "Regulation of Oxygen Affinity of Hemoglobin: Influence of Structure of the Globin on the Heme Iron," *Ann. Rev. Biochem.* 48:327-386, 1979.
424. Peskin, G. W., O'Brien, K., and Rabiner, S. F., "Stroma-Free Hemoglobin Solution; The 'Ideal' Blood Substitute?" *Surgery* 66:185-193, 1969.
425. Petersdorf, R. G., Adams, R. D., Braunwald, E., et al. (eds.), *Harrison's Principles of Internal Medicine*, 10th ed. (New York: McGraw Hill, 1983).

426. Peterson, T. E., Dudek-Wojciechowska, G., Scottrup-Jensen, L., et al., "Primary Structure of Antithrombin III (Heparin Co-Factor): Partial Homology Between Alpha-1-Antitrypsin and Antithrombin III," *The Physiological Inhibitors of Blood Coagulation and Fibrinolysis*, D. Collen, B. Wiman, B, Verstraete, and M. Verstraete (eds.) (Amsterdam: Elsevier, 1979), pp. 43-54.
427. Petrie, G. E., and Jonas, A., "Spontaneous Phosphatidylcholine Exchange Between Small Unilamellar Vesicles and Lipid-Apolipoprotein Complexes and Effects of Particle Concentrations and Compositions," *Biochemistry* 23:720-725, 1984.
428. Petska, S., "The Purification and Manufacture of Human Interferons," *Scientific American* 249:37-43, 1983.
429. Petz, L. D., and Swisher, S. N., *Clinical Practice of Blood Transfusion* (New York: Churchill Livingston, 1981).
430. Phillips, R. A., Gilder, R., Killough, J. H., et al., "The Results of Sixty-two Large Volume Hemoglobin Infusions in Man," *Res. Proj. NM 007-082.01.01*, U.S. Navy Medical Unit No. 3, Cairo, Egypt, 1951.
431. Pickering, J. W., and Gelder, F. B., "A Human Myeloma Cell Line That Does Not Express Immunoglobulin But Yields a High Frequency of Anti-Body-Secreting Hybridomas," *J. Immunol.* 129:406-411, 1982.
432. Pickering, L., "Roslyn Country Club Civic Association's First Drive a Success," *The Donor* (New York: Greater New York Blood Program, winter 1984), p. 1.
433. Piliavin, J. A., Callero, P. L., and Evans, D. E., "Addiction to Altruism? Opponent Process Theory and Habitual Blood Donation," *J. of Personality and Soc. Psych.* 43:1200-13, 1982.
434. Pindyck, J., Gaynor, S., Hirsch, R., et al., "Prevention of Infection Transmission by Transfusable Blood, Blood Components or Plasma Derivatives," contract No. 433-2900.0, submitted to the Office of Technology Assessment, Washington, DC, 1984.
435. Pittiglio, D. H., Baldwin, A. J., Sohmer, P. R. (eds.), *Modern Blood Banking and Transfusion Practices* (Philadephia, PA: F. A. Davis Co., 1983).
436. Plapp, F. V., and Sinor, L. T., "Nonisotopic Immunoassays in Blood Group Serology," *A Seminar on Antigen-Antibody Reactions Revisited*, C. A. Bell (ed.) (Arlington, VA: American Association of Blood Banks, 1982).

437. *Plasma Quarterly*, "About ABRA" 5(2):35, spring 1983.
438. *Plasma Quarterly*, "Red Cross to Pay Taxes" 4(1):17, winter 1982.
439. *Plasma Quarterly*, "Understanding Plasma" 6(2):36-38, summer 1984.
440. Poindexter, B., Office of Food and Drug Administration, Public Health Service, U.S. Department of Health and Human Services, personal communication, February 1984.
441. Polisky, B., Bishop, R. J., and Gelfand, D. H., "A Plasmid Vehicle Allowing Regulated Expression of Eukaryotic DNA in Bacteria," *Proc. Natl. Acad. Sci.* 73:3900-3904, 1976.
442. Pool, J., Hershgold, E., and Pappenhagen, A., "High-Potency Antihaemophilic Factor Concentrate From Cryoglobulin Precipitate," *Nature* 203:312, 1964.
443. Pool, J., and Shannon, A., "Production of High-Potency Concentrates of Antihemophilic Globulin in a Closed-bag System," *N. Engl. J. Med.* 273:1443-1447, 1965.
444. Popovic, M., Sarngadharan, M. G., Read, E., and Gallo, R. C., "Detection, Isolation, and Continuous Production of Cytopathic Retroviruses (HTLV-III) From Patients With AIDS and Pre-AIDS," *Science* 224:497-500, 1984.
445. Power, E. J., "AIDS and the San Francisco Blood Supply," contract No. 433-4520.0, submitted to the Office of Technology Assessment, Washington, DC, April 1984.
446. Prasanna, H. R., Edwards, H. H., and Phillips, D. R., "Interaction of Platelet Plasma Membranes With Thrombin-Activated Platelets," *Blood* 57:305-312, 1981.
447. Prince, A., Stephan, W., and Brotman, B., "Inactivation of Non-A, Non-B Virus Infectivity by a Beta-Propiolactone/Ultraviolet Irradiation Treatment and Aerosil Adsorption Procedure Used for Preparation of a Stabilized Human Serum," *Vox Sang.* 46(2):80-85, 1984.
448. Prochownik, E. V., Markham, A. F., and Orkin, S. H., "Isolation of a cDNA Clone for Human Antithrombin III," *J. Biol. Chem.* 258:8389-8394, 1983.
449. Proffitt, R. T., Williams, L. E., Presant, C. A., et al., "Liposomal Blockage of the Reticuloendothelial System: Improved Tumor Imaging With Small Unilamellar Vesicles," *Science* 220:502-505, 1983.
450. Prottas, J. M., "Encouraging Altruism: Public Attitudes and the Marketing of Organ Donation," *Milbank Mem. Fund Q.* 61(2):278-306, spring 1983.
451. Prottas, J. M., Visiting Professor, Center for Health Policy Analysis and Research, Brandeis University, personal communication, Jan. 5, 1984.
452. Pura, L., et al., "Directed Donor Program: A Three-Fold Benefit," paper presented at the AABB 36th Annual Meeting, New York, Nov. 1, 1983.
453. Quick, A. J., Goergotsos, M. S., and Hussen, C. B., "The Clotting Activity of Human Erythrocytes: Theoretical and Clinical Implications," *Am. J. Med. Sci.* 2208:207-213, 1954.
454. Rabiner, S. F., and Friedman, L. H., "The Role of Intravascular Haemolysis and the Reticulo-Endothelial System in the Production of a Hypercoagulable State," *Brit. J. Haematol.* 14:105-118, 1968.
455. Rabiner, S. F., Helbert, J. R., Lopas, H., et al., "Evaluation of a Stroma-Free Hemoglobin Solution for Use as a Plasma Extender," *J. Exp. Med.* 126:1127-1142, 1967.
456. Racker, E., and Stoeckenius, W., "Reconstitution of Purple Membrane Vesicles Catalyzing Light-Driven Protons Uptake and Adenosine Triphosphate Formation," *J. Biol. Chem.* 249:662-663, 1974.
457. Randolph, H. B., "The Future Shocks to Blood Banking Economics," paper presented at the South Central Association of Blood Banks Annual Meeting, Albuquerque, NM, Feb. 19-22, 1984.
458. Reijngoud, D. J., and Phillips, M. C., "Mechanisms of Dissociation of Human Apolipoproteins A-I, A-II, and C From Complexes With Dimyristoylphosphatidycholine As Studied by Thermal Denaturation," *Biochem.* 13:726-734, 1984.
459. Reilly, R. W., Executive Director, American Blood Resources Association, Annapolis, MD, personal communications, Dec. 9, 1983, and Jan. 5, 1984.
460. Rettig, R. A., testimony before Subcommittee on Investigations and Oversight, House Committee on Science and Technology, U.S. Congress, hearings on organ transplants, Apr. 13, 14, and 27, 1983.
461. Rijken, D. C., and Collen, D., "Purification and Partial Characterization of Plasminogen Activator Secreted by Human Melanoma Cells in Culture," *J. Biol. Chem.* 256:7035-7041, 1981.
462. Rixon, M. W., Chan, Y. W., Davie, E. W., et al., "Characterization of a Complementary Deoxyribonucleic Acid Coding for the Alpha Chain of Human Fibrinogen," *Biochem.* 22:3237-3244, 1983.
463. Robin-Tani, M., "Kidneys for Sale: The Con-

troversy Surrounding Dr. H. Barry Jacobs and the National Organ Transplant Act," *Contemporary Dialysis* 4(11):21-41, 1983.

464. Rodell, M. B., Vice-president, Regulatory and Technical Affairs, Ethical Products Division, Revlon Health Care Group, personal communication, Dec. 27, 1983.

465. Romano, M., Public Affairs Director, Broward County Blood Center, Lauderhill, FL, personal communication, August 1984.

466. Rosen, J., Vice President and General Manager, Sera-Tec Biologicals, North Brunswick, NJ, personal communication, 1984.

467. Rosenoer, V., Oratz, M., and Rothschild, M. (eds.), *Albumin Structure, Function, and Uses* (Oxford: Pergamon Press, 1977).

468. Roshenshein, M. S., Farewell, V. T., Price, T. H., et al., "The Cost Effectiveness of Therapeutic and Prophylactic Leukocyte Transfusion," *N. Engl. J. Med.* 302(19):1058, 1980.

469. Rossiter, E., "Technologies for Blood Collection," contract No. 433-4500.0, submitted to the Office of Technology Assessment, May 31, 1984.

470. Rossiter, E., President, Regulatory Resources, Inc., Richmond, VA, personal communication, June 1984.

471. Rougeon, F., Kourilsky, P., and Mach, B., "Insertion of a Rabbit B-globin Gene Sequence Into *E. coli* Plasmid," *Nuc. Acid. Res.* 2:2365-2375, 1975.

472. Ruoff, S., Supervisor, Component Laboratories, Blood Services Division, Los Angeles Region American Red Cross, personal communication, Feb. 23, 1984.

473. Russell, P. S., and Cosini, A. B., "Transplantation," *N. Engl. J. Med.* 301(9):470-79, 1979.

474. Sala-Trepat, J. M., Dever, J., Sargent, T. O., et al., "Changes in Expression of Albumin and Alpha-fetoprotein Genes During Rat Liver Development and Neoplasia," *Biochem.* 18:2167-2178, 1979.

475. Salvaggio, J., Arquembourg, P., Bickers, J., and Bice, D., "The Effect of Prolonged Plasmapheresis on Immunoglobulins, Other Serum Proteins, Delayed Hypersensitivity, and Phytohemagglutinin-Induced Lymphocyte Transformation," *Arch. Allergy* 41:883-894, 1971.

476. Sarngadharan, M. G., Popovic, M., Bruch, L., et al., "Antibodies Reactive With Human T-Lymphotropic Retroviruses (HTLV-III) in the Serum of Patients With AIDS," *Science* 224:506-508, 1984.

477. Savitsky, J. P., Doczi, J., Black, J., et al., "A Clinical Safety Trial of Stroma-Free Hemoglobin," *Clin. Pharmacol. Ther.* 23:73-80, 1978.

478. Saxton, P., Cable, R., and Katz, A., "Hemophilia Home Care: Distribution of Concentrate to Home Care Patients With Direct Reimbursement by Third Party Payer," presented at the annual meeting of the American Association of Blood Banks, New York, NY, November 1983.

479. Scannon, F. J., "Molecular Modification of Hemoglobin," *Crit. Care Med.* 10:261-269, 1982.

480. Scheller, R., Dickerson, R., Boyer, H., et al., "Chemical Synthesis of Restriction Enzyme Recognition Sites Useful for Cloning," *Science* 196:177-180, 1977.

481. Schiffer, C. A., and Aisner, J., "Platelet and Granulocyte Transfusion Therapy for Patients With Cancer," *Clinical Practice of Blood Transfusion*, L. D. Petz and S. N. Swisher (eds.) (New York: Churchill Livingston, 1981).

482. Schiffer, C. A., Aisner, J., Daly, P. A., et al., "Alloimmunization Following Prophylactic Granulocyte Transfusion," *Blood* 54:766-774, 1979.

483. Schiffer, C. A., and Slichter, S. J., "Platelet Transfusions From Single Donors," *N. Engl. J. Med.* 307(4):245-248, 1982.

484. Schmeck, H. M., Jr., "Substance Vital to Clot Blood Created in Lab," *New York Times*, Apr. 26, 1984, p. A-1.

485. Schmidt, P. J., "National Blood Policy, 1977: A Study in the Politics of Health," *Progress in Hematology*, vol. 10, E. B. Brown (ed.) (New York: Grune & Stratton, Inc., 1977), pp. 151-172.

486. Schmitt, V. W., Associate Director, Plasma Products Management, Blood Services, American Red Cross, Washington, DC, personal communication, Dec. 12, 1983.

487. Schoeppner, S. L., Ennis, K., and Mallory, D., "Evaluation of Routine ABO and Rh Typing by Microplates in Regional Blood Centers," abstract of poster presentations, MAABB/PABB Joint Meeting, Baltimore, MD, Mar. 1-3, 1984.

488. Schupbach, J., et al., "Serological Analysis of a Subgroup of Human T-Lymphotropic Retroviruses (HTLV-III) Associated With AIDS," *Science* 224:503-505, 1984.

489. Schwartz, S., "Elicitation of Moral Obligation and Self-Sacrificing Behavior," *J. Personality and Soc. Psych.* 15:283-93, 1970.

490. Sehgal, L. R., Rosen, A. L., Noud, G., et al., "Large-Volume Preparation of Pyridoxylated

Hemoglobin With High P_{50}," *J. Surg. Res.* 30: 14-20, 1981.

491. Sell, K. W., statement before Subcommittee on Investigations and Oversight, House Committee on Science and Technology, U.S. Congress, Apr. 13, 14, and 27, 1983.

492. Sellards, A. W., and Minot, G. R., "The Injection of Hemoglobin in Man and Its Relation to Blood Destruction With Special Reference to the Anemias," *J. Med. Res.* 34:469-494, 1916.

493. Seto, B., Coleman, W., Jr., Iwarsen, S., and Gerety, R., "Detection of Reverse Transcriptase Activity in Association With the Non-A, Non-B Hepatitis Agent(s)," *Lancet* ii(8409):941-945, 1984.

494. Sgouris, J. T., and Rene, A. (eds.), *Proceedings of the Workshop on Albumin February 12-13, 1975, Bethesda, MD*, DHEW publication No. (NIH) 76-925 (Washington, DC, U. S. Government Printing Office, 1975).

495. Sharom, F. J. D., Bonratt, D. G., and Grant, C. W. M. "Glyophorin and the Concanavolin A Receptor of Human Erythrocytes: Their Receptor Function in Lipid Bilayers," *Proc. Natl. Acad. Sci.* 74:2751-2755, 1977.

496. Sherman, L., "New Plasma Components," *Clinics in Hematology*, W. Bayer (ed.), in press (1984).

497. Sherman, L. A., "Fresh Frozen Plasma, Cryoprecipitate, Factor Concentrates," *American College of Surgeons 69th Annual Clinical Congress October 16-21, 1983, Postgraduate Course 1: Pre- and Postoperative Care: Blood and How to Use It*, G. S. Moss, Chair, American College of Surgeons, Chicago, IL, 1983.

498. Shinowara, G. Y., "Enzyme Studies on Human Blood. XI: The Isolation and Characterization of Thromboplastic Cell and Plasma Components," *J. Lab. Clin. Med.* 38:11-22, 1951.

499. Sie, P., Gillois, M., Boneu, B., et al. "Reconstitution of Liposomes Bearing Platelet Receptors for Human von Willebrand Factor," *Biochem. Biophys. Res. Comm.* 97:133-138, 1980.

500. Simon, E. R., "Whole Blood vs Red Blood Cells vs No Blood!" *Boswell Hospital Proceedings* 9:10-14, 1983.

501. Slichter, S. J., "Efficacy of Platelets Collected by Semi-Continuous Flow Centrifugation (Haemonetics model 30)," *Br. J. Haemotology* 38: 131-140, 1978.

502. Slovitar, H. A., Yamada, H., and Ogashi, S., "Some Effects of Intravenously Administered Fluorochemicals in Animals," *Fed. Proc.* 29: 1755-1757, 1970.

503. Sloviter, M. A., "Perfluoro Compounds as Artificial Erythrocytes," *Fed. Proc.* 34:1484-1487, 1975.

504. Smith, P., and Levine, P., "The Benefits of Comprehensive Care of Hemophilia: A Five-Year Study of Outcomes," *Am. J. Pub. Health* 74: 616-617, June 1984.

505. Snyder, E. L., Associate Professor of Laboratory Medicine, Yale University, personal communication, Feb. 6, 1984.

506. Solomon, J., "A Federal View: An Examination of Five Years of FDA Licensure of Source Plasma Manufacturers," *Plasma Forum, February 26-27, 1979: A Public Exchange of Views Regarding Plasmapheresis*, W. L. Warner (ed.) (Annapolis, MD: American Blood Resources Association, 1979).

507. Solomon, J., Clinical Center Blood Bank, National Institutes of Health, personal communication, March 1984.

508a. Solomon, J., "Contribution of the National Institutes of Health to Research on Acquired Immunodeficiency Syndrome (AIDS)," National Institutes of Health, Clinical Center Blood Bank Department, 1984.

508b. Solomon, J., "Legislation and Regulations in Blood Banking," *Federal Legislation and the Clinical Laboratory*, M. Schaeffer (ed.) (Boston: G. K. Hall Medical Publishers, 1981).

509. Solomon, J., "Regionalization of Blood Services in the Washington, D.C. Area," case study prepared for the Office of Technology Assessment, Washington, DC, March 1984.

510. Spector, J. I., and Crosby, W. H., "Coagulation Studies During Experimental Hemoglobinemia in Humans," *J. Appl. Physiol.* 38(2): 195, 1975.

511. *Spohn, R.B., Director of the Department of Consumer Affairs for the State of California v. Irwin Memorial Blood Bank of the San Francisco Medical Society*, Deposition of Bernice M. Hemphill, June 7, 1978.

512. Stackhouse, R., Chandra, T., Robson, K. J. H., et al., "Purification of Antithrombin III mRNA and Cloning of Its cDNA," *J. Biol. Chem.* 258: 703-706, 1982.

513. Stanier, R. Y., Duodoroff, M., and Adelberg, E. A., *The Microbial World*, 3rd ed. (Englewood Cliffs, NJ: Prentice-Hall, Inc., 1970).

514. Steger, L. D., and Desnick, R. J., "Enzyme Therapy. VI: Comparative in Vivo Fates and Effects on Liposomal Integrity of Enzyme Entrapped in Negatively and Positively Charged Liposomes," *Biochem. Biophys. Acta.* 464:530-546, 1977.

515. Steinitz, M., and Klein, E., "Human Mono-

clonal Antibodies Produced by Immortalization With Epstein-Barr Virus," *Immunol. Today* 13:38-39, 1981.

516a. Stel, H. V., Veerman, E. C. I., and van der Kwast, T., "Detection of Factor VIII/Coagulant Antigen in Human Liver Tissue," *Nature* 303: 530-532, 1983.

516b. Suggs, S. V., Wallace, R. B., Hirose, T., et al., "Use of Synthetic Oligonucleotides as Hybridization Probes: Isolation of Cloned cDNA Sequences for Human B_2-microglobulin," *Proc. Natl. Acad. Sci.*, 78:6613-6617, 1981.

517. Surgenor, D. M., President, Center for Blood Research, Boston, MA, personal communication, December 1983.

518. Surgenor, D. M., and Schnitzer, S. S., American Blood Commission, "The Nation's Blood Resource 1979 and 1980: A Summary Report," unpublished, 1983.

519. Sutcliffe, J. G., "Complete Nucleotide Sequence of the *Escherichia coli* Plasmid pBR322," *Cold Spring Symp. Quant. Bio.* 43:77-90, 1980.

520. Swisher, S. N., and Petz, L. D., "An Overview of Blood Transfusion," *Clinical Practice of Blood Transfusion*, L. D. Petz and S. N. Swisher (eds.) (New York: Churchill Livingston, 1981).

521. Switalski, R. W., "American Society of Anesthesiologists Blood Transfusion Practices Survey, 1981, Preliminary Survey Results," Arlington, VA, American Blood Commission National Blood Data Center, unpublished, no date.

522. Szoka, F. C., and Papahadjopoulos, D., "Comparative Properties and Methods of Preparation of Lipid Vesicles (Liposomes)," *Ann. Rev. Biophys. Biol.* 9:467-543, 1980.

523. Tait, R. C., and Boyer, H. L., "On the Nature of Tetracycline Resistance Controlled by the Plasmid pSC 101," *Cell* 13:73-77, 1978.

524. Tall, A. R., and Green, P. H., "Incorporation of Phosphatidyochoiine Into Spherical and Discarded Lipoproteins During Incubation of Egg Phosphatidycholine Vesicles With High Density Lipoproteins or With Plasma," *J. Biol. Chem.* 256:2035-2044, 1981.

525. Tarn, S. C., Blumenstein, J., and Wong, J. T., "Soluble Dextran-Hemoglobin Complex as a Potential Blood Substitute," *Proc. Natl. Acad. Sci.*, 73:2128-2138, 1976.

526. Tarn, S. C., Blumenstein, J., and Wong, J. T., "Blood Replacement in Dogs by Dextran-Hemoglobin," *Can. J. Biochem.* 56:981-984, 1978.

527. Teague, W. T., Executive Director, Gulf Coast Regional Blood Center, Houston, TX, personal communication, March 1984.

528. Temin, H. M., and Mizutani, S., "Viral RNA-Dependent DNA Polymerase," *Nature* 226: 1211-1213, 1970.

529. Thomas, W., International Patent Application No. WO82/03871 (1983).

530. Till, J. E., and McCulloch, E. A., "A Direct Measurement of the Radiation Sensitivity of Normal Bone-Marrow Cells," *Radiat. Res.* 14:213-219, 1961.

531. Tomasulo, P., "Blood Service Delivery in South Florida, 1978-1984," prepared for the Office of Technology Assessment, Washington, DC, April 1984.

532. Tomasulo, P. A., President, South Florida Blood Service, Miami, FL, personal communication, April 1984.

533. Tomasulo, P. A., "Platelet Transfusions for Nonmalignant Diseases," L. D.Petz and S. N. Swisher (eds.), *Clinical Practice of Blood Transfusion* (New York: Churchill Livingston, 1981).

534. Tomasulo, P., "Regional Blood Center Perspective," paper presented at the Annual Meeting of the American Association of Blood Banks, New York, NY, November 1983.

535. Toole, J., Genetics Institute, Boston, MA, personal communication, February 1984.

536. Toole, J., Knopf, J., Wozney, J., et al., "Molecular Cloning of a cDNA Encoding Human Antihaemophilic Factor," *Nature* 312 (5992): 342-347, 1984.

537. Tremper, K. K., Friedman, A. E., Levine, E. M., et al., "The Preoperative Treatment of Severely Anemic Patient With a Perfluorochemical Oxygen-Transport Fluid, Fluosol-DA," *N. Engl. J. Med.* 307:277-283, 1982.

538. Tullis, J. L., "Albumin: 2. Guidelines for Clinical Use," *J.A.M.A.*, 237:460-463, 1977.

539. Tullis, J., "Methods of Plasma Collection and Fractionation," contract No. 433-5310.0, submitted to the Office of Technology Assessment, Washington, DC, April 1984.

540. Tye, R. W., Medina, F., and Bolin, R. B., "Modification of Hemoglobin-Tetrameric Stabilization," *Advances in Blood Substitute Research*, R. B. Bolin, R. P. Geyer, and G. J. Nemo (eds.) (New York: Alan R. Liss, Inc., 1983), pp. 41-50.

541. Tyrell, D. A., Health, T. D., Colley, C. M., et al., "New Aspects of Liposomes," *Biochem. Biophys. Acta.* 457:295-302, 1976.

542. Ullrich, A., Shine, J., Chirgwin, J., et al., "Rat

Insulin Genes: Construction of Plasmids Containing the Coding Sequences," *Science* 196: 1313-1319, 1977.
543. Urdea, M. S., Merryweather, J. P., Mullenbach, G. T., et al., "Chemical Synthesis of a Gene for Human Epidermal Growth Factor Urogastrone and Its Expression in Yeast," *Proc. Natl. Acad. Sci.* 80:7461-7465, 1983.
544. U.S. Congress, Congressional Budget Office, *Changing the Structure of Medicare Benefits: Issues and Options* (Washington, DC: U.S. Government Printing Office, March 1982).
545. U.S. Congress, Congressional Budget Office, *The Effect of PSROs on Health Care Costs: Current Findings and Future Evaluations* (Washington, DC: U. S. Government Printing Office, June 1979).
546. U.S. Congress, General Accounting Office, *Actions Needed to Stop Excess Medicare Payments for Blood and Blood Products*, HRD-78-172 (Washington, DC: Feb. 26, 1979).
547. U.S. Congress, General Accounting Office, *Problems in Carrying Out the National Blood Policy*, GAO/HRD-77-150 (Washington, DC: 1978).
548. U.S. Congress, Office of Technology Assessment, *Assessing the Efficacy and Safety of Medical Technologies*, OTA-H-75 (Washington, DC: U.S. Government Printing Office, stock # 052-003-00593-0, September 1978).
549. U.S. Congress, Office of Technology Assessment, *Commercial Biotechnology: An International Analysis*, OTA-BA-281 (Washington, DC: U.S. Government Printing Office, stock # 052-003-00939-1, January 1984).
550. U.S. Congress, Office of Technology Assessment, *Diagnosis Related Groups (DRGs) and the Medicare Program: Implications for Medical Technology—A Technical Memorandum*, OTA-TM-H-17 (Washington, DC: U.S. Government Printing Office, stock #052-003-00919-6, July 1983).
551. U.S. Congress, Office of Technology Assessment, "Medical Technology and Diagnosis-Related Groups: Evaluating Medicare's Prospective Payment System," project proposal, Mar. 8, 1984.
552. U.S. Congress, Office of Technology Assessment, *The Safety, Efficacy, and Cost Effectiveness of Therapeutic Apheresis*, OTA-HCS-23 (Washington, DC: U.S. Government Printing Office, stock #052-003-00918-8, 1983).
553. U.S. Congress, Office of Technology Assessment, *Variations in Hospital Length of Stay: Their Relationship to Health Outcomes*, OTA-HCS-24 (Washington, DC: U.S. Government Printing Office, stock #052-003-00922-6 August 1983).
554. U.S. Department of Health, Education, and Welfare, National Institutes of Health, National Heart, Lung, and Blood Institute, Division of Blood Diseases and Resources, *Study to Evaluate the Supply-Demand Relationships for AHF and PTC Through 1980*, DHEW publication No. (NIH) 77-1274, Bethesda, MD, 1977.
555. U.S. Department of Health, Education, and Welfare, National Institutes of Health, National Heart and Lung Institute, National Blood Resource Program, *Summary Report: NHLI's Blood Resource Studies*, DHEW publication No. (NIH) 73-416, Bethesda, MD, June 30, 1972.
556. U.S. Department of Health, Education, and Welfare, National Institutes of Health, National Heart, Lung, and Blood Institute, Division of Blood Diseases and Resources, *Ten-Year Review and Five Year Plan, Section 5: Blood Resources*, final draft, revised November 1982.
557. U.S. Department of Health and Human Services; National Heart, Lung, and Blood Institute; *Directory of Federally Supported Research Projects in Lung and Blood Diseases and Blood Resources (FY 79)*, NIH publication No. 81-2183, Bethesda, MD, 1980.
558. U.S. Department of Health and Human Services; National Heart, Lung, and Blood Institute; *Tenth Report of the Director, National Heart, Lung, and Blood Institute, Volume 4: Blood Diseases and Resources*, NIH publication No. 84-2359, Bethesda, MD, 1984.
559. U.S. Department of Health and Human Services, Public Health Service, Centers for Disease Control, "Update: Acquired Immunodeficiency Syndrome (AIDS) Among Patients With Hemophilia—United States," *Morbidity and Mortality Weekly Report* 32(47):613-615, 1983.
560. U.S. Department of Health and Human Services, Public Health Service, Food and Drug Administration, *FDA Blood Products Advisory Committee Annual Report*, July 13, 1982.
561. U.S. Department of Health and Human Services, Public Health Service, Food and Drug Administration, FDA Blood Products Advisory Committee Meeting, Summary Minutes, Oct. 6-7, 1983.
562. U.S. Department of Health and Human Services, Public Health Service, Food and Drug

Administration, Office of Biologics, *FDA Panel on Review of Blood and Derivatives Final Report*, unpublished, Nov. 15, 1979.

563. U.S. Department of Health and Human Services, Public Health Service, Food and Drug Administration, *Working Relationships Agreement Among the Bureaus of Medical Devices, Radiological Health and Biologics*, April 1982.

564. U.S. Department of Health and Human Services, Public Health Service, Food and Drug Administration, National Center for Drugs and Biologics, *Memorandum to All FDA Registered Blood Establishments on Approval of Two New Blood Preservative Systems*, Bethesda, MD, Oct. 14, 1983.

565. U.S. Department of Health and Human Services, Public Health Service, Food and Drug Administration, Office of Biologics, *Guidelines for the Collection of Platelets by Mechanical Pheresis*, March 1981.

566. U.S. Department of Health and Human Services, Public Health Service, Food and Drug Administration, Office of Biologics, *Recommendations to Decrease the Risk of Transmitting Acquired Immunodeficiency Syndrome (AIDS) From Blood Donors*, Mar. 24, 1983.

567. U.S. Department of Health and Human Services, Public Health Service, National Institutes of Health, "Announcement of Consensus Development Conference on Fresh Frozen Plasma: Indications and Risks," Bethesda, MD, Apr. 17, 1984.

568. U.S. Department of Health and Human Services, Social Security Administration, Health Care Financing Administration, *Your Medicare Handbook*, Social Security Administration publication No. 05-10050, Baltimore, MD, 1983.

569. Valenzuela, P. Chiron Corp., Emeryville, CA, personal communication, February 1984.

570. Vehar, G., Keyt, B., Eaton, D., et al., "Structure of Human Factor VIII," *Nature* 312(5992): 337-342, 1984.

571. Veltkamp, J. J., "What Is the Prospective Impact of the Recombinant DNA Technique on the Production of Human Plasma Derivatives? What Are the Derivatives Where Donor Plasma Could Be Replaced?" *Vox Sang.* 44:390-395, 1983.

572. Vercellotti, G. M., Hammerschmidt, D. E., Craddock, P. R., et al., "Activation of Plasma Complement by Perfluorocarbon Artificial Blood: Probable Mechanism of Adverse Pulmonary Reactions in Treated Patients and Rationale for Corticosteroid Prophylaxis," *Blood* 59:1299-1304, 1982.

573. Villa-Komaeoff, L., Efstatiades, A., Broome, S., et al., "A Bacterial Clone Synthesizing Proinsulin," *Proc. Natl. Acad. Sci.* 75:3727-3731, 1978.

574. Virmani, R., Warren, D., Rees, R., et al., "Effects of Perfluorochemical on Phagocytic Function on Leukocytes," *Transfusion* 23:512-515, 1983.

575. Voak, D., and Lenox, E., "Principles of Monoclonal Antibodies in Blood Transfusion Work," *Biotest Bulletin* 4:281-290, 1983.

576. Wallace, E. L., and Wallace, M. A., American Blood Commission, *Hospital Transfusion Charges and Community Blood Center Costs*, prepared under contract with the Division of Blood Diseases and Resources of the National Heart, Lung, and Blood Institute of the Department of Health and Human Services, unpublished, July 1982.

577. Wallace, J., *Blood Transfusions for Clinicians* (London: Churchill Livingstone, 1977).

578. Wallen, P., Ranby, M., and Bergdorf, N., *Progress in Fibrinolysis* 5:16-23, J. R. Davidson, I. M. Nilsson, and B. Astedt (eds.) (New York: Churchill-Livingstone, 1981).

579. Watson, J. D., Tooze, J., and Kurtz, D. T., *Recombinant DNA: A Short Course* (New York: Scientific American Books, Freeman & Co., 1983).

580. Weimar, W., Van Seyden, A. J., Stebbe, J., et al., "Specific Lysis of an Ileofemoral Thrombus by Administration of Extrinsic (Tissue-type) Plasminogen Activator," *Lancet* i:1018-1020, 1981.

581. Weinstock, G. M., Rhys, C., Berman, M. R., et al., "Open Reading Frame Expression Vectors: A General Method for Antigen Production in *E. Coli*, Using Protein Fusions to Beta-galactosidase," *Proc. Natl. Acad. Sci.* 80:4432-4436, 1983.

582. Wessan, L., "Advances in Recombinant DNA Reach Blood Clotting Market," *Genet. Engineering News* 2(6):22, 1982.

583. Widmann, F. K. (ed.), *Technical Manual* (Washington, DC: American Association of Blood Banks, 1981).

584. Wield, D., "Alfa-laval Emerging as a Global Force in Industrial Biotechnology Scale-up," *Genet. Engineering News* 3(3):5, 1983.

585. Wigler, M., Sweet, R., Sim, G. K., et al., "Transformation of Mammalian Cells With

Genes From Procaryotes and Eucaryotes," *Cell* 16:777-785, 1979.
586. Williams, B. G., and Blattner, F. R., "Bacteriophage Lambda Vectors for DNA Cloning," *J. Virol.* 29:555-561, 1980.
587. Wilson, B. S., Teodorescu, M., and Dray, S., "Enumeration and Isolation of Rabbit T and B Lymphocytes by Using Antibody Coated Erythrocytes," *J. Immunol.* 116:1306-1311, 1976.
588. Wilson, K., "Options in Compatibility Testing," in M. Treacy and J. Bertsch (eds.), *Selecting Policies and Procedures for the Transfusion Service*, AABB Workshop, American Association of Blood Banks, Arlington, VA, 1982.
589. Wilson, W. A., and Thomas, E. J., "Activation of the Alternative Pathway of Human Complement by Haemoglobin," *Clin. Exp. Immunol.* 36:140-141, 1979.
590. Winston, D. J., Ho, W. G., and Gale, R. P., "Prophylactic Granulocyte Transfusions During Chemotherapy of Acute Nonlymphocytopic Leukemia." *Ann. Int. Med.* 94:616-22, 1981.
591. Wolf, C., Director of Blood Bank, New York Hospital, personal communication, Apr. 18, 1984.
592. Wood, W., Capon, D., Simonsen, C., et al., "Expression of Active Human Factor VIII From Recombinant DNA Clones," *Nature* 312(5992): 330-337, 1984.
593. World Health Organization, "Meeting of Experts on the Utilization and Supply of Human Blood and Blood Products," *Vox Sang.* 32:367-373, 1975.
594. World Health Organization, *The Collection, Fractionation, Quality Control, and Use of Blood and Blood Products* (Geneva, Switzerland: World Health Organization, 1981).
595. World Health Organization, *Official Records of the World Health Organization, Twenty-Eighth World Health Assembly, Part I*, WHA28.72, and Annex 14, Geneva, 13-30, May, 1975.
596. Wu, A. M., Till, J. E., Siminovitch, L., et al., "A Cytological Study of the Capacity for Differentiation of Normal Hemopoietic Colony-Forming Cells," *J. Cell Physiol.* 69:177-184, 1967.
597. Wu, P. S., Tin, G. W., and Baldeschwiller, J. D., "Phagocytosis of Carbohydrate-Modified Phospholipid Vesicles by Macrophage," *Proc. Natl. Acad. Sci.* 78:2033-2037, 1981.
598. Yankee, R. A., "Improvements in Transfusion Safety: Past, Present, and Future" (abstract), Council of Community Blood Centers 22d Annual Meeting, St. Petersburg, FL, Feb. 26-29, 1984.
599. Yokoyama, K., Naito, R., Tsuda, C., et al., "Selection of 53 PFC Substances for Better Stability of Emulsion and Improved Artificial Blood Substitutes," *Advances in Blood Substitute Research*, R. B. Bolin, R. P. Geyer, and G. J. Nemo (eds.) (New York: Alan R. Liss, Inc., 1983), pp. 189-196.
600. Zimmerman, T. S., Department of Molecular Immunology, Scripps Clinic and Research Foundation, La Jolla, CA, personal communications, February and March 1984.
601. Zuelzer, W., Emeritus Director, Division of Blood and Blood Resources, National Heart, Lung, and Blood Institute, National Institutes of Health, personal communication, Dec. 27, 1983.
602. Zwaal, R. F. A., "Membrane and Lipid Involvement in Blood Coagulation," *Biochem. Biophys. Acta.* 515:163-205, 1978.

Index

Index

Alpha Therapeutics, 21
AIDS, 10-17, 37, 44, 99-107
    directed donations, 17
    evaluation of donor screening criteria, 14
    identification of suspected AIDS-carrying donors, 16
    laboratory tests for AIDS, 16
alternatives and substitutes for blood products, 20
    impact on consumers, 22
    impact on the plasma derivatives industry, 21
    impact on the voluntary whole blood sector, 22
alternative technologies, 133-172
    alternative sources of blood products, 133-151
        platelet substitutes, 150
            liposomes as platelets, 151
        red blood cell substitutes, 136
        stem cell culturing, 134
            hemoglobin solutions, 141
            liposomes, 146
            perfluorochemicals, 138
    alternative source for plasma products—use of recombinant DNA technology, 152-172
    application of recombinant DNA technology to large-scale production of plasma-proteins, 159
American Association of Blood Banks, 4, 9, 23, 35, 52, 54, 112
American Blood Commission (ABC), 3, 9, 24, 34, 55, 108
American Blood Resources Association (ABRA), 6
American Council on Transplantation, 187
American Red Cross (ARC), 4, 8, 9, 19, 23, 24, 35, 52, 53, 60, 61, 65, 114
appropriate use of blood products, 22
    direct attempts to improve use, 23
    indirect effects on improved use, 23

blood and blood products, 36-38
    risks for donors, 39
blood services complex, 4, 51-75
    commercial plasma and plasma derivatives sector, 63-73
        sources of raw plasma, 65
        finished products licensed for use in the United States, 67
            coagulation factors, 69
            costs of major plasma derivatives, 72
            immune globulins, 70
            normal serum albumin and plasma protein fraction, 67
            reagent products, 72
    voluntary, whole blood, and blood components sector, 51-62
        blood collecting organizations, 52
        blood collections in the voluntary sector, 57
        costs of blood and blood components, 59
        costs and charges for blood products, 59
blood technologies, 79-95
    plasma fractionation technologies, 91
        fractionation methods and products, 93
        new and emerging technologies, 95
        plasma collection, 91
    technologies for blood collection and processing, 79-91
        blood collection, 80
        blood component preparation, 84
        pre-transfusion testing techniques, 90
        testing and labeling of blood from doctors, 85

containment of health care costs, 18
    DRG method of payment, 19
    financing of blood center operations, 19
    supply and distribution systems, 20
coordination of blood resources, 23
    American Blood Commission, 24
    regionalization, 24
    sharing and the blood credit system, 24
costs of blood products, 7, 17
Council of Community Blood Centers (CCBC), 4, 52, 54
current issues, 99-129
    appropriate use of blood products, 121-129
        albumin and plasma protein fraction, 126
        cryoprecipitate, 125
        Factor VIII, 127
        fresh-frozen and single-donor plasma, 126
        granulocytes, 125
        methods to change usage patterns, 127
        platelets, 124
        red cell concentrates, 122
        whole blood, 121
    coordination of blood resources, 107-117
        American Association of Blood Banks, 112
        American Red Cross, 114
        regionalization, 108
        resource sharing, 111
        volume of sharing, 115
    impact of AIDS on blood collection and use, 99-107
    impact of health care cost containment, 117-121

Clearinghouse Lifeline Program, 111, 112, 113
Congress:
   House Committee on Energy and Commerce, 4
Canadian Red Cross, 25
Centers for Disease Control (CDC), 13, 41, 100

Department of the Army, 44
Department of Health and Human Services (DHHS), 3, 14, 15, 33, 43, 103
Department of Justice, 9, 111
diagnosis-related groups (DRGs), 118

Factor VIII, 64, 72, 92, 93, 95, 101, 126, 127, 164, 165
Factor IX Complex, 95, 101
Federal activities, 41-48
   Food and Drug Administration (FDA), 45-47
   National Institutes of Health (NIH), 43
   payment for blood products and services, 42
      Health Care Financing Administration, 42
      payment for hemophilia care, 43
Food and Drug Administration (FDA), 5, 10, 12, 13, 15, 33, 34, 41, 45, 100, 103
future directions, 175-188
   organ and tissue banking, 181
      American Council on Transportation, 187
      compatibility, 186
      current scene, 182
      procurement system, 183
      supply and demand, 184
   voluntary v. commercial approaches, 175-181
      prospects for further voluntary sector involvement in plasma operations, 179
      voluntary efforts in the plasma sector, 176

Genentech, 20
General Accounting Office (GAO), 35, 36, 59
Genetics Institute, 20
Green Cross of Japan, 21
Gulf Coast Regional Blood Center, 62, 107

Hastings Center, 16
Health Care Financing Administration (HCFA), 36, 41, 42, 59, 120
history of Federal interest, 33-36

Irwin Memorial Blood Bank, 14, 104
issues, 12

League of Red Cross Societies, 40
legislation:
   National Heart Act, 43
   National Heart, Blood Vessel, Lung, and Blood Act of 1972, 43
   Public Health Service Act of 1975 (Public Law 94-63), 34, 43
   Senate Bill, S. 140, 35
   Senate Bill, S. 1610, 35
   Social Security Amendments of 1983, 41

Massachusetts Biologics Laboratory, 9
Mississippi Blood Services (MBS), 62

National Blood Policy (NBP), 3, 12, 33
National Cancer Institute, 43
National Gay Task Force, 13, 100
National Heart, Lung, and Blood Institute, 16, 33, 34, 36, 43, 44
National Hemophilia Foundation, 13, 101
National Institutes of Health (NIH), 13, 41, 43, 100
Netherlands Red Cross, 38
New York Blood Center, 5, 6, 9, 14, 52, 65, 109
Nixon, President Richard M., 33

Puget Sound Blood Center, 23

Rite-Aid Corp., 5

safety, 10
Stanford Medical Center, 11
Stanford University Blood Bank, 14

Titmuss, Prof. Richard, 33
Truman, President Harry S., 33

voluntary v. commercial blood sources, 25

World Health Organization (WHO), 40, 175